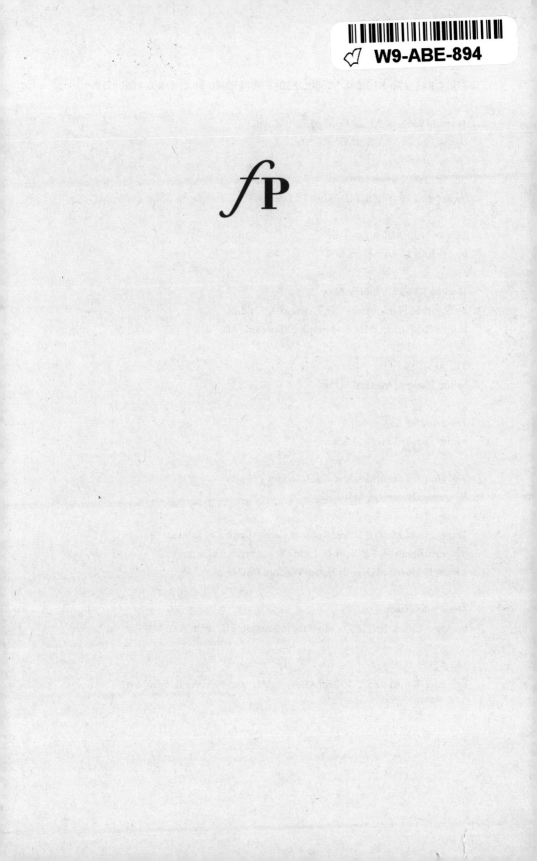

EAT, DRINK, AND BE HEALTHY

The Harvard Medical School Guide to Healthy Eating

A HARVARD MEDICAL SCHOOL BOOK

CO-DEVELOPED WITH THE HARVARD T.H. CHAN SCHOOL OF PUBLIC HEALTH

WALTER C. WILLETT, MD, DrPH

with Patrick J. Skerrett

Contributions by Edward L. Giovannucci, MD, DSc
Recipes by Maureen Callahan, other food writers, and chefs
Harvard Healthy Eating Pyramid illustration by Christopher Bing and Heather Foley

FREE PRESS

NEW YORK • LONDON • TORONTO • SYDNEY • NEW DELHI

To Gail

———

*f*P

Free Press
An imprint of Simon & Schuster, Inc.
1230 Avenue of the Americas
New York, NY 10020

This Free Press trade paperback edition September 2017

FREE PRESS and colophon are trademarks of Simon & Schuster, Inc.

For information about special discounts for bulk purchases, please contact Simon & Schuster Special Sales at 1-866-506-1949 or business@simonandschuster.com.

The Simon & Schuster Speakers Bureau can bring authors to your live event. For more information or to book an event, contact the Simon & Schuster Speakers Bureau at 1-866-248-3049 or visit our website at www.simonspeakers.com.

Manufactured in the United States of America

10 9 8 7 6 5 4 3 2

Library of Congress Cataloging-in-Publication Data

Names: Willett, Walter, author. | Skerrett, P. J. (Patrick J.), 1953– author. | Giovannucci, Edward L., author.
Title: Eat, drink, and be healthy : the Harvard Medical School guide to healthy eating / Walter C. Willett, M.D., Dr., P.H. with Patrick J. Skerrett ; contributions by Edward L. Giovannucci, M.D., D.Sc. ; recipes by Maureen Callahan ; new healthy eating illustrations by Christopher Bing and Heather Foley.
Description: Revised and expanded [edition]. | New York : Free Press Paperbacks, 2017. | "A Harvard Medical School book co-developed with the Harvard School of Public Health." | Includes bibliographical references and index.
Identifiers: LCCN 2017035108 | ISBN 9781501164774 (paperback)
Subjects: LCSH: Nutrition—Popular works. | BISAC: HEALTH & FITNESS / Diets. | HEALTH & FITNESS / Nutrition. | HEALTH & FITNESS / Healthy Living.
Classification: LCC RA784 .W635 2017 | DDC 618.97/689—dc23 LC record available at https://lccn.loc.gov/2017035108

ISBN 978-1-5011-6477-4
ISBN 978-1-4391-3481-8 (ebook)

Contents

Acknowledgments

THE CONCEPTS IN THIS BOOK owe much to the work and ideas of many predecessors, present colleagues, postdoctoral fellows, and doctoral students. In particular, I am grateful for the encouragement, support, and thoughts of my colleagues Ed Giovannucci, Meir Stampfer, Graham Colditz, Bernard Rosner, Laura Sampson, JoAnn Manson, Frank Sacks, David Hunter, Charles Hennekens, Sue Hankinson, Eric Rimm, Frank Hu, and Alberto Aschiero of the Channing Laboratory and Harvard T.H. Chan School of Public Health. Frank Speizer provided strong support over many years for the study of diet and disease within the Nurses' Health Study.

The vast majority of the research described in this book, by my group and by others, would not have been possible without the funding of research grants through the National Institutes of Health. My colleagues and I are most appreciative of the strong public support for health-related research in the United States. I hope that the information in this book will be deemed worthy of this investment.

I am grateful for the support of Dr. Anthony L. Komaroff and his team at Harvard Health Publications for helping to bring the first edition of the book to life.

Meir Stampfer, Susan Roberts, Frank Sacks, Eric Rimm, and Mollie Katzen, who reviewed the entire book or specific chapters of it, provided many helpful suggestions. Emily Graff offered important support and encouragement in the development of this update, and Hilary Farmer, Liz Lenart, and Debbie Flynn assisted in many aspects of the production. At home, my wife, Gail, assisted in many experiments in new ways of eating, and in this edition she compiled the new recipes from our friends and colleagues. Our sons, Amani, who managed to trade the apples in his lunch for Twinkies at day care, and Kamali, who showed me that a vegetarian diet could mean Coca-Cola, ice cream, and pizza, helped me stay in touch with reality.

Preface

D URING THE DARK AGES OF dietary advice—from which we were just emerging in 2000—guidelines for good nutrition were based on guesswork and good intentions. I wrote the first edition of this book to share with others what solid science was teaching us about the long-term effects of diet on health. The lessons were exciting. They showed that a delicious, satisfying diet based on whole grains, healthy oils, fruits, vegetables, and good sources of protein can help you stay healthy and active to an old age.

Another reason for writing this book was to challenge the misleading advice embodied in the U.S. Department of Agriculture's Food Guide Pyramid, which focused on avoiding all types of fat and loading up with starch. When the USDA announced in 2005 that it was considering revising its pyramid, my colleagues and I were delighted. I sent the USDA a copy of the first edition of *Eat, Drink, and Be Healthy* and said it was welcome to use the evidence-based Healthy Eating Pyramid my colleagues and I had developed, and which I had described in the book. As usual, though, politics and business trumped science—the USDA's new MyPyramid offered even less guidance on healthy eating than its predecessor. Five years later, in 2010, the USDA abandoned its pyramids and replaced them with MyPlate. This infographic also conveniently failed to convey the real information needed to make healthy food choices, so my colleagues and I developed the Healthy Eating Plate.

During the development of the 2015–2020 Dietary Guidelines for Americans, the influence of the beef, soda, and dairy industries on Congress and the USDA was on even clearer display. In its passage of the final national budget for 2015, Congress took the highly unusual step of saying that the USDA could not consider the chapter on diet and climate change that had been written by the USDA's Dietary Guidelines Scientific Advisory Committee. Going further, the USDA distorted the conclusions of that expert committee in the final Dietary Guidelines.

In this update of *Eat, Drink, and Be Healthy*, I examine the USDA's pyramids and plate and show where they have misled the public. The fundamental principles of healthy eating that I described in the first edition have not changed. However, in this edition I incorporate additional, important details that have emerged, including new information on weight-loss strategies; the benefits of specific fruits, vegetables, and vitamin D; the harms of trans fats; and other elements of healthy eating. Because the urgency of addressing climate change has become more apparent since 2001, I have devoted a chapter to the information censored by Congress.

Over the past thirty-five years, my colleagues and I have been continually surprised by the impact of diet on the risks of a host of chronic diseases. That dietary decisions could significantly affect the chances of contracting heart disease, various cancers, cataracts, and even serious birth defects was not appreciated by the nutrition community until relatively recently. And many aspects of diet that were off the nutrition science radar screen, such as trans fat intake, glycemic load, and low intakes of folic acid and vitamin D, have emerged as important factors in long-term health. This book will guide you to make better dietary decisions for yourself and your family.

My efforts to understand the long-term effects of diet on health began in the late 1970s when I realized that people were being given strong advice about what to eat and what to avoid, but that the direct evidence to support these recommendations was often weak or nonexistent. A key missing element was data based on detailed dietary intakes from many individuals that could be examined in relation to their future development of heart disease, various cancers, and other health problems. Of course, information on medical history, smoking, physical activity, and other lifestyle variables would be needed to isolate the effects of diet. Fortunately, at that time I was already investigating the relation of cigarette smoking to heart disease within the Nurses' Health Study, an ongoing study of over 121,000 women across the United States, and this appeared to be an ideal group in which to investigate the long-term consequences of various diets.

The first step was to develop a standardized method of dietary assessment for such a large population; many colleagues were skeptical that this was possible. Borrowing on work done at Harvard in the 1940s, we developed a series of self-administered dietary questionnaires and were able to document their validity in a series of detailed evaluations. Since 1980 we have been following women in this study with periodic updating of dietary and other information and have also added other large cohorts of men and women.

Although our large prospective studies have provided a unique and powerful flow of information about diet and health, the best understanding of a topic this complex should incorporate evidence from all available sources. This book attempts to do this, giving special weight to studies of actual disease risk in humans.

My own interest in food and health actually goes back much further than the studies described above. The Willett family has been involved in dairy farming in Michigan for many generations, so it was only natural that I joined a 4-H club when I was growing up. Vegetable growing was one of my major activities, and I was the Michigan winner of a National Junior Vegetable Growers Association contest. As an undergraduate at Michigan State University, I studied physics and food science, and paid my tuition by growing vegetables during the summers. In medical school at the University of Michigan, I had the opportunity to conduct a nutrition survey in a Native American community, my first experience in epidemiologic research and standardized methods of dietary assessment that were later developed for much larger-scale use.

For internship and residency, I joined the Harvard Medical Unit of Boston City Hospital, where I had the good fortune to meet individuals, many of whom remain colleagues today, who were interested in understanding the environmental and cultural origins of disease, rather than just its treatment. As a result, I enrolled in Harvard T.H. Chan School of Public Health, where I studied more about nutrition. After completing a residency in internal medicine, I taught community medicine for three years at the Faculty of Medicine in Dar es Salaam, Tanzania. While there, I studied the relation between parasitic infections and malnutrition in children, and became even more impressed with the power of epidemiologic approaches to understanding the occurrence of disease and to guiding both prevention and treatment. Returning to Boston, I enrolled in a doctoral program in epidemiology at Harvard School of Public Health and began work on the Nurses' Health Study, which had begun one year earlier.

Since then, the central theme in my work has been to develop and use epidemiologic approaches to study the relation of diet to the occurrence of disease. This has resulted in a textbook, *Nutritional Epidemiology*, and the publication of more than seventeen hundred scientific articles. As we have seen the results from our research emerge, most of my colleagues and I have taken advantage of this information and substantially modified our activity levels and diet. This book is my attempt to assemble this information in a cohesive manner that is directly accessible to everyone. I hope that this information will empower you and others to enjoy healthier, longer, and more interesting lives.

In creating this edition of *Eat, Drink, and Be Healthy*, I have been joined by Patrick J. Skerrett, an experienced and highly skilled science writer who also worked with me on prior editions, as well as on many other projects. He has helped to create a text that departs from my usual terse, scientific style. Maureen Callahan, a well-known dietitian and food writer, contributed many recipes to the first edition that reflect the earlier evidence presented in the book. For this edition, new recipes were contributed by my wife, Gail, as well as by friends, who include some of the world's leading chefs, cookbook writers, and healthy food advocates.

Perhaps one of the most important conclusions of our work is that healthy diets—and there is no single healthy diet—do not mean deprivation or monotony. In fact, the opposite is true. The classic Midwestern American diet centered on mashed potatoes, roast beef, and gravy—besides being among the world's unhealthiest fares—was terribly dull compared to what I describe in this book. And the recipes included here represent just a sampling of the tremendously varied possibilities for healthy and exciting eating.

CHAPTER ONE

Healthy Eating Matters

YOU EAT TO LIVE.

It's a simple, obvious truth. You need food for the basics of everyday life—to pump blood, move muscles, think thoughts. But what you eat and drink can also help you live well and live longer. By making the right choices, you can avoid some of the things we think of as inevitable penalties of getting older. Eating well—teamed with keeping your weight in the healthy range, exercising regularly, and not smoking—can prevent 80 percent of heart attacks, 90 percent of type 2 diabetes, and 70 percent of colorectal cancer.[1] It can also help you avoid stroke, osteoporosis, constipation and other digestive woes, cataracts, and aging-related memory loss or dementia. And the benefits aren't just for the future. A healthy diet can give you more energy and help you feel good today. Making poor dietary choices—eating too much of the wrong kinds of food and too little of the right kinds, or too much food altogether—can send you in the other direction, increasing your chances of developing one or more chronic conditions or dying early. An unhealthy diet during pregnancy can cause some birth defects and may even influence a baby's health into adulthood and old age.

When it comes to diet, knowing what's good and what's bad isn't always easy. The food industry spends billions of dollars a year to influence your choices, mostly in the wrong direction. Diet gurus promote the latest fads, most of which are less than healthy, while the media serves up near daily helpings of flip-flopping nutrition news. Supermarkets and fast-food restaurants also offer conflicting advice, as do cereal boxes and thousands of websites, blogs, Facebook pages, and tweets. The federal government, through its Food Guide Pyramid, MyPyramid, and MyPlate images, aimed to cut through the confusion but ended up giving misleading and often unhealthy recommendations (see chapter two) that benefit American agriculture and food companies more than Americans' health.

While the average American diet still has a long way to go before it can be called healthy, it has improved over the past decade or so in spite of the babel of nutrition information. Several of my colleagues and I looked at the diets of almost 34,000 Americans who took part in the National Health and Nutrition Examination Survey between 1999 and 2012. This survey, conducted every year, gauges the diet, health, and nutritional status of a sample of adults and children in the United States. We rated the diet of each participant using a tool we developed that assigns higher points to healthy components of the diet, like eating whole grains and unsaturated fats, and lower points to unhealthy components, like eating red meat and drinking sugar-sweetened beverages. The highest score, 110, indicates the healthiest diet possible. We were delighted to report that the quality of the American diet improved between 1999 and 2012.[2] Consumption of artery-damaging trans fats declined by 80 or 90 percent, and Americans drank about 25 percent fewer sugar-sweetened beverages. On average, people ate slightly more fruit, whole grains, and healthy unsaturated fats. Our study showed that the average American diet still wasn't very healthy— rating 48 points out of 110—and that poorer individuals and those with less education have poorer diets than wealthier and better-educated individuals. And this gap looks like it is increasing over time.

Yet, these modest improvements in diet quality had an astounding impact on the health of the nation. Between 1999 and 2012, we estimated that these changes prevented 1.1 million premature deaths from heart attacks, strokes, cancer, and other causes, and 3 million cases of type 2 diabetes. But there's more work to be done, since the "average American diet" in this study wasn't that great. The eating strategies described in this book will help you make a great diet and reap not only the benefits described in this study but many more as well.

SIMPLE STEPS

I wrote *Eat, Drink, and Be Healthy* in 2001 to cut through the confusion about diet. Basing the book on the most reliable scientific evidence available then, I offered recommendations for eating and drinking healthfully. Sixteen years and thousands of scientific papers later, the recommendations in this edition of the book are fundamentally the same, though supported with more extensive evidence and enhanced with important new details. That's encouraging, because it means that, with careful attention to the types and strength of studies, we can make conclusions about healthy eating that withstand the test of time and deep scientific scrutiny. However, the book needed to be updated, because far too many Americans are still confused about what constitutes a healthy diet and are looking for the best available information.

Even more encouraging is that national recommendations on healthy eating, called the Dietary Guidelines for Americans,[3] have been inching closer to what I advised in 2001 and still advise today.

I can't quite rival the brevity of food writer Michael Pollan's seven-word dietary credo, "Eat food. Not too much. Mostly plants."[4] That's a decent general overview, but it doesn't offer much real guidance. That's exactly what this book provides.

Here is the outline of my simple, actionable advice for healthy eating, which I describe in detail later in the book:

- Eat plenty of vegetables and fruits, but limit fruit juices and corn, and hold the potatoes.
- Eat more good fats (these mostly come from plants) and fewer bad fats (these mostly come from meat and dairy foods).
- Eat more whole-grain carbohydrates and fewer refined-grain carbohydrates.
- Choose healthy sources of protein, limit your consumption of red meat, and don't eat processed meat.
- Drink more water. Coffee and tea are okay; sugar-sweetened soda and other beverages aren't.
- Drink alcohol in moderation, if at all.
- Take a multivitamin for insurance, just in case you aren't getting the vitamins and minerals you need from the foods you eat. Make sure it delivers at least 1,000 international units of vitamin D.

Since the last edition of the book, many studies have supported the benefits of a primarily plant-based diet. This doesn't mean you must go vegan or vegetarian. Even a partial shift away from a meat- and dairy-centered diet and toward more plant sources of protein is a big step in the direction of long-term good health for you and planet Earth (see chapter twelve). If swearing off meat isn't for you, think about trying the "vegan till 6" plan favored by *New York Times* food writer Mark Bittman. Or experiment with the popular Meatless Monday movement and one day a week—choosing Monday makes it easy to remember, but it could be any day—not eat any meat.

While many food experts (Pollan, Bittman, and myself among them) agree with a plant-based diet, the USDA hasn't been entirely on board with it. You can see that in MyPlate, a less-than-healthy infographic the USDA cooked up to summarize the dietary recommendations in the 2010 *Dietary Guidelines for Americans* (see chapter two).

To counter that flawed information, I and several of my colleagues at the Harvard T.H. Chan School of Public Health, in collaboration with Harvard Health Publications, distilled the best evidence about healthy eating into the Harvard Healthy Eating Plate. This visual, evidence-based guide makes it easy to choose the healthiest options. It's also an important alternative to the USDA's misleading My Plate (see chapter two).

The main message of the Healthy Eating Plate, like its older sibling, the Healthy Eating Pyramid, is to focus on diet quality.

- Celebrate vegetables and fruits: Cover half of your plate with them. Aim for color and variety. Keep in mind that potatoes don't count (see "The Spud Is a Dud" on page 167).

THE HARVARD HEALTHY EATING PLATE

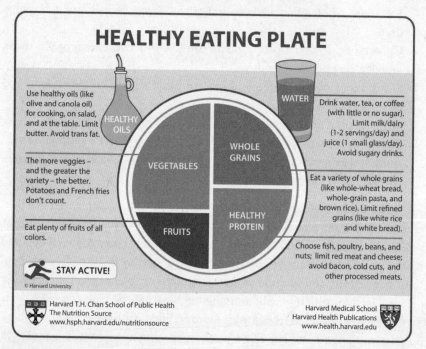

Figure 1. The Harvard Healthy Eating Plate was created to address deficiencies in the USDA's MyPlate. It provides simple but detailed guidance to help people make the best eating choices.

- Go for whole grains—about one-quarter of your plate. Intact and whole grains, such as whole wheat, barley, wheat berries, quinoa, oats, brown rice, and foods made with them, have a milder effect on blood sugar and insulin than white bread, white rice, and other refined grains (see chapter six).
- Choose healthy protein packages—about one-quarter of your plate. Fish, chicken, beans, soybeans, and nuts are all healthy, versatile protein sources. Limit red meat, and try to stay away from processed meats such as bacon and sausage (see chapter seven).
- Use healthy plant oils, such as olive, canola, soy, corn, sunflower, and peanut, in moderation. Stay away from foods containing partially hydrogenated oils, which contain unhealthy artificial trans fats (see "Trans fats," page 83). If you like the taste of butter or coconut oil, use them when their flavor is important but not as primary dietary fats. Keep in mind that low-fat does not mean healthy (see chapter five).
- Drink water, coffee, or tea. Skip sugary drinks. If you enjoy milk, don't have more than two glasses a day (see chapter nine). If you drink alcohol, keep it moderate—no more than two drinks a day for men, no more than one a day for women.
- Exercise. It's good for overall health and controlling weight.

Using the blueprint laid out in the Harvard Healthy Eating Plate is a good way to improve your diet. But I also want you to see the evidence on which it was built. This is detailed in chapters four through eleven. In them, I describe the classic and cutting-edge research that has defined and refined eating patterns that will help keep you healthy, including new information on slowly digested carbohydrates; what kinds of fruits and vegetables are particularly important to include in your diet; what protein can and can't do; how to put the omega-3 fats found in fish and some plants to work for you; the potential hazards of consuming too much milk and other dairy foods; and why it makes sense to take a daily multivitamin.

This book helps you incorporate this information into your snacks and meals with practical tips on buying healthy foods and eating defensively in a food environment that entices you to eat in ways that can prematurely end your life. It offers extra information to help individuals with special nutritional needs get the most benefit from what they eat. These include pregnant women, frail older individuals, those with celiac disease, and those with or at high risk of heart disease, diabetes, high cholesterol, high blood pressure, or some other chronic conditions. It ends with more than seventy tasty tested recipes.

This information isn't meant to replace the advice you get from your physician, especially if you have a condition that requires a specific diet. Instead, I encourage you to talk with your health care provider about your diet and share with him or her what you've learned from this book to make sure you are talking the same language about healthy eating. Keep in mind that most physicians-to-be get little education about nutrition in medical school or beyond. And the pressures of modern medicine and health care often make it difficult for clinicians to keep up with the field of nutrition, let alone spend time talking with their patients about healthy food choices. You may find yourself teaching your health care provider.

Not long ago my cholesterol began creeping up. Much to my dismay, my doctor recommended that I start a low-fat diet—a recommendation from the 1980s that we now know doesn't work for lowering cholesterol.

This book will help you stay healthy and educate your doctor if you need to.

CHAPTER TWO

Of Pyramids, Plates, and Dietary Guidelines

T HROUGHOUT MOST OF HUMAN HISTORY, the relatively brief life span of our species (during the Roman Empire, the average life expectancy at birth was under thirty years) meant that it didn't much matter what you ate as long as you took in enough calories to survive. Most Romans didn't live long enough for diet-related conditions like heart disease, type 2 diabetes, and cancer to take root.

That's changed. Today the average American lives for nearly eighty years, so *what* you eat matters as much as *how much* you eat.

We aren't born knowing how to choose healthy foods. Most of us need some help, especially in this era when food, food ads, and dietary advice are everywhere. *Consider this book as your personal guide for navigating the sea of information, misinformation, and disinformation that surrounds all of us.*

AN ABUNDANCE OF ADVICE

Actually, advice on healthy eating has never been in short supply. More than two thousand years ago, Greek physician and philosopher Hippocrates made diet (and exercise) the centerpiece of good health and the basis for treating disease. Here's just one of his recommendations that sounds familiar today: Suitable vegetables, cooked or raw, must be eaten in abundance.

Fast-forward fifteen hundred years and the human life span was increasing. Soon after the invention of the printing press in the mid-1400s, Bartolomeo Platina's *De honesta voluptate et valetudine* (*On Honorable Pleasure and Health*) became a bestseller throughout Europe. Aiming to combine health with the pleasure of eating, it melded medical advice with recipes taken from other published works.[1] In the 1860s a low-carb diet devised by London undertaker William Banting[2] became so wildly successful that the term "Banting" was used for years in Europe and the United States as a synonym for "dieting."

Today, hundreds of diet books are published each year, along with innumerable diet-related websites, Facebook pages, and blogs. Much of the advice they offer is misleading or erroneous.

You'd think you could turn to the federal government for accurate, safe recommendations about healthy eating. You'd be wrong.

"OFFICIAL" ADVICE

The United States government got into the dietary recommendation business in 1894. That's when the U.S. Department of Agriculture (USDA) published *Foods: Nutritive Value and Cost* by W. O. Atwater.[3] The department continued to churn out a steady stream of recommendations throughout the 1900s.

In the 1960s and 1970s, two different trends in the United States sparked renewed interest in diet and nutrition. One was the growing concern about hunger and malnutrition, highlighted in part by the 1968 television broadcast of *Hunger in America*, a powerful CBS News special report. The other was the growing number of Americans who were developing and dying from cardiovascular disease.

In response, Senator George McGovern of South Dakota created the United States Senate Select Committee on Nutrition and Human Needs. In 1977 the committee issued a report called *Dietary Goals for the United States* (also known as the McGovern Report) that urged Americans to eat less fat, less cholesterol, less refined and processed sugars, and more complex carbohydrates and fiber. That set the stage for the first official *Dietary Guidelines for Americans* in 1980. According to the USDA, this document provided "authoritative advice for people two years and older about how good dietary habits can promote health and reduce risk for major chronic diseases."[4] The law authorizing the *Dietary Guidelines for Americans* fortunately understood that science is an ongoing process and that evidence changes, and so mandated that the guidelines must be revised every five years.

Each five-year update starts with the appointment of a scientific advisory committee made up of diet and nutrition experts from around the country. They are charged with reviewing the available data on diet. In theory this review should provide an unbiased summary of the scientific evidence. But the beef and dairy industries have worked hard to ensure that some committee members represent their interests.

After the committee issues its report, the USDA and the U.S. Department of Health and Human Services work behind closed doors to "translate" this review into the official guidelines. This leaves open numerous back channels through which economic and political influences can twist and recast the scientific evidence. In the 2015–2020 update, for example, the advisory committee recommended limiting the consumption of red meat. But the guidelines presented to the American public didn't say that and instead recommended consuming lean meat.

What should be a scholarly and scientific process is often a free-for-all among lobbyists for agribusinesses, food companies, and special interest groups.

The *Dietary Guidelines for Americans* are supposed to help us choose foods that will keep us healthy and stay away from those that don't. Unfortunately, their advice has often been murky or downright misleading. The 2010 guidelines, for example, told Americans to avoid "solid fats" but didn't come out and say that the way to do this was by eating less red meat and dairy foods.

The failings of the guidelines are a shame, because millions of people look to them as a model for healthy eating. Their reach goes even further than helping individuals choose healthy diets: they also form the basis for federal food policies such as the Special Supplemental Nutrition Program for Women, Infants, and Children, school lunches, and food served in government facilities, such as military bases and prisons.

UNDUE INFLUENCE

One of the big problems with the *Dietary Guidelines for Americans* and the highly popular and influential icons derived from them (more about that later) is that they come from the USDA—the agency responsible for promoting American agriculture—with some input from the Department of Health and Human Services. What's good for American farmers isn't necessarily good for Americans' health. Just look at their reluctance to say "Eat less red meat," which would be terrific for health but bad for ranchers and the influential beef industry. (This oversight of competing interests isn't unique to the USDA. The Nuclear Regulatory Commission, for example, is charged with the often contradictory tasks of promoting nuclear power and regulating its use.)

The influence of the USDA—not to mention that of powerful lobbies operating through Congress as well as directly targeting the USDA—has shaped federal recommendations on what we should eat as much as, if not more than, science has.

In Rudyard Kipling's classic children's story "The Elephant's Child," el-

Fast Fact: How the U.S. Constitution Affects Diet

I once had lunch in Rome with George McGovern, then the U.S. representative to the World Food Programme, whose work in the U.S. Senate paved the way for the *Dietary Guidelines for Americans*. He pointed out to me that the U.S. Constitution, by giving every state two senators, is a powerful influence on agriculture policy. The sparsely populated Western states, with large ranching and other agricultural interests, play a disproportional role in Congress, which controls the USDA budget and leadership appointments. It's no wonder that the *Dietary Guidelines for Americans*, which is inexplicably under the USDA's leadership, don't promote plant-based diets.

ephants didn't originally have trunks, only bulging blackish noses as big as a boot. That changed when the curious elephant's child ended up in the middle of a terrific tug-of-war with a crocodile clamped onto its nose and a python wrapped around its legs.

A tug-of-war is pretty much how the *Dietary Guidelines for Americans* and their representative icons get their shapes—yanked this way and that by competing powerful interests, few of which have your health as a central goal. These include the National Dairy Council, the Soft Drink Association, the American Beverage Association, the North American Meat Institute, the National Cattlemen's Beef Association, the Salt Institute, the Wheat Foods Council, and others. The end result of this tug-of-war between the food industry and nutrition science is generally a set of positive, feel-good, all-inclusive recommendations that distort what should be an important tool for improving your health and the health of the nation—guidelines on healthful eating.

THE PYRAMID ARISES

I N 1992 THE USDA UNVEILED the influential Food Guide Pyramid. The goal was to make the *Dietary Guidelines* more accessible. It was built with the help of public relations giant Porter Novelli, whose current and former clients include McDonald's, the Snack Food Association, Krispy Kreme, Johnnie Walker, and Masterfoods USA, maker of M&M's. The Food Guide Pyramid was supposed to simply and visually convey the elements of the *Dietary Guidelines for Americans*, which were inherently flawed. The pyramid highlighted those flaws. It recommended:

THE USDA'S ORIGINAL FOOD GUIDE PYRAMID

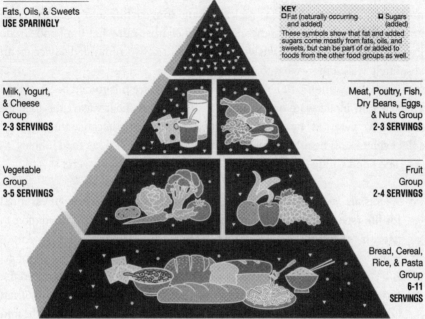

Fats, Oils, & Sweets
USE SPARINGLY

KEY
☐ Fat (naturally occurring and added)   ◪ Sugars (added)
These symbols show that fat and added sugars come mostly from fats, oils, and sweets, but can be part of or added to foods from the other food groups as well.

Milk, Yogurt, & Cheese Group
2-3 SERVINGS

Meat, Poultry, Fish, Dry Beans, Eggs, & Nuts Group
2-3 SERVINGS

Vegetable Group
3-5 SERVINGS

Fruit Group
2-4 SERVINGS

Bread, Cereal, Rice, & Pasta Group
6-11 SERVINGS

SOURCE: U.S. Department of Agriculture/U.S. Department of Health and Human Services

Use the Food Guide Pyramid to help you eat better every day. . .the Dietary Guidelines way. Start with plenty of Breads, Cereals, Rice, and Pasta; Vegetables; and Fruits. Add two to three servings from the Milk group and two to three servings from the Meat group.

Each of these food groups provides some, but not all, of the nutrients you need. No one food group is more important than another — for good health you need them all. Go easy on fats, oils, and sweets, the foods in the small tip of the Pyramid.

Figure 2. USDA Pyramid, 1992–2005. Despite sweeping changes in the science of healthy eating, this initially flawed pyramid went unchanged for thirteen years.

- eating lots of carbohydrates, most of which were unhealthy, highly processed carbohydrates such as white bread and white rice
- eating some fruits and vegetables, including potatoes (which are mostly a starchy carbohydrate)
- choosing meat, milk, and cheese as sources of protein
- not eating any types of oils or fats (including healthy ones).

Using a pyramid to convey dietary advice was a stroke of marketing genius. It placed "good" foods, which should be consumed in larger quantities, on the bottom; "bad" ones, which should be consumed in smaller quantities, on the top; and everything else in between. A pyramid also sends the subliminal message that the advice is rock solid and long-lasting and rises above the jungle of misinformation and contradictory claims. But what the Food Guide Pyramid really offered was wishy-washy, scientifically unfounded advice on an absolutely vital topic—what to eat.

Some recommendations on diet and nutrition are misguided because they are based on inadequate or incomplete information. That wasn't the case for the USDA's pyramid. Its recommendations were wrong because they ignored solid evidence on healthful eating and aimed to please various food lobbies.

The Food Guide Pyramid's most health-damaging faults were:

- *All fats are bad.* Wrong: some fats are good for you and are even essential for life (see chapter five). The Food Guide Pyramid's recommendation to use fats "sparingly" helped foster the phobia about fat that led many Americans to throw out the baby with the bathwater.
- *All "complex" carbohydrates are good.* The Food Guide Pyramid ignored the fact that some kinds of carbohydrates are significantly less healthy than others (see chapter six). Eating too much of the wrong kinds of carbs and too little of the right kinds can set you up for weight gain, type 2 diabetes, and heart disease.
- *All protein sources are equally good.* True: protein from steak and salmon is quite similar. But the protein *package* is vastly different (see chapter seven). Some high-protein foods deliver a lot of things that aren't so healthful, like saturated fat, cholesterol, and salt. Others provide healthy fats and additional good-for-you nutrients like fiber, vitamins and minerals, and a host of beneficial phytochemicals (literally, chemicals made by plants).
- *Dairy foods are essential.* Not true: you need calcium, not milk. Dairy foods are good sources of this mineral but also deliver plenty of calories and saturated fat. If you need extra calcium, there are cheaper, easier, and healthier ways to get it than dairy foods (see chapter eleven).
- *Silence on weight, exercise, alcohol, and vitamins.* Like the Sphinx, the Food Guide Pyramid was silent on four things you need to know about: the importance of weight control, the necessity of daily exercise, the potential health benefits of a daily alcoholic drink, and what you can gain by taking a daily multivitamin.

AN INJECTION OF SCIENCE AND THE CRUMBLING OF THE PYRAMID

As soon as the Food Guide Pyramid was unveiled, research from around the globe began to erode it at all levels. Results from scores of large and small studies chipped away at its foundation (carbohydrates), middle (meat and milk), and top (fats).

Back in the late 1970s, several colleagues and I realized that there was little solid evidence available on which to base recommendations for healthy eating. We saw an opportunity to change this through the Nurses' Health Study (see "Praise for Nurses and Health Professionals," page 33) which had been started in 1976 to investigate the long-term consequences of oral contraceptives. A few years later we created a similar long-term study of male health professionals. Thanks to both of these long-term cohort studies, we have been able to follow the eating patterns, lifestyle habits, and health of thousands of women and men for several decades (for more details, see chapter three). The treasure trove of data from this work has let us discover the benefits and harms of different eating patterns and find links between various foods and cancer, diabetes, cardiovascular disease, osteoporosis, and other chronic conditions. What emerged fairly early from this work, and from studies by others around the world, was that the picture of a healthy diet was quite different from that portrayed by the USDA pyramid.

We decided to test whether people who followed the *Dietary Guidelines for Americans* and its Food Guide Pyramid actually experienced better health and greater life expectancy than those who didn't. To do this, my colleagues and I used the Healthy Eating Index.[5] This scale was devised by the USDA's Center for Nutrition Policy and Promotion "to measure how well American diets conform to recommended healthy eating patterns." The index assigns scores of 0 to 10 for each of ten dietary components that were the focus of the original Food Guide Pyramid and the 1995 *Dietary Guidelines for Americans*: the number of daily servings of grains, vegetables (including potatoes), fruits, meat, and dairy products; lower intakes of total fat, saturated fat, dietary cholesterol, and sodium; and variety of the diet. A score of 100 meant perfectly following the USDA's recommendations, while a score of 0 meant totally disregarding them.

We extracted information on eating patterns from questionnaires that more than 135,000 female nurses and male health professionals had been completing every four years for more than a decade. Using this information, we calculated a Healthy Eating Index score for each individual. Those with the highest scores—meaning they closely followed the USDA's advice—were just as likely to have developed a major illness or to have died over a twelve-year period as those with the lowest scores. Heart attacks were only slightly less common among those with high Healthy Eating Index scores than they were among those with low scores.[6]

This dismal result shouldn't come as a surprise, since the USDA consistently ignored the extensive body of evidence linking certain eating patterns with long-term health. Take it as a warning that following the Department of Agriculture's advice may not help you eat to live well or live longer.

A MEDITERRANEAN EXPERIMENT

One strand of this evidence came from Greece. In the 1980s, Greek men lived four years longer than American men and had remarkably low rates of heart disease despite a relatively basic health care system. Their diet was thought to have something to do with this. (Note: The term "heart disease" encompasses a wide range of conditions ranging from chest pain to electrical problems in the heart and failure of the heart muscle to pump blood. In this book, the term heart disease refers to coronary artery disease, which stems from a blockage in one or more arteries that supply blood to the heart.)

My colleagues and I began working with other scientists who were deeply knowledgeable about traditional Greek cuisine as well as with experts with Oldways, an organization focused on creating healthier, tradition-based alternatives to the USDA's Food Guide Pyramid. Together we created in 1993 a pyramid to represent the traditional Mediterranean diet.[7] It was built on a base of healthy whole grains, fruits, vegetables, beans, and healthy fats. At the time it was widely criticized by many in the nutrition community because it was high in fat, mainly olive oil. Since then, various streams of evidence have confirmed that olive oil is a healthy source of calories (see chapter five).

Antonia Trichopoulou and her husband, Dimitrios Trichopoulos, the Greek colleagues and friends who helped us create the Mediterranean Diet Pyramid, then embarked on a more formal study of the Greek diet. They created a simple score to describe the traditional eating pattern of Greece. Points were given to higher intakes of olive oil, vegetables, legumes, fruits and nuts, cereal, and fish; lower intakes of meat, poultry, and dairy foods; and moderate alcohol consumption. They tested the score in a population of 22,000 Greek men and women whose diets and health were followed from 1994 to 1999. Those who most closely stuck with a traditional diet were less likely to have died prematurely and to have died from heart disease and cancer.[8] Later evaluations of the Mediterranean dietary score in populations around the world have confirmed its correlation with the development of many chronic diseases and lower risks of death.

Ten years later, Spanish colleagues of ours put the Mediterranean diet to the test in a randomized trial called PREDIMED.[9] They assigned nearly 7,500 men and women to either a Mediterranean diet with added nuts or extra-virgin olive oil or to a low-fat diet. After an average of five years, those who had been following the Mediterranean diet had a 30 percent lower rate of cardiovascular disease compared with those in the low-fat group. Further analyses showed that those following the Mediterranean diet also had lower rates of diabetes and breast cancer, and better cognitive function.

IN WITH THE NEW: THE HEALTHY EATING PYRAMID

Americans deserve more accurate, more helpful, and less biased information than what's offered by the federal government. To right the wrongs of the Food Guide Pyramid, my colleagues and I used the data we had, bolstered by the work in Greece, to create the Healthy Eating Pyramid (page 16) in 2000. It sits on a foundation of daily exercise and weight control. We then added the building blocks of a healthy diet, with each block supported not just by our own studies but also by the best of science from around the world. The blocks of the Healthy Eating Pyramid include:

- vegetable oils such as olive and canola oil as the primary sources of fat
- an abundance of vegetables and fruits, not including potatoes or corn
- whole-grain foods at most meals
- healthy sources of protein such as beans, nuts, seeds, fish, poultry, and eggs
- a daily calcium supplement or dairy foods one to two times a day
- a daily multivitamin
- for those who choose to drink, alcohol in moderation
- red meat, white bread, potatoes, soda, and sweets only occasionally if at all.

The Healthy Eating Pyramid, unlike the USDA's Food Guide Pyramid, didn't specify how many ounces or cups of specific foods you should have each day. That depends on your body size and physical activity. It also didn't describe percentages of calories from fat, carbohydrate, or protein, because there is no scientific basis for setting specific numbers. Also, in reality, it is very difficult for anyone to know if they are exceeding a specific percentage. These changes made the Healthy Eating Pyramid easier to use than the USDA pyramid.

There was just one key guideline to remember: Choose more foods from the lower parts of the pyramid than from its upper levels. Eating mostly minimally processed, whole foods from the lower part of the Healthy Eat-

THE HARVARD HEALTHY EATING PYRAMID

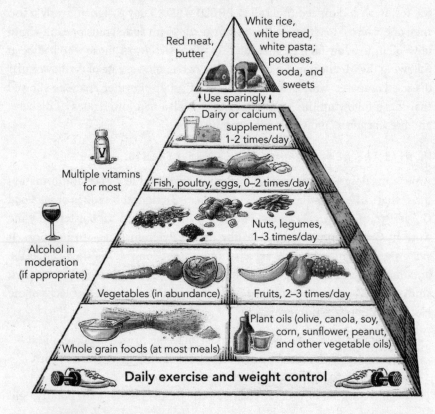

Figure 3. The Harvard Healthy Eating Pyramid. This pyramid, based on solid science, offers better guidance for healthy eating than the advice from the USDA.

ing Pyramid provides the balance of nutrients an individual needs and limits health-damaging foods.

We put the Healthy Eating Pyramid to the same test that we applied to the USDA Pyramid. We first created an Alternate Healthy Eating Index based on the Healthy Eating Pyramid. It included indicators such as intake of vegetables, fruits, nuts, cereal fiber, trans fats, and alcohol, multivitamin use, and the ratios of white to red meat and unsaturated fat to saturated fat. Using the same information from the 135,000 women and men described earlier, we calculated Alternate Healthy Eating Index scores for each individual. Women and men with high scores (those who followed the eating strategies embodied in the Healthy Eating Pyramid) had substantially lower risks of developing major chronic diseases, especially heart disease or stroke, than those scoring low on the index.[10]

My colleagues and I were pleased by these results. But we weren't entirely surprised, because each building block of the Healthy Eating Pyramid came from the finest possible quarry: solid evidence amassed by researchers from around the world. Seventeen years later, it is standing the test of time, as much new evidence has provided further support for it.

THE USDA PYRAMID GETS A MAKEOVER

Taking a cue from television reality shows, the federal government gave the Food Guide Pyramid an extreme makeover in 2005. In doing this, it squandered what could have been an opportunity to overhaul and correct the faults of the original. Working again with Porter Novelli, the USDA tipped the pyramid on its side, painted it in a rainbow of brightly colored bands running vertically from the tip to the base, and chiseled a jaunty stick figure running up stairs on its left side. That was it—no labels, no text, no key to help you decipher what it means. To understand what the new pyramid, dubbed MyPyramid, was saying, you needed a computer and a connection to the Internet.

MyPyramid didn't right the wrongs of its predecessor, nor did it offer any real information to help us make healthy choices. That was unfortunate, because the 2005 Dietary Guidelines themselves were inching closer to the dietary pattern described by our Healthy Eating Pyramid. The 2005 guidelines acknowledged the harmful effects of trans fat and the beneficial role of vegetable oils, and they emphasized the importance of whole grains. However, they still capped total fat intake and promoted consuming large amounts of starch.

At best, MyPyramid was a missed opportunity to improve the health of millions of people. At worst, the lack of information and misinformation it conveyed contributed to overweight, poor health, and unnecessary early deaths.

Once again, special interest lobbies took the lead, shoving science aside.

USDA'S NEW MYPYRAMID

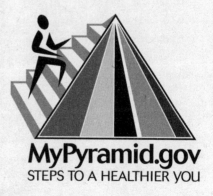

Figure 4. MyPyramid. In 2005, the USDA unveiled its catchy but information-free replacement for the familiar Food Guide Pyramid.

FROM PYRAMID TO PLATE

Bowing to criticism that MyPyramid was vague and confusing, the USDA replaced it in 2011 with MyPlate. This colorful image of a dinner plate divided into quarters makes an important and healthful point: Fill half your plate with vegetables and fruits. The other two quarters say little beyond "Eat more grains than protein." MyPlate says nothing about the quality of carbohydrates (grains). It makes no distinction between healthy sources of protein, such as beans, fish, and poultry, and less healthy sources such as red and processed meat. It recommends milk or dairy at every meal, even though there is little evidence that high dairy intake protects against osteoporosis and substantial evidence that consuming a lot of milk and dairy foods can be harmful. It offers no advice about healthy oils, which are good for the heart, arteries, and the rest of the body. And it is shockingly silent on sugary drinks, which provide far too many empty calories.

As we did with the Food Guide Pyramid, my colleagues and I created an alternative to MyPlate based on the most up-to-date research. The Harvard Healthy Eating Plate offers specific guidance for a healthy diet that comple-

MYPLATE

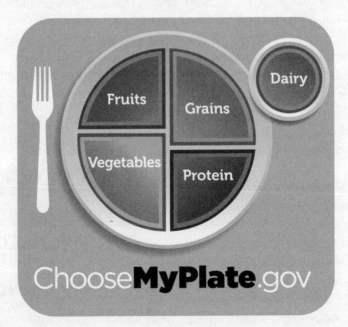

Figure 5. The USDA launched MyPlate in 2011.

THE HARVARD HEALTHY EATING PLATE

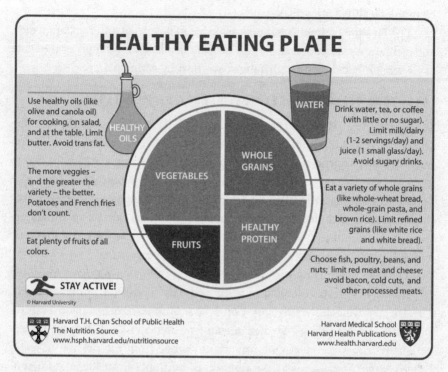

Figure 6. The Harvard Healthy Eating Plate offers simple guidance for making the best eating choices.

ments the Healthy Eating Pyramid and translates it to the context of a meal. As described in later chapters, it can help you improve the quality of your diet. Specifically, the Healthy Eating Plate recommends eating whole grains instead of refined grains, describes healthy sources of protein that don't include red meat, eliminates potatoes from the vegetable group, provides guidance about healthy sources of fat, and recommends water or other healthy beverages with every meal instead of milk.

Think of the Healthy Eating Plate as a simple guide for creating healthy, balanced meals, whether served on a plate or packed in a lunch box. It complements the Healthy Eating Pyramid, which can be used more as a grocery list. Fill your cart with items that populate its base, like vegetables, fruits, whole grains, healthy oils, and healthy sources of protein such as nuts, beans, fish, and chicken. Go easy on those near the top, such as red meat, white bread and other highly processed carbohydrates, sugar-sweetened beverages, and other sweets. Then, when you return home, prepare a meal that draws inspiration from the Healthy Eating Plate.

The Healthy Eating Plate is now available in dozens of different languages, and a children's version is also available. You can find all versions of the Plate at www.hsph.harvard.edu/nutritionsource/healthy-eating-plate/.

2015–2020 DIETARY GUIDELINES: PLENTY OF MEDDLING

To develop the 2015–2020 *Dietary Guidelines for Americans*, the USDA and the U.S. Department of Health and Human Services made an extra effort to minimize industry conflicts of interest. They appointed scientists without ties to lobbyists to serve on the Dietary Guidelines Advisory Committee. They also developed more specific rules for reviewing published studies to ensure that these scientists included all relevant evidence, a process called a systematic review. The committee members worked for two years, all as unpaid volunteers, to develop a comprehensive, science-based 571-page report.[11]

The recommendations in that report are very close to what *Eat, Drink, and Be Healthy* first recommended in 2001 and what it still recommends today. The Dietary Guidelines Advisory Committee emphasized healthy overall dietary patterns, including a Mediterranean-type diet, a vegan diet, and an eclectic healthy American diet. One important change from the previous *Dietary Guidelines for Americans* was the removal of an upper limit for total fat consumption, earlier set at 30 percent and then 35 percent of calories. I congratulate the advisory committee for correctly concluding that there was no evidence to support a specific upper limit. This is an important step, because the caps on total fat in the past led to promoting foods high in carbohydrates that were mostly refined starch and sugar.

After reviewing the abundant new evidence, the 2015–2020 Dietary Guidelines Advisory Committee explicitly recommended:

- limiting red meat consumption for both individual and planetary health
- reducing sugar intake to less than 10 percent of calories
- greatly reducing consumption of soda and other sugar-sweetened beverages.

The cattle and soda industries were furious about the recommendations. They put their powerful lobbies to work on Capitol Hill. The result was language embedded in the final government appropriations bill that forbade the USDA from including any statements in the final *Dietary Guidelines for Americans* about the environmental effects of dietary choices.

The lobbyists also had a supporter at the USDA, its head, Secretary Tom Vilsack. This former governor of Iowa has longstanding connections to the corn and pork industries. Even though Congress allowed the USDA to accept the recommendations of the Dietary Guidelines Advisory Committee to limit consumption of red and processed meat, the final *Dietary Guidelines for Americans* didn't mention that. Instead, it promoted consumption of red meat as long as it was lean, a finding not based on any evidence. The clear statement from the Dietary Guidelines Advisory Committee about reducing consumption of sugar-sweetened beverages was also considerably watered down.

The process of creating the 2015–2020 *Dietary Guidelines* vividly exposed the power of the agriculture and food industries in shaping dietary advice. The report of the advisory committee was censored. It was corrupted as it was "translated" into the official *Dietary Guidelines for Americans* that form the basis of federal food policy. These are the guidelines that our children learn in school.

The 2015–2020 Dietary Guidelines Advisory Committee report was a major advance in bringing advice on healthful eating in line with scientific evidence. But it still left some room for future improvements. The committee was told that its recommendations must meet the recommended dietary allowances (RDAs) for vitamins and minerals set by the Institute of Medicine (now called the National Academy of Medicine). That's a problem, because RDAs are often based on fragments of evidence and, for some nutrients, are seriously out-of-date.

Another problem with basing recommendations on RDAs is that the benefits of a food shouldn't be based simply on how much of a single nutrient it contains. This led to recommendations for high consumption of milk, which I discuss in chapters nine and ten.

The 2015–2020 advisory committee followed its predecessors by continuing to include potatoes as a vegetable despite substantial evidence that the health implications of eating potatoes are different than those of eating vegetables (see "The Spud Is a Dud" on page 167). Some experts challenged the advisory committee's decision to deemphasize the importance of limiting dietary cholesterol and eggs, a matter of judgment that I will talk about in chapter five.

That said, the committee deserves much credit for producing the most scientifically based report so far. It's highly unfortunate that their evidence-based recommendations weren't faithfully translated in the final dietary guidelines that guide policy and shape the eating habits of millions of Americans.

FURTHER TESTING OF THE PYRAMIDS, PLATES, AND DIETARY GUIDELINES

Back in 1995 the USDA created what it called the Healthy Eating Index. This ten-item score tried to measure how healthfully Americans were eating. The first five items checked how well a person's diet conformed to the Food Guide Pyramid for grains, vegetables, fruits, milk, and meat. The next four checked total fat in the diet, saturated fat, cholesterol, and sodium. The tenth measured the amount of variety in the diet. Each item was awarded 0 to 10 points: the higher the number, the more closely an individual was following the USDA's guidelines for healthy eating.

My colleagues and I, having highlighted the deep flaws in the USDA's dietary recommendations, put the Healthy Eating Index to the test among the participants of the Nurses' Health Study and the Health Professionals studies. Individuals with high scores were only slightly less likely to have had heart attacks or strokes, and there was no reduction in cancer. In other words, those who most closely followed the government's recommendations didn't fare much better than those who did.

What if such a diet-measuring tool made a distinction between healthful unsaturated fat and less-than-healthy saturated fat, or the main sources of carbohydrates or protein? So we devised the Alternate Healthy Eating Index in 2002.[12] It recorded nine diet items: servings of vegetables, fruits, and nuts or soy protein a day; grams of fiber from grains; the ratio of white to red meat; the amount of trans fat; the ratio of polyunsaturated to saturated fat; use of a multivitamin; and daily alcohol consumption. Like the Healthy Eating Index, points were awarded for each item, with higher points representing healthier choices.

When we compared the two indexes using diet data from the Nurses' Health Study and the Health Professionals Follow-Up Study, the Alternative Healthy Eating Index was far better at predicting the development of cardiovascular disease and other chronic conditions than the USDA's Healthy Eating Index.[13] That means we can further reduce the risk of cardiovascular disease, cancer, and other chronic conditions by following evidence-based dietary guidance rather than government-based guidance.

New evidence on diet and health prompted my colleagues and me to make small adjustments to our Alternative Healthy Eating Index. With the most recent update, in 2010, we added to the index, limiting soda and other sugar-sweetened beverages as a healthy eating strategy. We repeated our test to determine if women and men whose diets fit the pattern described by this index—which matches the recommendations in this book—have better long-term health and compared it to an updated version of the USDA's Healthy Eating Index that more closely resembles our Alternative Index.

As expected, both of these indices represent dietary advice and eating patterns that are in line with lower risks of dying prematurely or developing heart disease, type 2 diabetes, and other chronic conditions. Even so, our Alternative Healthy Eating Index did better than the USDA's.[14]

Other investigators have developed indices that include the same basic elements and have evaluated them in different populations and in relation to a variety of health outcomes. All of them predict better health. This convergence of evidence from many different sources makes me confident that what I recommend in this book will help you choose a diet that is healthy for a lifetime.

Despite a few naysayers who contend that nutrition scientists can't agree on anything,[15] the convergence of Harvard's Alternative Healthy Eating Index and the USDA's Healthy Eating Index suggest that a broad consensus has developed around the basic elements of a healthy diet.

The Healthy Eating Pyramid and Plate aren't set in stone, and additional fine details are likely to emerge with further research. For example, new findings about the health effects of vegetables in chapter eight are likely to surprise many readers. Yet we can have a high level of confidence that today's broad picture of a healthy diet will endure.

BETTER GUIDELINES AND BETTER DIETS PAY OFF

In spite of the back-and-forth of science, misleading dietary guidelines from the USDA, sensationalist reporting, and purposeful misinformation, the average American diet is getting better. Since the 1960s a doubling of polyunsaturated fat intake, a reduction in saturated fat intake, and a 40 percent decline in red meat consumption have contributed to a 60 percent reduction in deaths from heart disease and added years of life.

Curious about other potentially healthy changes in the American diet, my colleagues and I applied the Alternative Healthy Eating Index to the eating patterns of a national survey of Americans. We saw steady improvements between 1999 and 2012. The changes with the biggest effects on health were the near elimination of artery-damaging trans fats and a 25 percent drop in drinking sugar-sweetened soda. There were also modest increases in eating fruits, vegetables, whole grains, and unsaturated fat.[16] We estimated that these improvements in diet had prevented more than 1 million premature deaths and 12 percent of cases of diabetes between 1999 and 2012. Shortly after our report, the Centers for Disease Control and Prevention reported that new diagnoses of diabetes had declined for the first time, by a substantial 20 percent, consistent with reductions in trans fat and soda consumption.

Although the *trend* in diet quality was in the right direction, the average score was still less than 50 on a scale of 110, indicating the potential for far greater improvements in health. In the pages that follow, I will describe how to boost your score to be at or near the top of the scale, where the payoffs can be huge.

CHAPTER THREE

What Can You Believe About Diet?

RESEARCH ABOUT DIET AND NUTRITION seems to contradict itself with aggravating regularity. You stop using butter and start spreading margarine on your toast, only to learn later that margarine can be as bad for you, and then later that butter isn't as bad as it was once thought to be. After switching to bran muffins for breakfast because high-fiber diets supposedly prevent colon cancer, you hear about a big study showing that fiber doesn't prevent colon cancer. In an early study, coffee drinking appeared to increase the chances of developing pancreatic cancer, while later research shows that coffee drinking is harmless and may even have some benefits. Some studies find that eating fish prevents heart attacks; others don't. These flip-flops are so confusing and so common that a negative report on vitamin E and beta-carotene once goaded *Boston Globe* columnist Ellen Goodman to write, "There seems to be some sort of planned obsolescence now to medical news. Today's cure is tomorrow's poison pellet. Fresh research has a sell-by date that is shorter than the one on the cereal box."[1]

The sheer volume of information doesn't help. Fifty years ago nutrition was a quiet backwater of medical research. For example, the longest study of health in the United States, the legendary and ongoing Framingham Heart Study, collected hardly any data on diet when it was started in 1949. Over the years, though, the trickle of information on diet and health has swelled into a fast-flowing torrent.

It's only natural that people want to know the latest (often confused with the best) results, whether they are looking for ways to fine-tune their diets or for that single magic key—the right food or vitamin or supplement—that will open the door to the longest, healthiest life possible. The media cater to this interest and serve up a steady stream of nutrition news.

The problem is that newspapers, television, radio, blogs, websites, and apps tend to turn the baby steps of scientific research into "major advances," "breakthroughs," and "possible cures," or highlight the confusing contradictions when one study contradicts an earlier one. This makes following health news seem like reading pages torn at random from a book or, worse, reading the pages with misprints.

REPLACING EDUCATED GUESSES WITH EVIDENCE

Another reason for the flip-flops is that early recommendations about diet were often based on thin evidence. The thinking behind these early recommendations was that, since people were going to eat no matter what, guidelines based on intelligent guesses were better than no guidelines at all. That's actually a reasonable approach when there isn't much evidence. Unfortunately, these recommendations never carried warning labels like "Educated Guess, Subject to Change." Those educated guesses tend to be repeated thousands of times until they acquire the ring of truth.

When researchers began learning of the possible dangers of saturated fat, for example, many recommended that people switch from butter, which is high in saturated fat, to low-saturated-fat margarine. This recommendation made sense, even though there were no studies showing that people who ate margarine instead of butter had fewer heart attacks. Then along came studies showing that margarine eaters fared *worse* in the heart-attack department than butter eaters. That finding was reinforced by short-term studies showing that trans fat, which was high in many margarines, had far worse effects on blood cholesterol than saturated fat.

To a scientist, this is the normal path of scientific progress—a recommendation based on a good guess is tested and toppled by one based on better science. To the rest of the world, though, it is a frustrating contradiction.

The amount and quality of sound scientific information on diet and health have grown enormously over the past thirty years. That makes today's evidence-based recommendations more certain and less likely to undergo radical changes than those made three decades ago. As the quest for new and better knowledge about diet and health continues, rest assured that even today's recommendations will probably be subject to some fine-tuning, even though the big picture is unlikely to change appreciably.

CONTRADICTIONS ARE INEVITABLE

Nutrition research seems to generate more than its share of contradictory results. That's partly because the media pay special attention to nutrition—because of the public's interest—while inorganic chemistry, geology, and many other disciplines escape this daily scrutiny.

It's also because medical science has its own special rhythm, one that doesn't fit with the media's need to tell compelling but simple stories. Efforts to present "balanced" articles by quoting opposing views can sometimes confuse things even further.

For nutrition research, the rhythm is more a cha-cha—two steps forward and one step back—than a straight-ahead march. If you look at the day-to-day results, which are reported more like sports scores than scientific research, it's easy to wonder why researchers can't get it right the first time.

They can't because these conflicts and contradictions are the way science works. It happens this way in every field, from archaeology to zoology, nuclear physics to nutrition. Men and women carry out studies and report their results. Evidence accumulates. Like dropping stones onto an old-fashioned scale, the weight of evidence gradually tips the balance in favor of one idea over another. It is only when this happens that you should make changes in your life.

The size of the stone clearly makes a difference. As we describe on pages 30–35, most studies are like sand grains or small pebbles. Very few are like boulders.

WORKING WITH REAL PEOPLE POSES SPECIAL CHALLENGES

Nutrition scientists usually can't exert the same kind of control over their research subjects that chemists and zoologists can. Instead they must work with unpredictable, independent, mostly uncontrollable subjects: people.

Here are a few of the challenges that nutrition researchers face:

- *People don't eat "human chow" meal after meal after meal.* Instead, diets change from day to day, week to week, and season to season. What you usually eat now is probably a bit (or maybe a lot) different from what you used to eat two years ago or will eat two years from now. These changes are driven by personal taste, cultural changes, new developments in agriculture and technology, and changes in work and family life. Disease and aging can also change what people eat.
- *Many studies depend on people accurately reporting what they eat.* That's a

challenging task: Try remembering exactly what you ate one day last week. Despite this difficulty, people are fairly accurate about reporting their longer-term eating pattern. But because they aren't perfect, there's almost always some imprecision when linking diet and disease.

- *The foods you eat each day contain thousands of different natural chemicals, some known and well studied, some known and unstudied, many completely unknown and currently unmeasurable.* So far we've figured out what only a small percentage of them do in the body. And then there are the artificial compounds added as preservatives, stabilizers, flavor enhancers, and more. This makes it difficult to draw strong conclusions about a specific vitamin, mineral, or other molecule from studies of foods and diseases. Knowing exactly what is in different foods, how food compounds interact, and what they all do in the body are important jobs for the future.

- *Calculating the nutrients a person gets from the foods she or he eats—how much saturated fat, fiber, vitamin E, and so on—is tricky, since it depends on sometimes sketchy information about food composition.*

- *Almost everyone eats some fat, fiber, sugar, starches, fruits, vegetables, vitamins, and so forth.* That means nutrition researchers are faced with the difficult task of measuring how much of something is eaten, not just whether it is part of the diet.

- *Heart disease, cancer, diabetes, osteoporosis, cataracts, and other chronic diseases almost always develop over many years or even decades.* They also have other causes beside diet, including genes, physical activity, smoking, stress, and other factors yet to be identified.

DIFFERENT METHODS FOR DIFFERENT PROBLEMS

To get around these problems, nutrition scientists use a variety of research methods.[2]

Randomized Trials

These are often considered the gold standard by which other studies are usually judged. In these carefully controlled studies, half of a group of volunteers is randomly assigned to the experimental diet or treatment, and the other half is assigned to a comparison diet or treatment (called the control) or possibly to no treatment at all. After a preset time, the number of people in the experimental group who have developed the predetermined "endpoint"—death, heart attack, broken hip, and so on—is compared with the number in the control group.

For example, say you want to know if vitamin C prevents age-related memory loss. You would round up a large group of volunteers, then randomly assign some to take a daily vitamin C tablet, while the others take an identical tablet that contains an inactive ingredient that tastes like vitamin C (a placebo). After ten or twenty years you would compare the percentage of people in the vitamin C group who have experienced memory loss with the percentage in the placebo group.

This kind of study has plenty of advantages. If it is large enough, the randomization process does a good job of making sure the people in the experimental group are very similar to those in the control group in terms of age, health, exercise, and other possibly important factors. So the only thing different between the two groups is the diet or treatment.

Unfortunately, randomized trials are often impossible to do when it comes to nutrition. Getting people to prepare and eat special meals for a long time is difficult. So is getting people to take a vitamin pill or placebo for maybe a decade or more. Given the large number of volunteers needed, the cost of running a randomized trial can be astronomical. The Women's Health Initiative—which tested the effect of reducing dietary fat to 20 percent of calories and increasing consumption of fruits and vegetables on the development of breast cancer, heart disease, and other chronic conditions among almost 60,000 women in the 1990s—cost more than $2 billion and didn't yield clear answers on this important question, in part because there was actually very little difference in fat intake between women assigned to follow a low-fat diet and those following the comparison "usual diet."

A major limitation of randomized trials of vitamins and other nutritional supplements is that many or most of the participants may already be getting enough of the factor being studied in their normal diets. That could mean missing an important benefit in people with lower intakes. For example, randomized trials of folic acid supplementation conducted in the United States after the FDA required companies to fortify flour with this important B vitamin showed little overall effect on risk of cardiovascular disease. But a trial conducted in China, where folic acid levels were low, found an important reduction in strokes.[3] This makes it likely that at least some people in the U.S. with low folic acid intake would also benefit from getting more of this vitamin.

The ability of randomized trials to give misleading results is vividly illustrated by their failure to detect a benefit in stopping smoking, probably the single most important step a person can take to improve their health.[4] This happened in a classic trial called the Multiple Risk Factor Intervention Trial. The reason it didn't detect a benefit for quitting smoking is almost surely because many of the participants who stopped smoking took it up again, and the seven-year study wasn't long enough to see the full benefits for those who did quit permanently.

Cohort studies

Another effective method involves following large groups of "free-living humans"—regular people like you—for long periods of time. These cohort studies start with a group of people who often have something in common, like an occupation or place of residence. They are asked about their diets, smoking and drinking habits, education, occupation, medical conditions, and other possibly relevant things. The group is then followed for a period of time, ideally a decade or more, either directly with occasional checkups and mailed questionnaires or indirectly by monitoring death certificates. Once the study has gone on long enough, researchers can examine the accumulated information to test a variety of hypotheses. They can, for example, determine if people in the cohort who eat the most fiber have different rates of colon cancer from those who eat the least fiber, or if those who consume the most folate, an important B vitamin, have lower rates of heart disease than those who consume the least folate. Such long-term studies have yielded some of the best insights so far into the link between diet and health.

By gathering information at the beginning, before specific diseases have occurred, cohort studies avoid the skewed recall sometimes seen among people who develop a particular disease—and who would like to find an explanation for it. Cohort studies such as the Nurses' Health Study, the Health Professionals Follow-Up Study, the Adventist Health Studies, and others (see "Key Cohort Studies," page 31) use carefully tested questionnaires to determine what the participants eat. The Nurses' Health Studies and Health Professional's Follow-Up Study, both conducted by my research group, are unique because the participants fill out dietary questionnaires many times over the course of the study. This is important in long-term follow-up studies because diets change greatly over time due to individual preferences and changes in the food supply.

Randomized controlled trials are sometimes held up as the "best" evidence. But cohort studies can answer questions that aren't possible in such trials, such as long-term effects of diet. Trials can't evaluate the effects of diet or weight during childhood or adolescence on health during adulthood or old age. They also can't test something potentially harmful, like trans fats: it would now be unethical to do a trial in which half of the participants were given diets containing a high level of these artery-clogging fats.

Key Cohort Studies

Dozens of cohort studies of diet and health are in progress. They have already provided us with important information on connections between diet and disease, and will produce a flood of data over the coming years. They include:

- *American Cancer Society.* In 1992, the American Cancer Society launched the Cancer Prevention Study II–Nutrition Cohort, which has been following the health of 132,000 men and women to explore possible connections between alcohol use, exercise, diet, and other factors on the development of cancer. The Cancer Prevention Study-3, begun in 2006, adds another 300,000 participants with greater racial and ethnic diversity.
- *Adventist Health Studies.* These include studies of 27,658 male and female California Seventh-day Adventists, a group chosen because many members of this religion are vegetarians. The newer Adventist Health Study-2 is following 96,000 church members from the U.S. and Canada.
- *Black Women's Health Study.* This cohort, started in 1995, is following 59,000 black women to explore why they are more likely than other women to develop high blood pressure, breast cancer earlier in life, diabetes, stroke, and lupus.
- *European Prospective Investigation into Cancer and Nutrition and Study (EPIC).* This is a collaborative study started in 1993 in nine European countries. In all, 440,000 men and women have been enrolled.
- *Health Professionals Follow-Up Study.* A study of 51,529 male health professionals (dentists, veterinarians, pharmacists, optometrists, osteopathic physicians, and podiatrists) who were between the ages of forty and seventy-five in 1986. Like the participants of the Nurses' Health Study, these men have been completing health, diet, and lifestyle updates every other year.
- *Iowa Women's Health Study.* This is a study of 41,836 postmenopausal Iowa women who were between the ages of fifty-five and sixty-nine in 1986. It was designed to examine the effect of several dietary and other lifestyle patterns on the development of cancer.
- *Mexican Teachers' Cohort.* This study is following more than 115,000 female teachers living in Mexico, enrolled in the late 2000s, to investigate the effects of socioeconomic status, reproductive history, lifestyle, and dietary factors on the development of chronic diseases and mental illness.
- *Multiethnic Cohort Study of Diet and Cancer.* This is an ambitious study begun in 1993 that includes 215,000 men and women representing five

different ethnic groups: whites, African Americans, Japanese Americans, Latinos, and Native Hawaiians.

- *NIH-AARP Diet and Health Study.* A joint project between the National Cancer Institute and the AARP, this cohort was started in 1995 to investigate relationships between diet, lifestyle, and cancer.
- *Nurses' Health Study/Nurses' Health Study II.* These studies have been following the health and wellbeing of more than 200,000 female nurses since 1976 (see "Praise for Nurses and Health Professionals" on page 33).
- *Shanghai Women's and Men's Studies.* These cohorts consist of over 130,000 women and men living in Shanghai, China, who were between the ages of forty and seventy-five in 1986 and 1989. They focus on diet-related, environmental, and genetic factors that may cause cancer.

Studies in the U.S. that focus on racially and ethnically diverse populations will offer important information for all Americans. Those under way in Asia, and Mexico will provide valuable information on a wider range of dietary patterns. Africa and South America are still blank pages when it comes to diet and health, because large cohort studies haven't yet been launched.

Case-Control Studies

In this type of study, researchers gather information from a group of people who have developed a particular disease (the cases) and a similar group of people who are free of that disease (the controls). They then compare the two groups for differences in diet, exercise, or whatever variable they are interested in. Case-control studies are effective tools when the variable is clear-cut—say, cigarette smoking or occupation. They don't work as well for diet, when only small differences are likely to be seen from person to person. Case-control studies are also more prone to error and bias than cohort studies.

Because case-control studies can be done quickly and inexpensively, they supplied the evidence for many of the early recommendations about diet and health. As information emerges from cohort studies, though, we are finding that the conclusions from case-control studies were, not surprisingly, often off the mark.

Controlled Feeding Studies

These are a kind of short-term randomized trial done with volunteers, sometimes living in special clinic wards, who eat specially prepared meals. The controlled conditions make it possible to see how different foods or nutrients

Praise for Nurses and Health Professionals

Back in 1976, Dr. Frank Speizer at the Channing Laboratory of Brigham and Women's Hospital and the Harvard School of Public Health started the Nurses' Health Study. Its initial aim was to investigate the potential long-term consequences of oral contraceptives, which were then being taken by millions of women. Nurses were chosen as the study population because of their knowledge about health and their ability to provide complete and accurate information about various diseases, thanks to their nursing education. The research team signed up 121,700 female registered nurses between the ages of thirty and fifty-five. Since then, the aims of the Nurses' Health Study have broadened to look at the effects of diet and other lifestyle factors on cancer, cardiovascular disease, osteoporosis, mental health, and other conditions.

The participants complete follow-up questionnaires every two years to update information on a variety of health risk factors, and they complete diet questionnaires every four years.

Former secretary of the U.S. Department of Health and Human Services Donna Shalala called the Nurses' Health Study "one of the most significant studies ever conducted on the health of women." To recognize the fortieth anniversary of this study, the *American Journal of Public Health* devoted a whole issue to recount its many contributions.[5]

More studies are under way. The Nurses' Health Study II, started in 1989, includes 116,000 younger nurses. In addition, 15,000 of the children of these nurses are taking part in the Growing Up Today Study. The Nurses' Health Study 3 is now enrolling women and men and is also focusing on diet and lifestyle factors at younger ages; this study is being conducted entirely online.

Since the nurses' studies originally included only women, several colleagues and I started the Health Professionals Follow-Up Study in 1986 to examine the effects of diet on chronic disease in men. It initially included 51,529 male dentists, pharmacists, optometrists, osteopathic physicians, podiatrists, and veterinarians.

These dedicated nurses, their children, and male health professionals have made huge contributions to our understanding of the connections between diet and health. This book reflects their time and effort.

affect changes in blood cholesterol or other biochemical markers. But these studies are too small and don't go on long enough to measure the effect on disease risks. Nor can they measure how real diets affect people living in the far messier and less controlled real world.

Ecological Studies

Much of the motivation for research on diet and health, and some of the early clues about what might be important, have come from studies that compare diets and disease rates in various geographical areas. One of the seminal ecological studies was the Seven Countries Study, conducted by Dr. Ancel Keys and colleagues in the 1960s. These investigators enrolled about 1,000 men in fourteen different areas in seven countries and followed them for a decade to document their rates of heart attacks. They documented about a tenfold difference in rates of heart disease, with the lowest being on the Greek island of Crete and in Japan. Keys and colleagues also showed that, among the fourteen areas, there was a correlation between intake of saturated fat and heart disease rates.[6]

At the same time, other scientists were showing that men who migrated from areas like Japan, where heart disease rates were low, to the United States, where they were high, were more likely to develop heart disease than men who stayed put. These findings were profoundly important because they clearly showed that the high heart disease rates of the U.S. were not due to genetic factors and were not inevitable.

The central weakness of ecological studies is that many factors other than diet often differ between geographic regions. In the Seven Countries Study it wasn't possible to conclude that saturated fat was the key cause of heart disease. Clearly more research was needed, but evidence from these ecological studies provided the impetus to look at diet because, in principle, all populations might have been able to achieve the low rates of heart disease seen in Crete even without sophisticated medicine.

In parallel with the work of Keys and colleagues, other scientists were conducting ecological studies of breast and other major cancers. Similar findings emerged: large differences in rates from country to country, an increase in the breast cancer rate seen with migration to the U.S., and strong correlations with dietary factors.

Mendelian Randomization Studies

This approach, named after Gregor Mendel, the nineteenth-century monk known as the father of genetics, is a newcomer to study designs. It takes advantage of new technologies to identify DNA variations in almost every one of our 30,000 genes. If a large epidemiologic study links a genetic variant that's involved in metabolizing a specific dietary factor with a particular disease risk, it makes a strong case for a cause-effect relationship between the dietary factor and the disease.

Systematic Reviews, Meta-analyses, and Pooled Analyses

When many studies have been done on a particular topic—say, the effect of alcohol on cardiovascular health—it can be helpful to take a step back and look at all of them together. A *systematic review* combs through the medical literature to identify all the relevant studies and then offers conclusions based on them. A *meta-analysis* statistically combines the published results from a systematic review to provide an overall "bottom line."

One problem with meta-analyses is that they gather data only from published studies and so can't capture information from "negative" studies, which tend not to get published. Another is that almost anyone with a computer and Internet connection can do a meta-analysis. But to be done well for a complicated topic like diet and health, deep knowledge of the topic is also required. For example, investigators who conducted a headline-grabbing meta-analysis concluding that replacing saturated fat with unsaturated fat had no benefit for heart disease risk[7] were clearly unfamiliar with the published literature, the design of the studies they included, and even the definition of the dietary variables that they used.

In a *pooled analysis*, investigators contribute raw data, both published and unpublished, and analyze it altogether. This allows for more complete and detailed analysis because the raw data are used rather than just data from published studies. Pooled analyses also have their limits, as they are only as strong as the studies included. To combine studies, it is usually necessary to use only the variables that were included in all of the studies, such as just a single baseline assessment of diet.

DECIPHERING MEDICAL NEWS

Careful journalists try to put new research into perspective. But it's impossible to cram that kind of context into thirty seconds of air time or 250 words, so you often end up with little more than sound bites or headlines. Other than mastering the fine points of nutrition research, here are a few tips that can help you know what nutrition news is worth paying attention to:

- *Studies done on people.* How foods, nutrients, and food additives affect mice, dogs, and monkeys is an important thread in the fabric of nutrition research. But they may have completely different effects on people. Animal studies can pave the way for future research but are rarely the basis for changing your diet.

- *Studies done in the real world.* Diet studies done in hospitals or special research centers have given us important information about how the body responds to different nutrients and foods. But they don't look directly at disease risk, only intermediate markers of disease, so they can't reliably predict the consequences of different eating habits or strategies on what really matters: your health.

- *Studies that look at diseases, not markers for them.* Because it takes so long for chronic diseases to develop, many studies use intermediate markers like narrowing of the heart's arteries or changes in bone density as stand-ins. These changes don't necessarily translate into real diseases, though. Pay more attention to research that has looked at real health problems like broken bones or heart attacks.

- *Large studies.* In science, the play of chance is a real problem. The larger the study, the smaller the possibility that chance alone explains potentially important differences between two groups. Larger studies are also more likely to spot important connections that would be missed in smaller ones.

- *Weight of evidence.* The most persuasive evidence that an effect is real comes from a number of studies done by different researchers at different times using different methods and involving different groups of people. This is a bit like a court of law, in which multiple pieces of evidence are considered and weighed to determine whether someone is guilty with a high level of certainty. (The courtroom is an example of a situation in which important decisions, some of them literally matters of life or death, are made without randomized trials.) In diet and health, when data from randomized trials aren't available or feasible, the best evidence often comes when a link is seen between a dietary factor and disease in multiple well-designed cohort studies and controlled feeding studies. As described in chapter five, this is how trans fat was "convicted" for increasing the risk of heart disease.

A good example of consistent evidence is the link between moderate alcohol use and reduced risk of heart disease. Possible beneficial effects of alcohol have been suspected for more than two thousand years. In the late 1700s, William Heberden, the British physician who first described the chest pain known today as angina, wrote that "wine and spiritous liquors—afford considerable relief from angina."[8]

Sporadic reports appeared throughout the twentieth century suggesting that drinking alcohol prevented clogged arteries, but they were often balanced by reports of the detrimental effects of heavy drinking. Since 1974, though, dozens of case-control and cohort studies from different geographic regions with different alcoholic beverages have shown that people who have one or two alcoholic drinks a day are less likely to have a heart attack or die from heart disease than nondrinkers or heavy drinkers.[9] This relation persists even after the results have been statistically adjusted for smoking, exercise, and other variables that could differ between drinkers and nondrinkers. These observations have been further bolstered by evidence from laboratory, animal, and controlled feeding studies in humans showing that alcohol increases levels of protective HDL cholesterol and also makes blood less likely to clot, both of which would be expected to protect against heart disease. Using a Mendelian randomization approach, a genetic variant involved in metabolizing alcohol was shown to be associated with heart attack risk, and only in those consuming alcohol.[10]

This body of evidence points to a firm conclusion that drinking moderate amounts of alcohol reduces the risk of heart disease. A randomized trial just getting under way as this book goes to press should offer even more information about the benefits and risks of drinking alcohol.

Regardless of the results from all of these different streams of evidence, any decision about drinking should take into account alcohol's full range of risks and benefits (see chapter nine).

PUTTING IT INTO PRACTICE

Given the flood of information from nutrition research, I suggest that you not make big changes in what or how you eat based on a single study. If a result is on the right track, other studies will show the same thing. And it won't matter much in the long run whether you make a change today (like taking a vitamin or increasing the amount of monounsaturated fat in your diet) or six months from now.

In fact, Mark Twain's cynical, laconic view of health information is as good today as it was one hundred years ago: "Be careful about reading health books. You may die of a misprint."

In the following chapters, I describe the building blocks of evidence that support the key conclusions of this book and can make an important difference in your well-being.

CHAPTER FOUR

Healthy Weight

M Y AIM IN THIS BOOK is to offer straightforward, no-nonsense advice on health and nutrition based on the best information available. I'll start right here. If your weight is in the "healthy" range, keep it there (see Figure 7). If you are overweight, change your diet and exercise pattern so you won't add any more pounds and ideally will lose some. This isn't a new idea, and it certainly won't land me a spot as the next diet guru on *The Dr. Oz Show*. But the number that stares up at you from the bathroom scale is one of the most important measures of your future health. Keeping that number in the healthy range is more important for long-term health than the types and amounts of antioxidants in your food or the ratio of fats to carbohydrates.

The amount of food you eat is fundamentally important to whether you gain or lose weight. That will be the focus of this chapter. But the types of food you eat—the *quality* of your diet—influences how much you eat, so I will focus on the quality of what you eat, not just the amount. I hope you'll be relieved to know that the same diet that works for maximum health also helps control weight.

Weight sits like a spider at the center of an intricate, tangled web of health and disease. Three related aspects of weight—how much you weigh in relation to your height, your waist size, and how much weight you gain after your early twenties—strongly influence your chances of having or dying from a heart attack, stroke, or other type of cardiovascular disease; of developing high blood pressure, high cholesterol, or diabetes; of being diagnosed with postmenopausal breast cancer or cancer of the prostate, endometrium, colon, pancreas, esophagus, or kidney; of having arthritis; of being infertile or having trouble getting an erection; of developing gallstones or cataracts; of snoring or suffering from sleep apnea; of developing adult-onset asthma; and more. As shown in Figure 4, weight is directly linked with a variety of diseases in the Nurses' Health Study. These data indicate that with increasing body mass

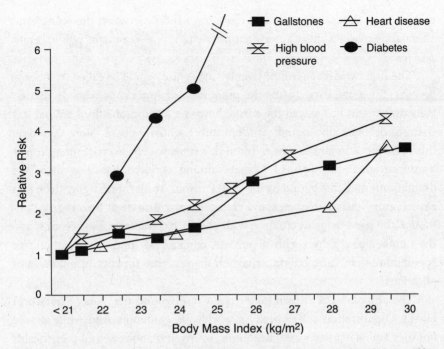

Figure 7. Weight and Disease. Among women in the Nurses' Health Study, the chances of developing any of four common conditions increases with increasing body mass index.

index—a measure that includes both weight and height—the risks of heart disease, high blood pressure, gallstones, and type 2 diabetes all steadily increase, even among those in the healthy weight category. Above a body mass index of 30, which is the boundary between overweight and obesity, the risks continue to increase. Similar trends are seen among men in the Health Professionals Follow-Up Study.

Given the importance of weight in staying healthy, no mention of weight in the USDA Food Guide Pyramid, MyPyramid, or MyPlate for two decades was a serious omission. And weight recommendations in the current *Dietary Guidelines for Americans* are set too high for many people and may mislead some into thinking that substantial weight gain within the "healthy" weight category is perfectly fine (see page 43). As the evidence shows, it's not.

THE OBESITY EPIDEMIC

Carrying too many pounds is a very personal problem. It can shape how you feel about yourself and how others treat you. It has a direct effect on your current and future health. It costs you (or at least your health insurance company) tens of thousands of dollars more in medical costs over the years.[1] And although excess weight is a personal problem, it is also a major public health problem.

The first two decades of the twenty-first century could be called the obesity decades. Since the early 1960s the proportion of Americans who are moderately overweight has stayed the same, hovering around one-third.[2] What has changed dramatically, though, is the number who are obese. More than one-third of American adults now fall into this category, almost triple the proportion from the early 1960s.[3] Obesity among children has also increased dramatically over this period by three- to fourfold, an alarming trend given that early obesity leads to diabetes and cardiovascular disease at a young age. Although the percentage of children with obesity has leveled off in recent years, the number of children with it remains dangerously high. As a nation, we spend more than $200 billion a year[4] on medical care for obesity and its complications.

The situation isn't much better elsewhere around the globe. The World Health Organization calls obesity a worldwide epidemic. And while deadly famines and starvation make headlines, overweight, obesity, and their health consequences have already replaced malnutrition and infection as the main causes of early death and disability in many developing countries.[5]

WHAT IS A HEALTHY WEIGHT?

What seems to be a simple question turns out to be remarkably difficult to answer. There are two parts of this problem. First, a weight that may be perfectly fine for someone who is six feet one—say 175 pounds—is way too much for someone who is five feet two. Another part is lingering confusion about the way healthy weight has been defined in the past.

A number called the body mass index (BMI), or Quetelet index, gets around the first problem. This measure of weight adjusted for height does a good job of accounting for the fact that taller people tend to weigh more than shorter people. If you like math, you can calculate your BMI like this: Divide your weight in pounds by your height in inches; divide that number by your height in inches; and multiply that number by 703. You can also just look it up in the table on page 41 or have it calculated for you by any number of online BMI calculators, such as the one on the Harvard Health Publications website (www.health.harvard.edu/bmi).

Setting guidelines for healthy BMIs has traditionally been done by examining death rates in large groups of people and then picking the BMIs with the

BODY MASS INDEX CHART

Body Weight (pounds)

Height (inches)																																			
58	91	96	100	105	110	115	119	124	129	134	138	143	148	153	158	162	167	172	177	181	186	191	196	201	205	210	215	220	224	229	234	239	244	248	253	258
59	94	99	104	109	114	119	124	128	133	138	143	148	153	158	163	168	173	178	183	188	193	198	203	208	212	217	222	227	232	237	242	247	252	257	262	267
60	97	102	107	112	118	123	128	133	138	143	148	153	158	163	168	174	179	184	189	194	199	204	209	215	220	225	230	235	240	245	250	255	261	266	271	276
61	100	106	111	116	122	127	132	137	143	148	153	158	164	169	174	180	185	190	195	201	206	211	217	222	227	232	238	243	248	254	259	264	269	275	280	285
62	104	109	115	120	126	131	136	142	147	153	158	164	169	175	180	186	191	196	202	207	213	218	224	229	235	240	246	251	256	262	267	273	278	284	289	295
63	107	113	118	124	130	135	141	146	152	158	163	169	175	180	186	191	197	203	208	214	220	225	231	237	242	248	254	259	265	270	278	282	287	293	299	304
64	110	116	122	128	134	140	145	151	157	163	169	174	180	186	192	197	204	209	215	221	227	232	238	244	250	256	262	267	273	279	285	291	296	302	308	314
65	114	120	126	132	138	144	150	156	162	168	174	180	186	192	198	204	210	216	222	228	234	240	246	252	258	264	270	276	282	288	294	300	306	312	318	324
66	118	124	130	136	142	148	155	161	167	173	179	186	192	198	204	210	216	223	229	235	241	247	253	260	266	272	278	284	291	297	303	309	315	322	328	334
67	121	127	134	140	146	153	159	166	172	178	185	191	198	204	211	217	223	230	236	242	249	255	261	268	274	280	287	293	299	306	312	319	325	331	338	344
68	125	131	138	144	151	158	164	171	177	184	190	197	203	210	216	223	230	236	243	249	256	262	269	276	282	289	295	302	308	315	322	328	335	341	348	354
69	128	135	142	149	155	162	169	176	182	189	196	203	209	216	223	230	236	243	250	257	263	270	277	284	291	297	304	311	318	324	331	338	345	351	358	365
70	132	139	146	153	160	167	174	181	188	195	202	209	216	222	229	236	243	250	257	264	271	278	285	292	299	306	313	320	327	334	341	348	355	362	369	376
71	136	143	150	157	165	172	179	186	193	200	208	215	222	229	236	243	250	257	265	272	279	286	293	301	308	315	322	329	338	343	351	358	365	372	379	386
72	140	147	154	162	169	177	184	191	199	206	213	221	228	235	242	250	258	265	272	279	287	294	302	309	316	324	331	338	346	353	361	368	375	383	390	397
73	144	151	159	166	174	182	189	197	204	212	219	227	235	242	250	257	265	272	280	288	295	302	310	318	325	333	340	348	355	363	371	378	386	393	401	408
74	148	155	163	171	179	186	194	202	210	218	225	233	241	249	256	264	272	280	287	295	303	311	319	326	334	342	350	358	365	373	381	389	396	404	412	420
75	152	160	168	176	184	192	200	208	216	224	232	240	248	256	264	272	279	287	295	303	311	319	327	335	343	351	359	367	375	383	391	399	407	415	423	431
76	156	164	172	180	189	197	205	213	221	230	238	246	254	263	271	279	287	295	304	312	320	328	336	344	353	361	369	377	385	394	402	410	418	426	435	443
BMI	19	20	21	22	23	24	25	26	27	28	29	30	31	32	33	34	35	36	37	38	39	40	41	42	43	44	45	46	47	48	49	50	51	52	53	54

Figure 8. BMI Tables. To use these tables, find your height in the left-hand column. Move across to a given weight. The number at the bottom of the column is your BMI.

lowest death rates as the "healthy range." Most studies have shown that range to be BMIs between 18.5 and 24.9.

In 2013, several statisticians at the Centers for Disease Control and Prevention (CDC) published an analysis showing that the healthy range (meaning the lowest death rate) was among people who were overweight (BMIs between 25 and 29.9). In their analysis, overweight people were less likely to have died over the study periods than those who were at healthy weights (BMI between 18.5 and 24.9). As in other studies, individuals who were very thin or seriously obese were also more likely to have died. The report, published in the *Journal of the American Medical Association*,[6] garnered widespread press coverage, spawning headlines like "How Love Handles Can Help You Stay Healthy," "Astonishing New Research Shows How Being Overweight Can Stop You from Dying Early," and "Carrying a Few Extra Pounds Could Protect the Heart."

These findings don't make sense. How can being overweight, which increases the likelihood of developing type 2 diabetes, heart disease, many cancers, and other chronic conditions—all of which are known to reduce life expectancy—be better than healthy weight when it comes to survival?

Although the CDC study was a large one, including more than 2.8 million people, it ignored key information that distorted the results. The problem with the study, and similar ones that came before it, is that they included smokers and people who were chronically ill but didn't fully account for the effects of these.

Cigarette smokers tend to be leaner than nonsmokers, in part because smoking blunts the appetite. People who smoke heavily are likely to be leaner than light smokers. Because smoking is such a powerful risk factor for death, this will tend to make being lean look unhealthy. Also, in any large population, the leanest people are a mix of a small number of thin people who have managed to strike a long-term balance between the number of calories they take in and the number they burn plus people who are thin because they have illnesses that are accompanied by weight loss (such as cancer, heart disease, emphysema, and frailty in the elderly). In other words, low weights don't necessarily *cause* premature death but are instead often the result of diagnosed or undiagnosed illnesses that eventually will be fatal. These confounding factors make the leaner group appear to be more likely to die prematurely. By comparison, then, the overweight group will appear to be less likely to die prematurely.

Two strategies can sidestep these limitations: (1) Look only at nonsmokers. (2) Ignore in the data crunching any deaths that occur during the first few years of follow-up to eliminate individuals with previously undiagnosed cancer or other conditions that would have accounted for their low weight.

My colleagues and I did just that in a 2016 analysis that combined data from 239 cohort studies that included more than 10 million men and women between the ages of 35 and 89 from all around the world. During a follow-up period averaging fifteen years, we saw that the lowest death rates were among people with BMIs between 18.5 and 24.9, much as we had expected.[7] Among those with BMIs above 25, the greater the weight, the greater was the risk of dying during the study period. The relation between weight and mortality was similar across all geographic regions of the world.

Another 2016 meta-analysis that included more than 30 million people[8] concluded the same thing.

CURRENT WEIGHT GUIDELINES CAN BE TOO GENEROUS

The 2015–2020 *Dietary Guidelines for Americans* sets healthy weights as those corresponding to BMIs between 18.5 and 25. BMIs above 25 are labeled as unhealthy (see Figure 9). In choosing these limits, the Scientific Advisory Committee for the 2015–2010 Dietary Guidelines for Americans tried to balance scientific evidence with public policy and perception. That's a difficult job, because there is no simple break point between healthy and unhealthy

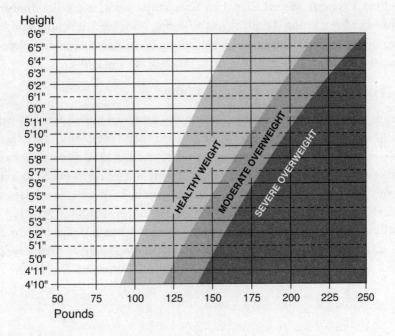

Figure 9. Dietary Guidelines for Americans: Healthy Weight Guidelines

weights. Panel members agreed that the risk of heart disease, diabetes, and high blood pressure begins to climb at a BMI of 22 or so. But they didn't feel justified choosing such a low number as the cutoff between healthy and unhealthy weights, because doing so would have labeled a large majority of the U.S. population as overweight. Instead they chose a BMI of 25 as the upper bound of healthy weights, based on clear evidence that the risk of dying prematurely increases above that point. (The guidelines committee didn't include the 2013 CDC study I described earlier [see page 42]). That means almost everyone with a BMI over 25—except for extremely muscular bodybuilders—would be healthier with a lower BMI, but many people with a BMI of 23 to 25 are not at their healthiest weight. Still, drawing the line at 25 means that two-thirds of adult Americans are overweight or obese.

Another problem with defining a range of BMIs from 18.5 to 25 as healthy is that this "allows" you to gain a fair amount of weight and still stay in the healthy range. For example, a perfectly healthy thirty-year-old woman who is five feet six and weighs 130 pounds (BMI of 21) could gain twenty-five pounds and still be in the healthy range (BMI of 25). Yet this much added weight poses clear health risks.

What about BMIs under 18.5, which the government's tables say isn't healthy? This can, indeed, signal an unhealthy weight, especially if an individual has been losing weight or has an eating disorder. But people who have maintained a low BMI for years while eating healthfully and being active are usually just fine and have no reason to increase their weight.

KEEP YOUR BMI IN THE HEALTHY RANGE

Here's the bottom line on BMI: If your weight corresponds with a BMI below 25, do all you can to keep it there by healthy eating and exercising. More specifically, try to keep from gaining weight, even if you could add some pounds and still stay within the healthy BMI range. If your weight corresponds to a BMI above 25, you will do yourself a huge health favor by keeping it from increasing and, if possible, by trying to bring it down. If you inhabit the low end of the BMI curve and your weight hasn't changed, great. But if you've been watching your weight slip downward and you aren't dieting or trying to lose weight, check with your physician to pin down why this is happening.

THE COLLEGE WEIGHT SCALE

If you could travel back in time and stand next to your twenty-year-old self, how would you measure up? Older and wiser, to be sure. But how about around the waist or on the bathroom scale? It's not an idle question: how much your weight and your waist have changed since your early twenties has a major bearing on your chances of staying healthy or developing a chronic disease.

Adding a few pounds here and a few there during adulthood seems innocuous enough. It has its own catchy moniker—middle-age spread—and was once considered a sign of prosperity and success. It also seems to be an inevitable part of aging, affecting most Americans. In reality, adult weight gain is neither inevitable nor innocuous. In many cultures, gaining weight during adulthood just isn't the norm. In Japan, for example, men and women—especially women—tend to stay the same weight throughout their adult years. On trips through Japan, I have often asked what would happen if a Japanese woman gained weight as she got older. The answer I usually get is a shocked "That would be one of the worst possible things for her." Women in Sweden and France have also stayed slim, with obesity rates below 10 percent, far lower than among American women, about 40 percent of whom are obese.

Even in the United States, we see clear differences in weight gain across different groups. For example, the less education people have, the more likely they are to be overweight or obese, especially men.[9] There are also big geographic differences in obesity rates across the country.

Gaining more than a few pounds after your early twenties can nudge you down the path toward chronic disease. The more weight, the harder the push. In the Nurses' Health Study and the Health Professionals Follow-Up Study, middle-aged men and women who gained between 8 and 35 pounds after age twenty were two to three times more likely to have developed heart disease, high blood pressure, type 2 diabetes, and gallstones than their counterparts who gained 5 pounds or less.[10] Larger weight gains meant even higher chances of developing these diseases.

These studies and others that examine the relationship between weight and aging underscore this conclusion about the "healthy range" for weight and BMIs: someone who was lean at age thirty—say, with a BMI of 20—can gain more than 25 pounds and still stay in the healthy range, even though this weight gain has serious health consequences.

APPLES AND PEARS

Some people store much of their fat around the waist and chest; others store it around the hips and thighs. These two different body shapes have been dubbed "apple" and "pear." Magazine articles and websites make a big fuss out of these arbitrary categories, and several websites use them as a key point in determining your health profile and risk of developing heart disease.

Fat that accumulates around the waist and chest (often called abdominal adiposity) may pose more of a health problem than fat around the hips and thighs. Abdominal fat has been linked with high blood pressure, high cholesterol, high blood sugar, and heart disease. This fat, especially the fat inside the abdomen, may be generating more hormones and other chemicals that affect health than fat stored elsewhere. It is also possible that it isn't doing this but instead is a signal about the harms of overall fatness that weight and height alone can't describe. In a pooled analysis of cohort studies that included 650,000 men and women, a larger waist predicted a higher risk of premature death at every BMI.[11]

Where, exactly, is your waist? For clothing designers, it's the narrowest part of the torso. For scientists studying the health effects of body fat, it's the region near the navel, where fat is typically deposited. The best way to measure your waist size is with the same two-step process used by researchers with the ongoing National Health and Nutrition Examination Survey: (1) Gently press your right hip bone to find its high point. (2) Place a tape measure just above that point and wrap the tape around your abdomen, keeping it parallel to the floor (see Figure 10). For most people, the top of the hip bone is generally in line with the navel. Others may need to pull the tape down a bit to the top of the hip bone.

Measuring your waist can be useful because many people—particularly men—find themselves converting muscle to abdominal fat as they go through midlife. Even though weight may remain stable, an expanding waistline can be a warning sign of trouble on the horizon. So use your waist as a kind of low-tech biofeedback device—a waist-wise expansion of two or three inches over the years should trigger a warning that you need to reevaluate your diet and physical activity level. A waist size of 35 inches for women and 40 inches for men is a worrisome signal. As is the case with weight, it's better to take action if your waist is increasing before you reach these limits.

Some researchers advocate calculating a waist-to-hip ratio. That means di-

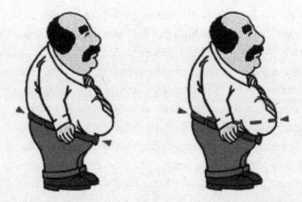

Figure 10. Measuring Your Waist. To measure your waist, wrap a flexible measuring tape around your midsection where the sides of your waist are narrowest. This is usually even with the navel. Make sure you keep the tape parallel to the floor.

viding the size of your waist by the size of your hips. A waist-to-hip ratio greater than 0.90 for men and 0.85 for women can indicate the potential for health problems. But simply measuring your waist is probably just as useful. Many studies have shown that this single number is just as powerful at gauging the chances of developing chronic disease as the waist-to-hip ratio. It's also a lot easier to do.

WHY WE GAIN WEIGHT

Your weight depends on a simple but easily unbalanced equation: weight change equals calories in minus calories out over time. Burn as many calories as you take in and your weight won't change. Take in more than you burn and your weight increases. Dieting explores the other end of the spectrum: burning more calories than you take in.

Chalk up why you're the weight you are to a combination of what and how much you eat, your genes, your lifestyle, and your culture.

- *Your diet.* What and how much you eat affects your weight. I will talk about this throughout the rest of the book.
- *Genes.* Your parents are partly to blame, or to thank, for your weight and the shape of your body. Studies of twins raised apart show that genes have a strong influence on gaining weight or being overweight, meaning that some people are genetically predisposed to gaining weight. Heredity plays a role in the tendency to store fat around the chest, waist, or thighs. It is

47

possible that some people are more sensitive to calories from fat or carbo-hydrates than others, although the evidence for this is thin. I must stress the phrase "partly to blame," however, because genetic influences can't explain the rapid increase in obesity seen in the United States over the last thirty years or the big differences in obesity rates among countries.

It's likely that our prehistoric ancestors shaped our physiological and behavioral responses to food. Early humans routinely coped with feast-or-famine conditions. Since it was impossible to predict when the next good meal might appear—like a patch of ripe berries or a catchable antelope—eating as much as possible whenever food was available might have been a key to surviving the lean times. This survival adaptation means that complex chemical interactions between body and mind that evolved eons ago in response to routine periods of starvation may drive us to eat whenever possible. In this era of plenty, that means all the time.

- *Lifestyle and physical activity.* If eating represents the pleasurable, sensuous side of the weight change equation, then metabolism and physical activity are its nose-to-the-grindstone counterparts. Your resting (basal) metabolism is the energy needed just to breathe, pump and circulate blood, send messages from brain to body, maintain your temperature, digest food, and keep the right amount of tension in your muscles. It typically accounts for 60 to 70 percent of your daily energy expenditure. Physical activity makes up most of the rest. If you work a desk job and do little more than walk from your car to your office and back again, you may burn ridiculously few calories a day.

- *Culture.* Ours is a culture of living large, of Texas-size appetites where quantity often edges out quality. Indulgence is tolerated, even revered. Love is food, and food is love: Imagine your grandmother urging you to have another helping or the pleasurable groans and belt loosening that end many holiday and regular meals. These are not universal tendencies. In France and throughout much of Asia, the cuisine emphasizes quality and presentation, not how much food can be crammed on a plate or into your belly. People in many cultures also believe it is inappropriate or downright rude to eat until you are full, and teach their children to eat to 70 percent of capacity.

- *Family and friends.* In a book called *Thinfluence*[12] that I coauthored with Dr. Malissa Wood, a cardiologist and health promotion expert, and Dan Childs, we described the many layers of our social environments that nudge us away from or toward better weight control. Our family and friends, where we work and play, and other social factors strongly influence what and how much we eat. Making healthy choices can be challenging when everyone around is filling up on sugary soda and pizza and no healthful foods are in sight. In *Thinfluence* we also describe how individuals can change or circumvent the factors working against them, for their own well-being and for those around them.

- *Your microbiome.* Billions of bacteria, fungi, viruses, and other microbes— collectively called your microbiome—live quietly inside your intestines. They help digest your food; protect you against microbes that can cause disease; make vitamins such as vitamin B_{12}, thiamine, and riboflavin; and more. It's possible but unproven that your microbiome helps regulate your weight.[13] Some types of gut bacteria seem to be better at releasing calories from food or causing inflammation, either of which can lead to weight gain. But we still don't know if the microbiome is causing weight gain or weight gain is changing the microbiome.

In addition to all of the above, we have what I call the overproduction problem. U.S. farmers produce about 4,000 calories' worth of food a day for every man, woman, and child in America.[14] That's nearly double what the average person needs. The almost inevitable consequence of this surfeit is a system that encourages full-tilt consumption. Producers and food manufacturers want us to eat more of their products, and they are competing with one another to exploit our weaknesses. The food industry spends billions of dollars a year learning the best ways to entice us to buy more and eat more, and then acts on that knowledge. The keen senses we have inherited for salt and sweetness that were once needed for survival (our taste for sweet things, for example, helped early humans sort through leaves to find the tender young ones with a ready supply of energy) are continually exploited. The sugar and salt content of products have been ratcheted up to increase our expectations for sweetness and saltiness and get us to eat—and buy—more.

Adding to the problem is the fact that food is sold everywhere: gas stations sell doughnuts and sandwiches, bookstores and department stores offer coffee and sweets, and you can get full, belly-busting meals at sporting events and concerts. Restaurants contribute by ratcheting up portion sizes. Modest servings of nouvelle cuisine have been overshadowed by supersizing, and it isn't uncommon to consume a meal that contains 1,500 to 2,000 calories, almost what you need for an entire day.

This incredible access to food and the nearly unlimited variety of choices test the willpower of even the most sensible eater. When combined with too little physical activity, it's a sure recipe for weight gain. And because weight control is the single most important factor in your good health after not smoking, overeating can pose serious health risks.

FOR ENERGY, A CALORIE IS A CALORIE

We eat food for two physiological reasons: to get energy and to get chemical building blocks. The amount of energy a particular food can deliver to mitochondria—the tiny engines that power your cells—is measured in calories. Technically, a food calorie is the amount of heat needed to raise the temperature of a liter of water (just over a quart) from 14.5° C to 15.5° C. Practically, a food calorie is about the amount of energy a 150-pound person burns each minute while sleeping.

If you read diet books or keep up with health and nutrition news, you've probably heard a lot about "fat calories" or "carbohydrate calories." The idea that fat calories are different from carbohydrate calories came from studies done under extreme conditions, such as consuming pure carbohydrate, protein, or fat. In these situations, the body converts dietary fat to body fat a bit more efficiently than it does carbohydrate or protein.

In a normal diet, though, your body converts all carbohydrate, fat, and protein to energy at the same rate. When it comes just to generating energy, a calorie is a calorie. (Calories from trans fat may be an exception; more on that later.)

This calorie blindness is the result of a neat solution to a vexing problem faced by some of earth's early inhabitants: how to run a body on different fuels. Instead of having completely different intracellular systems for fats, carbohydrates, protein, alcohol, and the like, the cells in your body use one of two energy sources: glucose and fat. Much of what you eat is (or can be if needed) converted to the energy coin of the realm, a six-carbon sugar called glucose. When you eat, some of the glucose dumped into your bloodstream is used immediately by your cells. Some is linked into long chains, called glycogen, and stored in your muscles and liver. Any leftovers are converted to fat and squirreled away in special fat storage cells and padded in between muscles. If glucose is like cash in your pocket, ready to be spent when needed, glycogen is money in the bank, available with a bit of effort, and fat is money tied up in stocks or mutual funds. However, the conversion of glucose to fat is a one-way street: fat can't be converted back to glucose. So while your cells typically run on glucose, when there isn't enough, you can switch over to burning fats, either directly from the fat you eat or by withdrawing fat from storage in your body. Brain cells are an exception: they run on glucose only.

CALORIE QUALITY MATTERS TOO

While a calorie *is* ultimately a calorie on the cellular level, the foods you eat for calories can have an important effect on your health.

The source of calories can influence how satisfied you feel after eating. Some foods, like an apple, can fill your stomach and leave you content for hours, while a can of soda with twice the calories will hardly ease your hunger. A good approach is to take in fewer calories by eating whole high-fiber foods like apples or carrots. In that way, the quality of your diet and the amount of food you consume are highly intertwined, improving both your weight and your long-term health.

Another way in which "calories" may differ is highlighted in the book *Always Hungry?* by my colleague David Ludwig. He highlights a longstanding paradox: some people have hundreds of thousands of surplus calories stored as body fat and yet can be just as hungry as thin people. How is it that over-weight and obese individuals aren't able to draw from their stored calories when they are hungry instead of eating more? Ludwig offers evidence that a higher insulin level, stimulated mainly by eating rapidly digested and ab-sorbed carbohydrates, is a key metabolic signal that shunts calories into stor-age as fat and keeps those calories locked up and inaccessible. That provides a rationale for following a diet with a lower glycemic load, which I describe in chapter six.

While carrying too many pounds is a key threat to health, it's important not to lose sight of the fact that diet affects health in many ways that aren't related to weight. Those need to be factored into planning a diet for long-term weight control. For example, among women in the Nurses' Health Study, low diet quality contributed as much to heart disease risk as excess weight.[15]

DOES FIDDLING WITH THE FORM OF CALORIES
HELP YOU LOSE WEIGHT?

Almost any kind of diet can lead to weight loss, at least for a few months. Some of the most absurd diets ever published have their champions who will tes-tify, complete with eight-by-ten glossy color photographs, that the diet helped them lose weight. That's because even the oddest diet makes people pay atten-tion to how much they are eating rather than eating willy-nilly throughout the day. This mindfulness is often enough to limit daily calories, the single most important key to controlling weight. It is aided and abetted by the monotony imposed by many of these diets and their inability to please the palate. Most fad diets fail in the long run. For that matter, so do many middle-of-the-road, commonsense diets.

The ultimate diet is one that offers meals and snacks that rapidly make you feel pleasantly full (technically called satiety), delay the return of hunger pangs (technically called satiation), are pleasing and satisfying, meet your body's needs for energy and nutrients, and work to prevent chronic disease. That's a tall order. Countless books have been written claiming they'll give you all or part of this dietary nirvana. Most promise far more than they deliver.

Diets usually fiddle with the form of calories by focusing on one particular dietary villain or hero. The most common ones are fat, carbohydrates, protein, the glycemic index, and energy density.

LOW-FAT DIETS AREN'T THE ANSWER

A common though absolutely false thread that runs through many diets is the idea that fat in food makes fat in the body. Limit "fat calories," so the thinking goes, and you'll be able to control your weight. Although there's a pleasant symmetry to that logic, there's no good evidence linking dietary fat with excess weight. In fact, there's plenty of evidence showing that a higher percentage of calories from fat doesn't lead to gaining weight or being overweight and the evidence is tending in the opposite direction.

That's why the Harvard Healthy Eating Pyramid and Healthy Eating Plate don't ban fats. Instead, they treat fats as important nutritional factors in your diet. I cover what fats to choose and how much to eat in chapter five.

To be sure, some countries with high fat intake have many overweight people. In the United States, for example, the average person gets about one-third of his or her daily calories from fat (a relatively high percentage), and almost two-thirds of the population is overweight or obese. But not long ago in parts of South Africa, where 60 percent of people were overweight, fat contributed barely one-quarter of calories. In other words, factors other than dietary fat influence overweight and obesity.

I am not trying to absolve dietary fat or downplay its potential contributions to weight or weight gain. Dietary fat affects energy, fat stores, and weight. But there is no evidence that calories from fat contribute more to weight gain than calories from carbohydrates or other sources.

But if you balance the number of calories you eat with the number of calories you burn, especially if part of the burn comes from exercise, then you won't gain weight on a diet that has 35 percent, 40 percent, or more calories from fat. And if you are eating the right kinds of fat, you will help protect yourself from heart disease and other chronic conditions.

A LOW-CARB DIET MAY HELP

For years, mainstream nutrition experts dismissed Dr. Robert Atkins's carbohydrate-shunning diet as an unhealthy fad. How in the world could a high-protein, high-fat, low-carbohydrate diet help with weight loss when everyone knew that fat was a dietary demon? Once the Atkins diet got its day in court—the court of careful scientific testing—the good doctor was proven to have a decent case, at least in part.

The low-carb idea isn't new. In the mid-1800s, the aforementioned William Banting, an obese British undertaker, happened on a low-carbohydrate diet. He tried it for a few months and watched with delight as the pounds slipped away without the gnawing hunger and cravings that other diets had caused him. Banting's *Letter on Corpulence, Addressed to the Public*, written in 1863,[16] became so popular that people began using the term "to bant" in place of "to diet."

Eating chicken, beef, fish, beans, and other high-protein foods that are the staples of low-carb diets slow the movement of food from the stomach to the small intestine. Slower stomach emptying means you feel full longer and it takes longer to get hungry. Second, protein's gentle, steady effect on blood sugar smooths out the blood sugar–insulin roller coaster caused by the digestion of rapidly digested carbohydrates like white bread, white rice, or a baked potato (see "Why Carbohydrates Matter" on page 112 and can stretch the time between hunger pangs.

Are bunless burgers the key to weight loss? Some solid studies, like the Dietary Intervention Randomized Controlled Trial (DIRECT) trial I describe on page 56, indicate that low-carb diets can help overweight people shed pounds. Low-carb diets like the Atkins diet seem to be easier to stick with than low-fat diets and, contrary to experts' warnings, generally don't cause harmful changes in blood cholesterol even when they contain fairly high amounts of fat, although that depends on the type and source of fat.

One concern in the nutrition community about low-carb, high-protein diets was that eating a lot of protein would be bad for the bones. The digestion of protein creates acid. Generating too much acid could, in theory, force the body to pull calcium from bone to neutralize it. But that doesn't appear to be the case.

High protein intake can also put extra demands on the kidneys. This probably isn't an issue for most people, but it may pose problems for those with mild kidney disease. People with high blood pressure are often in this category.

But eating unlimited amounts of beef, sausage, butter, and cheese, as promoted by the original Atkins diet, isn't a good idea for overall good health. There are better ways to cut back on unhealthy carbs. Eating more nuts, beans, soy foods, fish, poultry, nonstarchy fruits and vegetables, whole grains, and vegetable oils, as recommended by the Healthy Eating Pyramid and Healthy Eating Plate, can work for weight control even as it reduces the risks of heart disease, diabetes, and several cancers. Even Atkins was heading in that direction before his untimely death in 2003, as his final book had shifted toward this version of a low-carbohydrate diet.

LOW-GLYCEMIC DIETS MAY BE AN EXCELLENT OPTION

When you eat a carbohydrate-rich food like bread or rice, your blood sugar rises. How much it rises depends on the food, how much of it you eat, how much insulin your body produces in response to it, and if (or how much) you are resistant to the effects of insulin. White bread, cornflakes, and other highly processed carbohydrates, as well as white potatoes, trigger large, rapid increases in blood sugar (glucose). Intact or minimally processed grains, beans, and most fruits and vegetables generate smaller, slower increases (see chapter six).

Easily digested foods that cause sharp spikes in blood sugar also stimulate a matching production of insulin. The more insulin dumped into the bloodstream, the faster glucose is removed. A sudden drop in glucose, along with other hormonal changes, generates new hunger signals.

In an elegant study involving a dozen overweight boys at Boston Children's Hospital, those who ate specially prepared breakfasts enriched with easily digested carbohydrates snacked almost twice as much during the morning as those who ate breakfasts that delivered the same number of calories but included more slowly digested carbohydrates.[17]

The glycemic index and glycemic load (see page 118) measure how different foods affect blood sugar. People with diabetes have been using the glycemic index and glycemic load for years to plan meals and snacks that cause the smallest possible increases in blood sugar. These measures have become popular dieting tools. Both offer useful guides for choosing carbohydrates.

You don't need to religiously follow glycemic index and glycemic load tables in planning meals or snacks. There are simpler rules of thumb: Don't eat highly processed sources of carbohydrates such as breads, pastries, cereals, crackers, and other foods made with white flour; white rice; and sugar-sweetened beverages. Instead, eat more intact grains and foods made from them, in addition to fruits, vegetables, and beans.

ENERGY DENSITY ISN'T A RELIABLE GUIDE

Several popular diet books claim foods that deliver relatively few calories per mouthful, like soup or baked squash, fill you up faster than foods that pack more calories, like meat or nuts, and so help you lose weight. This concept is called energy density. Apples, potatoes, cooked rice, and lettuce have low energy densities, largely because they are mostly water. Nuts, bagels, cookies, Wasa bread, and other dry, high-fiber foods have high energy densities.

As a concept, energy density doesn't necessary help when it comes to dieting. Some foods with low energy densities, like white bread and white potatoes, do nothing for weight loss and plenty for weight gain, while some high-energy-density foods, like nuts and olive oil, can help control weight.

The strongest evidence against using energy density to control weight comes from the PREDIMED trial I mentioned earlier. In this trial, several thousand people did not gain weight even though they supplemented a Mediterranean-type diet with extra olive oil or nuts, two of the most energy-dense foods we know.

HEALTHY EATING AIDS WEIGHT LOSS

As I mentioned earlier, there's a solid connection between healthy eating and weight loss. Strong evidence showing that healthy eating contributes to weight loss comes from the Nurses' Health Study, the Nurses' Health Study II, and the Health Professionals Follow-Up Study. My colleagues and I looked at consumption of specific foods in relation to changes in weight over twenty-four years among 120,877 women and men in these cohorts who were not initially overweight.[18] The foods linked to greater weight gain included:

- soda (overall, the most important food or beverage for weight gain because it was consumed so often)
- potatoes in all forms
- red meat

- refined grains
- sweets
- fruit juice.

Foods related to *less* weight gain included:

- vegetables
- fruits
- whole grains
- nuts
- yogurt.

Milk (both whole and low-fat) and diet soda weren't appreciably linked to weight gain.

Unless you believe in magic, it shouldn't come as a surprise that no single food or beverage accounted for a large change in weight. But when we added up the contributions of these foods and beverages and others, diet quality had a large effect on weight gain. Interestingly, the pattern of foods related to the least weight gain corresponded quite closely with a Mediterranean-type diet and one matching our Alternative Healthy Eating Index, both of which are linked to long-term good health and weight loss or weight control.

GO MEDITERRANEAN

The most impressive evidence for the benefit of a Mediterranean-type diet on long-term weight control comes from the Dietary Intervention Randomized Controlled Trial (DIRECT). In this trial, 322 moderately obese men and women were randomly assigned to one of three diets: a low-fat diet with about 1,500 calories a day for women and 1,800 a day for men; a Mediterranean-type diet with the same calorie targets; and a low-carbohydrate diet with no calorie target but an aim to provide only 20 grams of carbohydrate a day for the first two months, then gradually increasing to a maximum of 120 grams a day.

Among the participants who finished the two-year trial, those who followed the low-fat diet lost an average of 7 pounds, those following the Mediterranean diet lost about 10 pounds, and those on the low-carb diet lost 12 pounds. The healthiest changes in cholesterol levels were seen in the low-carb and Mediterranean groups, while the healthiest change in blood sugar was seen in the Mediterranean group.[19] When the researchers checked in with the participants four years after the trial had stopped, those originally in the low-fat group had regained all the weight they had lost, while those in the Mediterranean-diet group had maintained their weight loss; the low-carbohydrate group was in between. Favorable metabolic changes had also persisted in the Mediterranean diet group.[20]

One likely reason the Mediterranean eating plan led to successful and long-term weight loss is that the participants reported being highly satisfied with the variety and flavors of their new way of eating and didn't feel deprived.

THREE STEPS TO WEIGHT CONTROL

Given how easy it is to add a few pounds here and there, and the food temptations that bombard us, how can you avoid gaining weight or lose weight if you need to? I recommend this three-pronged strategy:

1. If you aren't physically active, get moving. If you are, try to be even more active.
2. Find an eating strategy that works for you. Those offered in this book are a great place to start.
3. Become a mindful and defensive eater.

I wish I could give you a more precise set of instructions guaranteed to control weight. But I can't—and I don't think anyone else can, either. Chalk that up to the wonderful diversity of the human race. People are as unique as snowflakes. They come in different sizes and shapes, have different metabolisms, and like and dislike different tastes and textures. So no single weight-loss strategy can work for everyone. You need to find what works for you and stick with it using a scale and your waist size as guides.

What I *can* do is suggest different strategies that have worked for others and that may work for you.

1. Get Moving

Although I have focused on the intake side of the energy balance equation so far, the expenditure side is critically important.

Exercise counts most toward good health. Exercise is essential to getting healthy or staying healthy and keeping chronic diseases at bay. Exercise is far more than merely a way to lose or control weight. Regular physical activity:[21]

- improves your odds of living longer and living healthier
- helps protect you from developing heart disease or its handmaidens, high blood pressure and high cholesterol
- helps protect you from developing certain cancers, including colon and breast cancer

- helps prevent type 2 diabetes
- helps prevent arthritis and may help relieve pain and stiffness in people with it
- helps prevent the insidious bone loss known as osteoporosis
- reduces the risk of falling among older adults
- eases symptoms of depression and anxiety and improves mood
- helps prevent erectile dysfunction
- controls weight.

Build muscle, burn fat. Physical activity burns calories that would otherwise end up stored in fat. It also builds muscle or at least maintains it, an often ignored but absolutely essential ingredient in weight control.

Even when you are sleeping, your muscles are constantly using energy. When you walk, run, swim, lift weights, dance, play tennis, clean the house, or do anything active, your muscles burn even more calories. Physical activity stimulates muscle cells to grow and divide, prompting them to grow in strength and size. The more muscle you have, the more calories you burn, even at rest.

Without exercise, fat replaces muscle. If you don't exercise, your muscles gradually waste away. It's the same kind of atrophy that occurs when you wear a cast on an arm or leg only stretched out over years rather than weeks, so it's impossible to feel or see. The less muscle you have, the less energy your body uses at rest and the easier it is to gain weight. To make matters worse, lost muscle is usually replaced by fat (see Figure 11). This starts a vicious and tough-to-break cycle. For a fifty-year-old person who isn't physically active, a 10-pound weight gain over the years may really mean a loss of 5 pounds of muscle and gain of 15 pounds of fat.

Unlike muscle, fat uses little glucose and burns few calories. As the balance between muscle and fat shifts further and further in favor of fat, resting metabolism slows even more. And as the body needs less and less energy to take care of its basic needs, more and more food goes into fat stores. The extra weight can also act as a physical or mental barrier to activity, which further reduces resting metabolism. In other words, the shift from muscle to fat makes it easier to gain weight, makes it harder to maintain your weight, and increases your risk of heart disease and diabetes.

A colleague of mine once saw her physician for one of those "big birthday" physical exams. Everything was fine, with one exception: her blood pres-

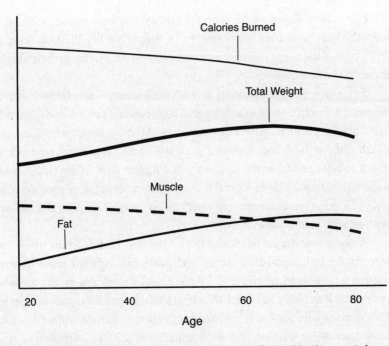

Figure 11. Age-Related Changes in the Absence of Physical Activity. Total weight, the amount of muscle and fat, and the number of calories the body burns at rest tend to change with age (assuming no increase in physical activity). Muscle mass declines, owing to decreased production of sex and growth hormones. Less muscle mass means the body uses less energy at rest and accumulates more fat. An increase in physical activity can break this vicious cycle.

sure was too high. When her doctor told her she needed to lose 30 pounds or so to get her pressure under control, she shot back, "Where were you when I was putting on those pounds?" It's a great question. The physical and physiological changes wrought by decreased muscle mass and increased weight are tough to reverse and in some cases may be irreversible.

Ounces of prevention are better than pounds of cure. It is easier to prevent weight gain than it is to lose weight. In fact, gaining weight makes your body more receptive to future weight gain and makes getting rid of extra pounds doubly difficult. To make matters worse, some of the effects of excess weight, such as diabetes, heart disease, or stroke, may not fully disappear even with successful weight loss.

The two big questions about exercise are these: How much exercise do we need each day? And what is the best kind of exercise?

Walk for health. Experts once thought that we needed vigorous exercise to keep the heart and circulatory system in shape. Not so. Brisk walking offers many of the same benefits as sweating it out in a noisy gym or jogging through your neighborhood.

For many people, walking is an excellent type of physical activity because it doesn't require any special equipment, can be done anytime and anyplace, and is generally quite safe. More vigorous exercise, such as running or bicycling, lets you pack the same cardiovascular workout into a shorter period and also gives you a higher level of physical fitness. Although activities more vigorous than brisk walking may provide some added benefits, you can achieve much in the way of chronic disease prevention with a good daily walk.

Among women participating in the Nurses' Health Study, there is a very strong link between walking and protection against heart disease: women who walked an average of three hours a week at a brisk pace were 35 percent less likely to have had a heart attack over an eight-year period than women who walked infrequently.[22] Vigorous exercise offered similar protection. Brisk walking also substantially cut the risk of diabetes; more vigorous exercise was associated with an even lower risk.

Exercise at least thirty minutes a day. You need to intentionally burn at least 2,000 calories a week to truly reap the benefits of physical activity. That's a difficult number to calculate. Most recommendations translate this into time: thirty minutes of physical activity on most, if not all, days of the week. There is no question that this much activity is far better than inactivity.

But thirty minutes of activity a day isn't much when you think about how active our farmer or laborer forefathers and foremothers were. Even someone who runs five miles a day usually sits for most of his or her other

Fast Fact: What, Exactly, Is "Brisk?"

The pace described as "brisk" means walking quickly enough so your heartbeat and breathing speed up, but not so fast that you can't carry on a normal conversation. It's moving as if you were late for an important meeting. If you are a counter or measurer, brisk walking is taking around one hundred steps a minute or walking at a clip of three to four miles per hour.

waking hours. So consider thirty minutes of physical activity as a daily minimum for maintaining your health and weight. And keep in mind that most people will benefit from more.

A word of caution here: The intensity of your activity also matters. Sauntering through the mall for fifteen minutes beats sitting—and it may help your bones and mood—but it won't do much for your heart, lungs, and blood vessels. For an activity to help your cardiovascular system, it must speed up your heartbeat and your breathing. Think brisk.

Quit sitting around. The average American spends more than half of his or her day sitting: working at a computer, commuting, watching television, or doing other in-activities. All that sitting isn't good for the body. A 2015 meta-analysis of forty-seven studies that included more than 800,000 participants showed that the longer people sat, the greater their risk for dying during the study period or developing cardiovascular disease, cancer, and type 2 diabetes.[23] That was true even for people who exercised regularly. If you sit much of the day, find ways to get up and move about. Pace while you are talking on the phone or when commercials are playing on television. Make a point of standing and walking around every hour you spend sitting. Or try working at a standing desk.

Make your day more active. There are many ways to inject more activity into your day. Some people choose to live close enough to their jobs so they can walk, run, or ride a bike to work. Not only does self-propelled commuting improve your health, it makes a small contribution to others' health by cutting down on traffic congestion and air pollution. Restructuring your day can add small "activity bits" that add up. Possibilities include walking up the stairs at work instead of taking the elevator; parking in a far corner of the lot and walking to your building; getting off your train or bus a stop or two early and walking the rest of the way; using a rake for leaves or a shovel for snow rather than a leaf or snow blower.

Have fun. Many people turn walking into a social activity, a chance to touch base with a partner or friends several times a week. Others enjoy the challenge of learning new skills, like rowing or tennis, and pushing themselves to improve. If you make exercise a fun priority, you'll find a way to fit in thirty minutes of activity a day, either in one long stretch or in several small bursts. It might help to consider this outlay of time as a solid investment that will offer an excellent return for your long-term health and the well-being of those who depend on you.

2. *Find a Diet that Works for You*

If your weight has been holding steady in the healthy range, you are clearly doing many of the right things as far as the amount of food you are eating. Even so, you can probably fine-tune your diet so it's even healthier. The Healthy Eating Pyramid and Healthy Eating Plate, and information in the following chapters, can help you choose the right foods to further improve your health.

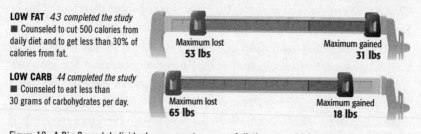

LOW FAT *43 completed the study*
■ Counseled to cut 500 calories from daily diet and to get less than 30% of calories from fat.

Maximum lost
53 lbs

Maximum gained
31 lbs

LOW CARB *44 completed the study*
■ Counseled to eat less than 30 grams of carbohydrates per day.

Maximum lost
65 lbs

Maximum gained
18 lbs

Figure 12. A Big Spread. Individual responses to a year of dieting vary widely. In one controlled trial, people lost—and gained—weight on both low-carb and low-fat diets.

But if your weight has been creeping upward or if you are already overweight, a new direction is in order. Its compass points are eating fewer calories and burning more of them. Many people get lost. Some ignore exercise, a crucial part of losing weight and keeping it off. Others are overwhelmed by the legions of diets and diet books, have trouble following a particular diet, or try one and it doesn't work. That's too bad, because there's a way for almost everyone to lose weight or at least stop gaining weight.

A diet must work for you. One finding buried in the data from diet trials is that individuals respond differently to weight-loss strategies. Take low-carb diets as an example. *Overall,* low-carb dieters lose an average of 10 to 15 pounds over the first year of dieting. That average hides what really happens to each individual. Some lose more than 25 pounds, some see smaller changes in weight, others don't lose any weight at all, and a few gain weight. These differences, which are probably due to a combination of genetic, environmental, and psychological or social factors, are actually good news. It shows that there is a route for just about everyone who wants to lose weight. Individual differences are one reason why this book doesn't define healthy eating by a rigid breakdown of calories into percentages from protein, carbohydrate, and fat. Instead, we provide a variety of information to help you find the best program for you.

If you are one of the lucky folks who have successfully controlled weight with the first diet you tried, thank your genes, your psyche, and your family. But if you try a diet and it doesn't work, don't give up! It may not have been right for your metabolism, eating habits, or social situation. Experiment with other weight control strategies as long as they emphasize healthy sources of fat, carbohydrate, and protein and include regular physical activity. You should be able to find the one that's right for you.

Diets low in refined carbohydrates often work best. For years we've been hearing that low-fat diets rich in carbohydrates are the best route to weight loss and improved cardiovascular fitness. For many people, probably most people, just the opposite is true. As I describe in chapter six, only people who are lean and active can tolerate a lot of carbohydrates. For others, too many carbohydrates promote weight gain.

The Atkins, South Beach, Dukan, and other low-carb diets ask you to take drastic measures, at least at first, and stop eating virtually all carbohydrates. As long as you aren't gobbling no- or low-carb foods packed with saturated and trans fats, limiting or eliminating refined carbohydrates is a good step to take. Keep in mind, though, that "crash" diets overemphasize short-term weight loss when the real goal should be finding a healthy eating pattern that can help you control your weight for years. The strategies described in this book are aimed at exactly that.

Giving up refined carbohydrates in favor of whole grains, vegetables, fruits, and healthy sources of protein and fat will reduce the spikes of glucose and insulin that provoke hunger while also supplying important vitamins, minerals, fiber, and other phytonutrients. Making that switch can also reduce your chances of developing high blood pressure, type 2 diabetes, or heart disease. Cutting out trans fats, cutting back on saturated fats, and getting more monounsaturated and polyunsaturated fats can improve your cholesterol levels, prevent blood clots, allow your arteries to work more effectively, and boost your muscles' response to insulin. Not eating red and processed meats and eating in their place fish, nuts, beans, and poultry will reduce the risks for colon cancer, prostate cancer, premenopausal breast cancer, diabetes, and heart disease, even if the total amount of fat you are eating remains high.

Choose a healthy global diet. An eating plan that borrows heavily from the Mediterranean and other traditional diets offers a healthy nutritional foundation. Plenty of vegetables, moderate amounts of intact and whole grains, and relatively little red meat can help you feel satisfied on fewer calories. The abundance of vegetables and whole grains, as well as the relatively high percentage of fat (30 percent or more of calories, mainly from olive and other vegetable oils), make for mild effects on blood sugar. Just as important, these kinds of diets are open to creative interpretation. You can incorporate cuisines from around the world, as well as your own creations, into an eating pattern with enough variety and pleasure to last a lifetime.

3. Practice Defensive Eating

Most people in our relatively sedentary society need to watch their calories as they age to avoid gaining weight. This involves more than just selecting certain types of foods or a particular kind of diet. It also means learning how to avoid overeating, which I call defensive eating. Here are some suggestions that can help you be a defensive eater:

> *Practice stopping before you are stuffed.* Recognize that we are victims of our culture, one that glorifies excess.
> *Be selective.* Don't eat just because food is put in front of you.
> *Choose small portions when eating out.* Restaurant portions are often oversized and a single meal can deliver a whole day's worth of calories. Think about sharing entrées, or order two appetizers instead of an entrée.
> *Slow down and pay attention to your food when you eat.* When you wolf down food, you effectively bypass the intricate set of *I'm full* signals that your digestive system is designed to generate. Eating at a moderate pace gives your stomach and intestines time to send these messages to your brain and for your brain to respond to them.
> *Beware of desserts.* A single slice of the Cheesecake Factory's Original cheesecake packs more than 700 calories and an incredible 29 grams of saturated fat, or nearly 50 percent more than the average person should take in each day. And that's one of the better choices: a serving of the carrot cake has twice as many calories (1,550) and just as much saturated fat. Many people consume calorie-laden desserts after eating an entire meal. If you want to order a rich dessert, share it with your dining companions. Better yet, have a healthy meal and finish it off with a piece of fruit or what I call the three pleasures: a few nuts, some fruit, and a bit of dark chocolate (see page 374).

Be creative with lower-calorie options to show you really care. Don't love your family and friends to death with calories they don't need.

Spoil your appetite. Have a snack, appetizer, or nibble of dark chocolate before eating a meal. Remember the dreaded line "It will spoil your dinner!" that your mother used to utter when you asked for a cookie or some popcorn late in the afternoon? She was right (of course). Use this principle to your advantage.

Minimize temptation. Many of us find it hard to ignore sweet chocolates, cookies, chips, ice cream, or other goodies when they are sitting on a shelf or in the refrigerator. Out of sight doesn't necessarily mean out of mind. Keeping calorie-laden snacks out of your home offers a much better deterrent. In their place, keep on hand a supply of low-calorie snacks such as apples, carrots, or whole-grain crackers for when you really want to munch on something.

Be vigilant. The food industry is out to exploit your weaknesses and destroy your defenses. You need to be smart to avoid their traps.

Keep it simple. Here's a truism from animal research: Rats fed "rat chow" or monkeys fed "monkey chow" don't weigh as much as animals that get to pick from a variety of foods. The same is probably true for humans. Think back to the last time you wandered through a cafeteria with great choices and you'll probably picture a tray piled with more food than you usually eat. There's no question that we need variety in our diets. Different foods offer different nutrients that are essential for good health. At each meal, though, simplicity may be a better strategy. You'll probably eat less if your entire meal is a chicken dish and vegetables than if you prepare several tempting recipes. Such simplification runs counter to trends in the marketplace, as the food industry offers an ever-growing and ever-beguiling variety of foods. But it may help reverse the ever-expanding trend of your waistline.

Beware of liquid calories. Sugary sodas and fruit drinks can be a big source of invisible extra calories that you can easily cut from your diet. A small glass of juice in the morning is perfectly good for you. It offers a refreshing way to start the day and provides some vitamins and minerals. But drinking juice throughout the day can add hundreds of extra calories. Keep in mind that you would have to eat two or three oranges to get the same number of calories as you do from a glass of orange juice. Sugar-sweetened soda is worse because it gives you nothing but calories.

Make healthy cooking or eating a social activity. Your social life influences what and how much you eat. Invite your friends to prepare a healthy meal together—trying some of the recipes in this book can provide a reason to get together—or join a group already organized for this purpose. Weight Watchers has created a major industry around the use of social support and interactions to improve eating habits.

Weight control isn't impossible, nor does it need to mean deprivation or a boring, repetitious diet. With conscious effort and creativity, most people can successfully control their weight over the long term with an enjoyable but reasonable diet and near daily exercise.

THE SKINNY ON POPULAR DIETS

Legend has it that King Arthur and his Knights of the Round Table searched fruitlessly for the Holy Grail. Today, millions of people are looking for its dietary equivalent: the one true combination of foods that will help them lose weight or stay healthy. Like Arthur, most search in vain. They are led astray by empty promises from dueling diet books and conflicting nutrition news. They try diets that work for a few weeks, then stop working, or ones that don't work at all. They end up frustrated—and still overweight.

Disappointment with diets shouldn't come as a surprise. Part of the problem is the notion that there's a single diet that is right for everyone or that a diet that worked for a friend will work for you—ideas as mythical as the Grail. Genes, family, friends, the environment, and many other factors influence how, why, what, and how much you eat. A bigger problem is that anyone can cook up a diet. You don't have to know anything about medicine, nutrition, or even physiology. All you need is an idea and the chutzpah to promote and sell it.

The graveyard of fad diets stands in silent testimony to their design flaws. Remember the cabbage soup diet, which claimed that the more cabbage soup you ate, the more weight you would lose? How about the rigid Scarsdale diet, which promised 1-pound-per-day weight loss by limiting daily intake to about 1,000 calories a day with the help of specified amounts of fruits, vegetables, and mostly lean sources of protein? The list goes on: the Hollywood 48-Hour Miracle Diet, the grapefruit diet, the Subway diet, the Russian Air Force diet, the apple cider vinegar diet, a host of forgettable celebrity diets, and countless others.

The fact is, almost any diet will work—at least for a short time—if it helps you take in fewer calories. Diets do this in two basic ways:

- defining "good" foods you should eat (like the grapefruit diet) and "bad" ones to avoid (think low fat or no carbs)
- changing how you behave and the ways you think or feel about food.

Most restrictive diets come with the seeds of failure planted and already germinating. Hunger from eating less, not to mention cutting back on common or once-favorite foods or giving them up altogether, creates cravings that can lead to "cheating." This can trigger feelings of failure and hopelessness. These, in turn, undermine the effort and enthusiasm needed to stick with a diet.

Weight loss is only one spoke in the wheel of good health. You could put yourself on a hot dog diet and almost certainly lose weight. But it won't last or be good for you in the long run. What's really needed is a plan you can sustain for years. It should be as good for your heart, bones, brain, colon, and psyche as it is for your waistline. Its hallmarks should be plenty of choices, few restrictions, and few "special" foods—exactly what I recommend in this book.

How do current diets measure up using this yardstick? Let's take a look at a few popular ones.

LOW-FAT DIETS

The two key ideas behind low-fat diets are: fat makes you fat and fat is bad for the heart. Neither of these is accurate.

One of the best-known low-fat diets is Dr. Dean Ornish's Eat More, Weigh Less plan. The "eat more" idea comes from the fact that fat contains 9 calories per gram while carbohydrates contain 4 calories. By switching from fatty foods to carbohydrate-rich ones, especially fruits and vegetables, you can double your food intake without taking in more calories.

The Ornish plan got a boost from a small study that Dr. Ornish conducted among forty-eight men and women with heart disease.[24] It showed that a very-low-fat vegetarian, whole-grain diet, along with exercise, stress management, and group support, reduced the narrowing of blood vessels in the heart better than less intensive changes. The improvement could have come from the low-fat diet. It could also have come from the other changes.

Keep in mind that "doing Ornish" means forgoing refined grains in favor of whole grains. It also means exercising. Eating carbohydrates without exercising can increase triglycerides and decrease protective HDL cholesterol, neither of which is good for the heart. Reducing stress is another essential part of the program.

There is no question that following a low-fat diet can aid weight loss, at least for the short term. Some people manage to stick with such a diet for the long haul. But that takes real commitment. Why? A low-fat diet tends to be less flavorful than other eating strategies and more restrictive about food choices, especially when dining out. It can also leave you feeling hungry, one reason why low-fat diets usually call for high-fiber foods that increase the sensation of fullness as well as between-meal snacks.

The reputation of low-fat diets as being good for the heart is a holdover from a time when many experts believed that all fats were bad for the heart. This belief has faded in light of findings that unsaturated fats can improve cholesterol levels, reduce blood pressure, and snuff out potentially deadly heart rhythm disturbances.

Bottom line: Some people lose weight and keep it off with a low-fat diet. Others lose weight then put it back on, or don't lose weight at all. On average, most people do worse over the long run on low-fat diets than on higher-fat diets (see "A Low-Carb Diet May Help" on page 53).[25] It can be difficult to stick with a low-fat diet for a long time because fats make food taste good and a low-fat diet limits the number and types of food you can eat. If you decide to follow a low-fat diet, choose intact or whole grains, fruits, vegetables, beans, and other slowly digested carbohydrate-rich foods.

LOW-CARB DIETS

In the 1990s, carbohydrates began to replace fats as the great dietary demon. Thanks to Dr. Robert Atkins (*Dr. Atkins' Diet Revolution*) and Dr. Arthur Agatston (*The South Beach Diet*), millions of Americans gave up bread, pasta, rice, and other carbohydrate unmentionables in their quest to lose weight. The more recent Wheat Belly diet books (by Dr. William Davis and others), *Grain Brain* (by Dr. David Perlmutter), and *The Dukan Diet* (by Dr. Pierre Dukan) have continued to fuel the anti-carb fires.

Low-carb diets tend to be better than low-fat diets at helping people lose weight. The main issue with them is what to eat in place of carbohydrates. Many people choose hamburger, steak, and sausage. These deliver a lot of saturated fat, which can counterbalance the metabolic benefits of reducing carbohydrate intake. High-protein and high-fat options based on plant foods, such as beans, soy, nuts, and liquid plant oils, are better choices, and fish and poultry are fine to include.

Shying away from whole grains, fruits, and vegetables can lead to low intake of fiber, healthy fats, vitamins, and minerals—deficits that supplements can't possibly overcome. In the Nurses' Health Study, the lowest risk of heart disease and diabetes was in women with diets lower in carbohydrates and higher in protein and fat from plant sources—good to keep in mind if planning to try a low-carbohydrate diet for weight control.[26]

Bottom line: A low-carb diet works for some people, helping them shed pounds faster than a low-fat diet and possibly keeping off the weight for longer. Low-carb diets can be expensive: following the portion sizes and ingredients in the Atkins and South Beach diets can nearly double your average grocery bill. A lower-carb diet based largely on plant sources of protein and fat can be gentler on your household budget.

RIGHT-CARB DIETS

Instead of banning carbohydrates, diets such as the Glucose Revolution, Wheat Belly, and Sugar Busters! embrace "correct" carbohydrates while shunning "harmful" ones. This means eating plenty of fruits, vegetables, and whole grains (no wheat in the case of the Wheat Belly diet) and cutting way back on refined sugars (white sugar, high-fructose corn syrup, honey, molasses, etc.) and processed grains.

Right-carb diets rely heavily on the glycemic index and glycemic load (see pages 118–122). These measure how strongly a particular food boosts blood sugar and insulin levels. Right-carb diets focus on foods that make blood sugar and insulin levels rise slowly. These foods include whole grains, beans, vegetables, and fruits. In theory, foods with a low glycemic index, which generate small but steady increases in blood sugar, help stave off hunger, while foods with a high glycemic index cause large but fleeting increases that quickly ring your internal hunger alarm. There isn't enough solid research to confirm the effectiveness of right-carb diets for weight control. A six-month trial showed that lowering the glycemic index offers modest benefits for weight loss.[27] It would be quite useful for a research team to mount a large two-year trial examining the effect of a lower glycemic diet on weight control.

Bottom line: In general, right-carb diets promote healthy eating by focusing on fruits, vegetables, and intact whole grains. Their reliance on the glycemic index can overly complicate choosing what to eat, especially when dining out. Diets that completely prohibit refined sugars also make dieting and healthy eating unnecessarily complex. Cutting back on foods made with refined carbohydrates and added sugars certainly makes sense.

Traditional Mediterranean diets have a relatively low impact on blood sugar because they use plenty of fruits and vegetables, are relatively high in healthy fats, and are relatively low in easily digested carbohydrates. So do diets like these that are in line with Harvard's Healthy Eating Pyramid and Healthy Eating Plate (see pages 16, 19). Their benefit on weigh control likely comes from multiple factors, including low glycemic effects.

PERFECT PROPORTIONS AND CORRECT COMBINATIONS

Several popular diets are based on the notion that specific proportions of nutrients or certain combinations of foods are essential to weight loss.

According to the Zone diet, for example, achieving the right balance of carbohydrates, proteins, and fats at every snack and meal creates a hormonal balance that will lead to weight loss, improved energy, and other health benefits. You reach "the Zone" by creating meals and snacks that contain 9 grams of carbohydrate for every 7 grams of protein and 1.5 grams of fat (40 percent carbohydrate, 30 percent fat, and 30 percent protein). This might result in a healthy diet, but it might not; it depends on the sources of carbohydrate, protein, and fat. What's more, there is little evidence that such a rigid approach to eating is necessary or even helpful for weight loss. This approach makes it difficult to eat with family members not on the program, or to dine out. But if you like structure and rules, then the Zone might be right for you.

The Eat Right 4 Your Type diet takes an odd and even less scientific tack: that your blood type determines what you should eat (not to mention how you should exercise, what supplements you need, and what type of personality you have). According to this plan, people with type O blood need a high-protein, low-carb diet that's light on wheat and beans, while those with type A blood need a high-protein, low-carb diet that contains plenty of fish and beans but steers clear of red meat, dairy foods, and wheat. Following this diet means remembering a lot of detailed information, including lists of good and bad foods for your blood type—and the blood types of your family. It isn't a balanced diet that gives you all the nutrients you need—something you can tell from the long list of recommended supplements. And it certainly isn't family friendly: most families encompass more than one blood type, which means different meals for different family members.

Bottom line: Exact proportions or specific food combinations may help you lose weight. Any success is almost certainly because such diets force you to focus on what you are eating and to eat less each day, not because of any nutritional or physiological secret the diet developers have uncovered. Their long-term health effects have not been studied.

WHAT ABOUT ENERGY DENSITY?

Another approach to losing weight takes aim at energy density, the concentration of calories in each portion of food (see "Energy Density Isn't a Reliable Guide" on page 55). The Volumetrics Weight-Control Plan tries to manipulate satiety, the body's signals that it has gotten enough food by recommending foods that fill the belly without adding too many calories. These tend to be water-rich foods such as fruits, vegetables, low-fat milk, cooked grains, beans, lean meats, poultry, and fish. Soups, stews, casseroles, pasta with vegetables, and fruit-based desserts get the thumbs-up, while high-fat foods like potato chips and dry, calorie-dense ones like pretzels, crackers, and fat-free cookies get the thumbs-down.

Bottom line: The strategy of eating foods that fill you up without delivering many calories probably helps people lose weight the same way most other diets do: it narrows your choices so you take in fewer calories each day. Although the Volumetrics idea is appealing, and many of the foods included would be part of a healthy diet, it is much too simplistic. For example, a can of Coca-Cola has a low energy density but it contributes plenty of calories that do little to fill you up or delay hunger. White bread made from highly processed wheat that has been stripped of many vitamins, minerals, and fiber has low energy density, while a high-fiber crisp bread has high energy density. But the energy density concept doesn't take into account how rapidly a food is digested and absorbed, which can have a big impact on the return of hunger.

EAT LIKE IT'S 100,000 B.C.

"Paleo" diets are a relatively new entry into the diet scene. They encourage you to eat as your Paleolithic ancestors did, thousands of years before the advent of agriculture. Following a paleo diet means eating anything that an early human could have found or hunted down—greens, root vegetables, berries and fruits, nuts, seeds, meat, birds, and fish—and staying away from processed grains, milk and dairy foods, refined sugar, processed foods and oils, and salt.

A diet that keeps you away from refined grains, sugar, and processed foods is a step in the right direction toward healthy eating. However, a "hunter" paleo approach that recommends you eat a lot of red meat isn't good for your long-term health or the health of the planet (see chapter twelve). If everyone tried to eat such a diet, most of the earth's 7.5 billion inhabitants would go hungry: it takes so much land and energy to produce meat that it would be impossible to feed even a billion earthlings on a paleo diet.

A "gatherer" plant-based approach that has you eating lower on the food chain—plenty of fruits, vegetables, whole grains, nuts, seeds, and the like—is far better than the average American diet. I was recently on a panel with S. Boyd Eaton, the radiologist whose 1985 paper "Paleolithic Nutrition—A Consideration of Its Nature and Current Implications" in the *New England Journal of Medicine* kicked off the concept of the paleo diet.[28] He said that the concept of a gatherer paleo diet—one based on food from plants rather than meat—would be a perfectly fine adaptation.

BEHAVIOR CHANGE

Some weight-loss strategies focus as much on *how*, *why*, and *when* you eat as on *what* you eat. The attention isn't entirely misplaced. Some people use food for comfort. They overeat because they are sad, lonely, frustrated, nervous, bored, depressed, or due to any number of other triggers. Breaking an unhealthy relationship with food can help such individuals lose weight.

Bottom line: There is no question that habits, behaviors, and relationships with other people and with food influence the ability to lose weight or maintain a steady weight. Some people can benefit from recognizing these issues and getting counseling for these underlying problems. But not all overweight people have dysfunctional habits or relationships. The truth is, everyone, overweight or not, needs to watch what and how much they eat and to exercise.

THE EVIDENCE ON DIETS

Although the glut of unsubstantiated diet plans shows no signs of abating, we have learned quite a bit over the last fifteen years about strategies for weight control. Two things we know for sure about weight-loss diets:

- Almost any type of diet works for a while.
- No single diet works for everyone.

As mentioned earlier, anyone can concoct and peddle a diet. No laws mandate that it be tested first. Some diet promoters try their plans on themselves, their families, and their friends. Those who lose weight become the success stories hyped in the books. But in most cases there's no hard-nosed evaluation of what percentage of people who start the diet stick with it or how many lose weight and keep it off.

Important clues about the individual nature of weight loss come from the National Weight Control Registry. This is a select "club" of more than 10,000 women and men who lost an average of 30 pounds and kept it off at least a year.

What's their secret? They don't have one.[29] An early look at registry participants showed that:

- 45 percent said they lost weight on their own; the others relied on some type of program. Interestingly, this is similar to the experience of those who quit smoking: most do it on their own by going cold turkey, presumably motivated by the accumulation of information about the dangers of continuing to smoke.
- 98 percent changed what they ate in some way, usually by cutting back on daily calories.
- 94 percent exercised more, usually by walking.

One of the main messages from the registry is that successful weight loss is very much a "do it your way" endeavor.

Consumer Reports once surveyed more than 32,000 dieters. Its findings echoed the findings from the registry. Nearly one-quarter of those surveyed lost at least 10 percent of their starting body weight and kept it off for at least a year. Most chalked up their success to eating less and exercising more.[30] The vast majority did it on their own, without resorting to commercial weight-loss programs or weight-loss drugs. Interestingly, the successful dieters in the *Consumer Reports* survey tended to adopt low-carb, high-protein rather than low-fat diets.

What the registry and *Consumer Reports* groups have in common is a focus on daily calories and exercise. In other words, successful dieters learn to manipulate energy in and energy out to lose or maintain weight.

A second thread of truly scientific evidence about dieting comes from randomized controlled trials like DIRECT (see page 56) and others. As I mentioned earlier, these are the gold standard of medical research. Such trials have shown that people who follow low-carb or Mediterranean diets tend to lose weight faster than those who follow low-fat diets. Interestingly, although some low-carb dieters who consume large amounts of meat and high-fat dairy foods have increases in harmful LDL cholesterol, low-carb dieters generally have larger reductions in potentially harmful triglycerides and increases in protective HDL cholesterol than low-fat dieters. The best long-term outcomes, both for weight and cholesterol and other metabolic variables, have been with the Mediterranean-type diet.

To see if we could learn more about the effectiveness of low-fat and higher-fat diets, several of my colleagues and I evaluated fifty-three randomized clinical trials that compared the impact of low-fat and higher-fat diets for at least a year. When the intensity of counseling and monitoring was the same in both diets, higher-fat, lower-carbohydrate diets helped people lose weight slightly more than low-fat diets did.[31]

But buried in the data from these trials is the finding that people respond differently to different diets. For some people, low-carb diets work well. For others, low-fat diets are the ticket. There's an important lesson here: It's okay to experiment on yourself. If you give a particular diet your best shot and it doesn't work after a few months, it's possible that it isn't the right one for you, your metabolism, and/or your situation. Don't get too discouraged or beat yourself up because a diet that "worked for everybody" didn't pay off for you. Try another. You'll do *all* of your body good if it is based on foods that deliver healthy fats, carbohydrates, and protein packages—precisely what the Harvard Healthy Eating Pyramid and Healthy Eating Plate recommend.

DO IT YOURSELF

Instead of following someone else's weight-loss diet, build your own. Base it on a Mediterranean-type diet, which is the one that works best for long-term weight control and overall good health. With the information provided in this book, you can swap in or out the basic elements of the traditional Mediterranean diet to incorporate the foods and flavors of other cuisines and cultures, including your own personal tastes.

A good diet should provide plenty of choices, relatively few restrictions, and no long lists of sometimes expensive special foods and supplements. It should be as good for your heart, bones, brain, and colon as it is for your waistline. And it should be something you can sustain for years.

The principles of healthy eating presented in this book can give you the foundation for such a plan. They won't give you a quick fix. Instead, they offer something better: a lifetime of savory, healthy choices that will be good for all of you, not just parts of you.

CHAPTER FIVE

Straight Talk About Fat

F
EW PUBLIC HEALTH MESSAGES HAVE been as powerful and as persistent as the false "Fat is bad" message that has dominated talk about the American diet for decades. Beginning in the 1970s, fat became dietary Public Enemy Number One, feared for its ability to cause disease and even kill. As a nation, we took that message to heart. The average American now eats a lower percentage of calories from fat than he or she ate four decades ago. We spend billions of dollars a year on low-fat cookies, no-fat salad dressing, pills that block the absorption of fat from the digestive system, and all manner of fat-busting diets and cookbooks.

But we aren't any healthier for it. In fact, we're worse off in many ways. An astounding two-thirds of adult Americans are overweight. And more than half of those are classified as obese.[1] The number of people with diabetes has greatly increased over this period. And the war on fat hasn't appreciably reduced rates of heart disease and obesity-related cancers—the two main reasons for it in the first place.

Fast Fact: Putting Fats to Work

Your body depends on fats for a host of functions. They are a major energy source for cells. They make up body fat (adipose tissue), which stores energy, cushions and protects vital organs, and provides insulation. Many people think of cholesterol as a fat, but it isn't, because it is made up of rings of carbon and hydrogen atoms, not simple chains (see "Types of Fat" on page 76). The body doesn't break down cholesterol for energy but instead uses it to make cell membranes, the critically important sheaths around nerves. It is also a building block from which the body makes vitamin D and many hormones.

Before exploring the health effects of dietary fat on health, let's take a look at the varieties of this important component of food.

What went wrong? The war on dietary fat ignored the simple fact that your body needs fat (see "Fast Fact: Putting Fats to Work," page 75). Some types are essential for you, and it's important to include them in your diet. These are the healthy unsaturated fats found in plant oils like olive, canola, soybean, and corn oils, and in fish. Cutting them from your diet is a bad idea. The true bad fats are trans and saturated fats. Trans fats, produced by the industrial process of partial hydrogenation, shouldn't be part of anyone's diet (see page 83). Saturated fat, from red meat, dairy foods and tropical oils, is better off being replaced with unsaturated fats whenever reasonably possible.

TYPES OF FAT

Chemically speaking, the family of fatty acids—the true and technical term for what most people just call fats—is part of the extended clan known as lipids. All members of the fatty acid family consist of a chain of carbon atoms bonded to hydrogen atoms with maybe a smattering of oxygen atoms. That's it—no

Types of Dietary Fat

Type of Fat	Important Sources	State at Room Temperature	Effect on Cholesterol Compared with Carbohydrates
Monounsaturated	Olives and olive oil, canola oil, peanut oil; cashews, almonds, peanuts, and most other nuts; peanut butter; avocados	Liquid	Lowers LDL; raises HDL
Polyunsaturated	Corn, soybean, safflower, and cottonseed oils; fish	Liquid	Lowers LDL; raises HDL
Saturated	Whole milk, butter, cheese, and ice cream; red meat; chocolate; coconuts, coconut milk, and coconut oil	Solid	Raises both LDL and HDL
Trans	Most margarines; vegetable shortening; partially hydrogenated vegetable oil; deep-fried fast foods; most commercial baked goods	Solid or semi-solid	Raises LDL*

* Compared to monounsaturated or polyunsaturated fat, trans fat increases LDL, decreases HDL, and increases triglycerides.

Fats and Cholesterol in the Bloodstream

For fats to get from your digestive system to the cells that need them, they must travel through your bloodstream. That isn't as simple as it sounds. Like oil and water, fats and blood don't mix. If your intestines or liver simply dumped digested fats into your blood, they would congeal into unusable globs. Instead, fat is packaged into protein-covered particles that mix easily with blood and flow with it. These tiny particles are called lipoproteins (lipid plus protein). During the packaging process, the body adds some cholesterol for delivery to cells and to help stabilize the particles.

Like a highway at rush hour, your bloodstream carries many sizes and shapes of fat-transporting particles. Lipoproteins are generally classified by the balance of fat and protein they contain. Those with a little fat and a lot of protein are heavier and more dense; those that contain more fat than protein are lighter, fluffier, and less dense. The proteins do more than help fat mix with blood. Those on the outside of the particles act like address labels that help the body route fat-filled particles to specific destinations. Once there, cells pull fats and cholesterol from the particles to use as energy or building blocks.

Cholesterol Testing

When you have your cholesterol checked, you usually get back several test results. *Total cholesterol* tells you how much LDL, HDL, and other lipoprotein particles are circulating in your blood. The ideal total cholesterol level is under 200 milligrams per deciliter (one-tenth of a liter) of blood. Borderline high cholesterol is a total cholesterol level between 200 and 239 milligrams per deciliter and high cholesterol is 240 milligrams per deciliter or higher.

Because total cholesterol is a mix of bad and good, it doesn't tell the whole story about what's happening in your bloodstream, arteries, and other tissues. That's why many physicians also check LDL and HDL levels. The lower the LDL the better, with anything under 130 milligrams per deciliter considered healthy. A level between 130 and 159 milligrams per deciliter is borderline high, and 160 milligrams per deciliter or above is high. For people with heart disease or at high risk for it, the thresholds are lower. The opposite is true for HDL: higher levels offer greater protection against heart disease. An HDL over 35 milligrams per deciliter is considered okay, although higher is better.

The exact role that triglycerides play in the development of heart disease is controversial, but recent studies show that a high level of them increases the odds of developing it. A normal triglyceride level is below 150 milligrams per deciliter. Borderline high is between 150 and 199, and high is anything above 200 milligrams per deciliter.

nitrogen, iron, or other elements. What makes one fatty acid different from another is the number of carbon atoms, how the carbon atoms are connected to each other, and the geometry of the carbon chain.

Almost all of the fatty acids in our diet are triglycerides: three fatty acids bound together by a "glue" called glycerol. There are four main categories of these: saturated, monounsaturated, polyunsaturated, and trans (see "Types of Dietary Fat" on page 76). From here on out I will refer to fatty acids simply as fats, which is how they are listed on food labels.

Until the middle of the twentieth century, fats were thought to play one main role in the body: serving as fuel for cells. We now know that they have many other important jobs. Fats provide the raw materials for building cell membranes, the delicate yet sturdy skin that surrounds cells and controls what gets in and what gets out. Fats make up the sheaths that surround and protect nerves. They provide raw materials that the body uses to make hormones and the chemicals that control blood clotting and muscle contraction.

The human body can build most of the different fats it needs from any other fat in the diet. If your body needs more of one type of monounsaturated fat for a specific function, it can make it out of saturated fat. It can also build fat from carbohydrates. However, a few fats can't be made from scratch. Called *essential fats*, these must come directly from food.

Here is a quick overview of the types of fat in food, and how they affect the body.

Saturated fat. The term "saturated" means that the carbon atoms in a chain hold the maximum number of hydrogen atoms they possibly can. This happens only when each carbon atom is connected to its carbon neighbors by single bonds. Saturated fats look like straight chains.

About two dozen different saturated fats exist in nature. They are abundant in meat and animal fat, milk and dairy foods, and a few vegetable oils like palm and coconut oil. At room temperature, saturated fats are solid rather than liquid, something you see if you let the drippings from cooked bacon or hamburger congeal in a pan.

When it comes to their effects on cholesterol and the artery-clogging process known as atherosclerosis, saturated fats come in gradations of bad. The saturated fats in butter and other dairy foods strongly increase harmful LDL cholesterol (see "Cholesterol Types and the Heart" on page 79). Those in beef fat aren't quite as powerful at boosting LDL, and those in chocolate and cocoa butter have an even smaller impact. The saturated

Fast Fact: Cholesterol Types and the Heart

Cholesterol moves through the bloodstream packaged in tiny particles called lipoproteins. The three key types, low-density lipoprotein (LDL), high-density lipoprotein (HDL), and very-low-density lipoprotein (VLDL), have the biggest effects on heart health.

LDL is often referred to as "bad" cholesterol. When there are too many LDL particles in circulation, they can build up inside of artery walls. This narrowing of the artery, called atherosclerosis, makes it difficult for blood to flow through the vessel. These cholesterol-laden buildups, called plaque, set the stage for heart attacks and strokes.

In contrast, HDL is often referred to as "good" cholesterol. These particles sponge up cholesterol from the bloodstream, the lining of blood vessels, LDL and VLDL particles, and elsewhere. They carry it to the liver for disposal. HDL also helps the liver recycle other lipoprotein particles.

Triglycerides make up most of the fat that you eat and most of the fat that circulates in your bloodstream. Triglycerides are essential for good health, since your tissues rely on them for energy. But, as is the case for cholesterol, too many triglycerides in circulation may be bad for the arteries and the heart.

fats in coconut oil give an extra boost to protective HDL. That has given a halo to this source of fat, which is often touted as being a wonder food for the heart, the skin, and more. But any HDL boost from coconut oil doesn't compensate for its LDL-raising effect.

Monounsaturated fat. The Greek prefix *mono-*, meaning one, hints at the structure of these fats. At one point along the carbon backbone, two carbons are connected by a double bond. This seemingly small change in structure leads to three key differences. It reduces the number of hydrogen atoms the carbon chain can hold by two. It changes the shape of the molecule from a straight chain to a bent stick. And it makes the fat a liquid at room temperature. Monounsaturated fats are the primary fat in plant oils, including olive oil, peanut oil, and canola oil. Avocados and most nuts are also good sources of this healthful fat. When eaten in place of carbohydrates or saturated fat, monounsaturated fats reduce harmful LDL.

Polyunsaturated fat. A fat with two or more double bonds is a polyunsaturated fat. A polyunsaturated fat holds even fewer hydrogen atoms than a monounsaturated fat with the same number of carbon atoms. Magnified thousands of times, a polyunsaturated fat would look like a stick with two or more bends. Polyunsaturated fats are also liquid at room temperature.

Polyunsaturated fats can be subdivided into the omega-3 and omega-6 groups. ("Omega" means end, and the number refers to whether the double bond is between the third and fourth carbon from the end of the chain or the sixth and seventh.) Each type plays different roles in the body. Our bodies don't make polyunsaturated fats, so we need to get these essential fats from eating plant oils like corn and soybean oil, seeds, whole grains, and fatty fish such as sardines, salmon, and tuna. Like monounsaturated fats, eating polyunsaturated fats in place of carbohydrates or saturated fat reduces harmful LDL. They are needed for cell growth, brain function, and proper functioning of the immune system, and also help the heart keep a steady rhythm.

Trans fats. More than one hundred years ago, food chemists discovered that they could solidify polyunsaturated vegetable oil by heating it in the presence of hydrogen gas and finely ground particles of nickel. During the process, called partial hydrogenation, hydrogen latches on to some— but not all—of the double-bonded carbons, changing them into single bonds. At the same time some of the remaining double bonds twist into a new straightened shape, which gives the fat new chemical and physical properties.

Why did anyone bother? It turns out that it's easier to ship and store solidified vegetable oil than liquid oil. Partially hydrogenated vegetable oil can be used in place of butter or lard in baking. A lesser degree of hydrogenation yields a still-liquid oil that doesn't become rancid as quickly as unprocessed vegetable oils. Without hydrogenation, we wouldn't have had margarine or vegetable shortenings such as Crisco. We'd also have less heart disease and thousands of fewer deaths from it each year (see "Trans Fats—A Special Concern" on page 83).

OMEGA-3 FATS: A SPECIAL BENEFIT

One type of polyunsaturated fat deserves extra attention, even though it makes up a small part of the fat in our diet. These are the omega-3 fatty acids (also called n-3 fats). They are essential fats, which means your body needs them for normal functions but can't make them from scratch. There are three key types of omega-3 fats in our diet. Since their names are a mouthful, I'll use their abbreviations: ALA (alpha-linolenic acid), EPA (eicosapentaenoic acid), and DHA (docosahexaenoic acid).

As polyunsaturated fats, they have two or more extra-strong double bonds joining neighboring carbon atoms. The first double bond is on the third carbon from the end. ALA, with eighteen carbons, is sometimes called a medium-chain omega-3 fat; EPA and DHA are sometimes called long-chain omega-3 fats because EPA contains twenty carbons and DHA contains twenty-two.

ALA is the main omega-3 fatty acid in most Western diets. It's found in a variety of vegetable oils (especially soybean and canola oils) as well as walnuts, leafy vegetables, and some animal fat, especially from grass-fed animals (see the table on page 82). EPA and DHA come mainly from fish and so are sometimes referred to as the marine omega-3s. Your body uses ALA primarily for energy. It can also transform this polyunsaturated fat into EPA and DHA, although it can't do the reverse.

What makes omega-3 fatty acids so special? For one thing, they are necessary to make cell membranes throughout the body. Membranes hold the contents of cells together, and determine what comes in and what goes out. DHA, for example, is the most abundant fatty acid in the human brain.[2] For another, they provide the starting point from which some hormones are made. These omega-3–derived hormones perform functions such as regulating blood clotting, helping artery walls contract and relax, and turning inflammation on and off. Equally important, omega-3 fats have been shown to help prevent or treat heart disease and stroke. They may help control lupus, eczema, and rheumatoid arthritis. They may also help prevent dementia, loss of vision from macular degeneration, and other chronic conditions.

The strongest evidence for a beneficial effect of omega-3 fats is in preventing death from heart disease. These fats help the heart beat at a steady clip and keep it from lapsing into dangerous, sometimes fatal erratic rhythms. These arrhythmias, as they are called, cause many of the nearly 300,000 sudden cardiac deaths that occur each year in the United States—half of which happen to people with no history of heart disease.

Omega-6 Confusion

Several popular books are based on the idea that eating too much omega-6 fats from good sources such as corn, sunflower, and soybean oils is bad for health. Omega-6 worriers claim that higher intakes of these increase inflammation throughout the body and increase the risk of asthma, heart disease, many types of cancer, autoimmune disease, neurodegenerative diseases, and more. But this is merely a theory, which has not been borne out by the many studies that have examined it. In fact, several dozen studies have looked at the effects of

Alpha-Linolenic Acid in Various Foods

Food	Serving	Weight grams	Alpha-linolenic acid grams
Flaxseed oil	1 tbsp.	13.6	6.91
English walnuts	1 ounce	28	1.90
Canola oil	1 tbsp.	14	1.30
Soy oil	1 tbsp.	13.6	0.95
Mayonnaise	1 tbsp.	14	0.85
I Can't Believe It's Not Butter!	1 tbsp.	14	0.76
Generic soy margarine	1 tbsp.	14	0.49
Italian salad dressing	1 tbsp.	14	0.45
Shedd's Spread Country Crock	1 tbsp.	14	0.44
Olivio Spread	1 tbsp.	14	0.43
Beef	6 ounces	170	0.38
Benecol Light	1 tbsp.	14	0.38
Brussels sprouts, raw	1 cup	88	0.18
Corn oil	1 tbsp.	13.6	0.14
Promise Soft Margarine	1 tbsp.	14	0.11
Almonds	1 ounce	28	0.11
Kale, raw	1 cup	67	0.09
Olive oil	1 tbsp.	13.5	0.08
Hazelnuts	1 ounce	28	0.06
Cashews	1 ounce	28	0.06
Safflower oil	1 tbsp.	13.6	0.05
Whole milk	1 cup	244	0.05
Cheddar cheese	1 ounce	28	0.05
Chocolate	1 bar	44	0.04
Spinach, raw	1 cup	30	0.04
Peanuts	1 ounce	28	trace

Source: Connor, W. "Alpha-Linolenic Acid in Health and Disease." *American Journal of Clinical Nutrition* (May 1999): 827–28; and analyses performed at Harvard School of Public Health.

omega-6 fats on inflammation. Remarkably, none show an increase and about half show a reduction in chronic inflammation, which is a good thing.

Proponents of the idea that omega-6 fats are harmful focus on the benefits of a lower ratio of omega-6 to omega-3 fats. There's no doubt that many Americans could benefit from getting more omega-3s. But there is also strong evidence that omega-6s, which make up the majority of the polyunsaturated fats in our diet, help shape healthy cholesterol levels and reduce heart disease. In the Nurses' Health Study, the ratio of omega-3 to omega-6 fatty acids wasn't linked with risk of heart disease because both of these were beneficial.[3] In 2016, our group examined consumption of different types of fat in relation to deaths from all causes. We found that omega-6 fatty acids were more strongly linked to lower death rates than omega-3 fats. This suggests that a *higher* ratio of omega-6 to omega-3 fats is desirable if this can be achieved by increasing omega-6 fats, not by decreasing omega 3 fats.[4]

Of course, too much of a good thing can pose problems, and we really don't know the upper limit of healthy omega-6 or omega-3 fat intake for optimal health. We do know, though, that reducing omega-6 fatty acids from the current amounts in the average American diet is likely to wipe out many of the gains we have made in preventing deaths from heart disease over the last fifty years.

TRANS FATS—A SPECIAL CONCERN

There's a family of fats you should definitely stay away from: the trans fats. These are mostly man-made fats that almost invisibly became a substantial part of the American diet. Thanks to long-awaited FDA rulings, that has changed in the past fifteen years.

A century ago, the average American ate a minuscule amount of trans fats, which naturally occur in meat and milk. By the early 1990s, however, trans fats contributed an average of 2 to 3 percent of total calories, with many people taking in double or triple this amount. That's because the food industry had found hundreds of uses for partially hydrogenated oils, the main source of artificial trans fats. These included margarines, vegetable shortenings, doughnuts, commercial baked goods such as packaged pastries and cookies, powdered creamer, and the fats used for deep-frying fast food in restaurants.

How bad are trans fats for us? Like saturated fats, trans fats raise levels of harmful LDL cholesterol. They are particularly good at boosting levels of small, dense LDL particles, the kind that are most damaging to arteries. They elevate levels of triglycerides and lipoproteins, both unhealthy trends that have been linked with heart disease. They lower the level of protective HDL cholesterol, something that saturated fats don't do. They promote the formation of blood clots inside blood vessels, which can trigger heart attacks and strokes. They cause inflammation, an overactivity of the immune system that plays key roles in the development of heart disease, diabetes, and other leading causes of death and disability. They also increase insulin resistance, a precursor of diabetes and its complications.

The rise in the amount of trans fats made and eaten in the United States suspiciously paralleled the rise in heart disease throughout much of this century. In the Nurses' Health Study, women who ate the most trans fats (about 7 grams of trans fats a day, or about 3 percent of daily energy) were more than 50 percent more likely to have developed heart disease over a fourteen-year period than those who ate the least (slightly over 1 percent of daily calories).[5] The risk of diabetes also increased steadily with greater consumption of trans fat.[6] Higher intake of trans fat has also been associated with greater risk of gallstones and dementia.

For the longest time, trans fats existed as stealth fats because food makers didn't have to list them on food labels. The only way you could have known that trans fat was in a particular food was to scrutinize the ingredients list and recognize "partially hydrogenated vegetable oil" or "vegetable shortening," the giveaways for trans fats. But even then you couldn't tell how much trans fat was present.

After a long campaign led by Fred A. Kummerow, now professor emeritus of food science and human nutrition at the University of Illinois, along with the Center for Science in the Public Interest and members of our Department of Nutrition, the FDA in 2003 ruled that trans fats were even more harmful than saturated fats and had to be included on the Nutrition Facts label by 2006. This let consumers know which foods contained trans fats and also provided a strong incentive for manufacturers to remove them from their products.

The FDA took an even bigger step in 2015 when it ruled that partially hydrogenated oils, which are the main source of harmful trans fats in food, are no longer "generally recognized as safe."[7] At the time, Susan Mayne, the director of the FDA's Center for Food Safety and Applied Nutrition, wrote in the FDA Voice blog that "it has become clear that what's good for extending shelf-life is not equally good for extending human life."[8]

By the time of the FDA's 2015 decision, earlier educational efforts and bans on trans fats by many cities and states had already driven the vast majority of trans fats out of the U.S. food supply. (We weren't the first, though, as Denmark and other countries had banned trans fat years earlier.)

In the 2015 ruling, food companies were given until 2018 to stop using trans-containing partially hydrogenated oils. Any companies wanting to continue to use them after 2018 must get the FDA's special approval to do so, which is unlikely to happen.

We have estimated that eliminating trans fats from our food supply would prevent between 72,000 and 220,000 heart attacks or heart disease deaths per year.[9] The Center for Science in the Public Interest projected that this would save $50 billion in medical costs a year.

SOME FATS ARE GOOD FOR YOU

There's a good reason we haven't seen a payoff from recommendations to reduce fat in the diet. In spite of the scorn heaped upon dietary fat and the anti-fat recommendations that once came from the country's leading health organizations, the truth is that some fats are good for you, and it is important to include these good fats in your diet. In fact, eating more good fats—and staying away from bad ones—is high on the list of healthy nutritional strategies.

Dietary fat gets much of the blame for causing heart disease and stroke, the leading killers in the United States and around the world. In the United States alone, more than 1.5 million people have heart attacks or strokes each year, and these two conditions account for about one-third of all deaths. The cost of heart disease and stroke is close to $320 billion a year, including the costs of lost productivity.[10]

Dietary fats aren't the only factors that affect the risk of heart disease. Smoking, being overweight or obese, and inactivity contribute a substantial share of deaths and disability. But managing the type of fat you eat is an important way to prevent heart disease.

HOW DIETARY GUIDELINES HAVE DISTORTED THE FAT FACTS

The traditional link between diet and heart disease goes like this: (1) Too much fat in the diet increases cholesterol levels in the blood. (2) Too much cholesterol in the bloodstream increases the chance of having a heart attack or stroke or developing some other form of cardiovascular disease. (3) Eating less fat should decrease rates of heart disease.

Except it doesn't work that way.

Dietary Fat and Body Fat

You may be thinking, Hold on a second. Won't eating more fat make me fatter, something I know is definitely bad for my health? True, but only if you add extra fat to your diet *without cutting anything out of it*. Remember, the goal here isn't adding more fat to your diet. It's cutting back on bad fats (eliminating trans fat and limiting saturated fat) while increasing good fats (monounsaturated and polyunsaturated fats) *and keeping the number of daily calories constant*. Do that and you won't gain weight.

If you follow a low-fat diet and your level of protective HDL is low, your triglyceride level is high, or you are having trouble controlling your weight, think about cutting back on carbohydrates—especially highly processed ones—and adding in foods that deliver unsaturated fat.

Even though there's a nice, intuitive feel to the notion that eating more fat makes you fatter, for most people, there's little evidence to confirm it. For example, randomized trials comparing low-fat diets against higher-fat (low-carb) diets show that both can help people lose weight.[11] On average, though, most people do better on lower carbohydrate, higher fat diets (see "A Low-Carb Diet May Help," page 53).[12]

In the United States, the gradual reduction in the fat content of the average diet—from over 40 percent of calories in the 1960s to about 33 percent today—has been accompanied by a gradual increase in average weight and a dramatic increase in obesity.

In short, the amount of fat in your diet doesn't necessarily make you fat. If you usually eat more calories than you burn, you're going to gain weight regardless of whether your calories mostly come from fat, carbohydrates, or protein. If you keep your calories constant, though, you won't gain weight if you cut back on saturated fat, refined carbohydrates, and sugar and eat more unsaturated fat.

The relatively simple diet-heart hypothesis leaves out a lot. An important omission is that different fats have different effects on cholesterol. What's more, there are many ways that dietary fat can affect heart disease other than through the single channel of total cholesterol. Dietary fats influence how much harmful LDL and protective HDL are in your bloodstream, how your blood clots, how susceptible your heart is to erratic rhythms, and how the inner lining of your blood vessels responds to stress—and probably affects other pathways to heart disease we haven't yet discovered.

Tragically, public policy based on the oversimplified diet-heart hypothesis doesn't cover these alternate pathways. For years we have been urged to use fats and oils "sparingly" and to choose diets low in saturated fat and cholesterol. Only recently have our *Dietary Guidelines for Americans* provided any guidance about the proven benefits of unsaturated fats.

None of the overly simplistic advice tells you that eating unsaturated fats instead of saturated fats can improve the levels of cholesterol and other fats in your bloodstream, fortify your heart against erratic heartbeats, or help counteract a number of processes that underlie atherosclerosis, the gradual clogging and narrowing of arteries.

SIMPLER GUIDELINES AREN'T ALWAYS BETTER

Back in 1957, with only a limited amount of hard data at hand, the American Heart Association (AHA) set out its first dietary guidelines.[13] Although the AHA hedged its bets with liberal use of the word "may," its first guidelines were remarkably on target. They said: (1) Diet may play an important role in the development of heart disease. (2) Both the fat content and the total calories in the diet are probably important. (3) The ratio between saturated and unsaturated fats may be the basic determinant, and people should get more unsaturated fat and less saturated fat. (4) A wide variety of other factors besides fat, both dietary and nondietary, may be important.

Four years later the AHA was still suggesting that people increase their intake of unsaturated fat.

Over the years, though, as expert panels discussed and sometimes fought over the most effective public health message, the AHA, the National Cholesterol Education Program, and other influential groups decided that Americans couldn't grasp a concept as nuanced as good fat/bad fat. Instead they settled on the simpler "Fat is bad" message.

There's no question that the public heard and heeded this message. Today, fats and oils make up about 33 percent of the calories in the average diet, compared with 40 percent in the 1960s. If this reduction meant we were eating less potentially harmful saturated fat, that would be great news and would show up as lower rates of heart disease. But we've thrown out the baby with the bathwater, mainly cutting back on beneficial unsaturated fats.

REPLACING FATS WITH CARBOHYDRATES CREATES A NEW PROBLEM

Reducing the amount of fat in the diet almost always means adding something else. If you follow the standard dietary guidelines, that "something else" has traditionally been carbohydrates, usually foods rich in simple or highly processed carbohydrates, such as sugar, white bread, white rice, and potatoes. Replacing foods rich in saturated fat with those rich in refined carbohydrates lowers total cholesterol levels a bit. But it also lowers levels of protective HDL cholesterol. (Replacing saturated fat with whole grains is a much healthier option.)

The two trends encouraged by the standard dietary guidelines—decreasing the intake of all fats and increasing the intake of carbohydrates—have other troubling consequences beyond their harmful impact on HDL. Carbohydrates can and do increase weight every bit as effectively as fats if you consume more calories than you burn off. Equally harmful, white bread and other foods made from white flour, potatoes, pasta, and white rice cause large spikes in blood sugar (glucose) and insulin, something that doesn't happen with fat, protein, and slowly absorbed carbohydrates like those from intact whole grains, beans, fruits, and non-starchy vegetables (see chapter six).

Spikes in blood sugar and insulin place a constant and heavy demand on the pancreas to make more insulin. This is a key ingredient for adult-onset diabetes, now called type 2 diabetes, especially when paired with lack of exercise. Eating carbohydrates instead of unsaturated fats also tends to increase blood pressure.[14] Finally, following a low-fat diet usually means forgoing foods such as nuts, avocados, salad dressings made with unsaturated oils, and other foods that contain beneficial monounsaturated and polyunsaturated fats. Less unsaturated fat also means less vitamin E and other valuable nutrients that travel along with fats.

THE BENEFITS OF EATING UNSATURATED FATS IN PLACE OF SATURATED FATS

Eating less saturated fat and more unsaturated fat improves cholesterol levels across the board. It also helps prevent heart disease in other ways. It is this message I hope to hammer home against the "All fat is bad" drumbeat. Since the first edition of *Eat, Drink, and Be Healthy* was published in 2001, the message that some fats are healthy has been slowly spreading. Many people have experienced the benefits of making this swap, and it has now finally become part of mainstream dietary advice, as seen by its inclusion in the 2015–2020 *Dietary Guidelines for Americans.*

By steering clear of all fats, you eliminate a number of foods that can improve your long-term health. Don't get me wrong: I wholeheartedly agree with pruning out saturated and trans fats from your diet. But the same doesn't apply to unsaturated fats. Eating unsaturated fats instead of saturated fats or carbohydrates:

Eggs

Once upon a time, eggs were seen as a healthy, eat anytime food, the centerpiece of solid breakfasts and the hearty garnishes atop salads and side dishes. The discovery of a link between blood cholesterol levels and risk of heart disease sullied that reputation. With more than 200 milligrams of cholesterol in each yolk, eggs were branded as unhealthy, to be eaten sparingly. Per capita egg consumption tumbled from more than four hundred per year in the late 1940s to under two hundred per year today[15] and many people eat them with a side order of guilt.

The dangers of eggs aren't all they're cracked up to be. Adding an extra 200 milligrams of cholesterol a day to the diet barely increases blood cholesterol levels in most people and boosts, *in theory*, the risk of heart disease by only a small amount. But eggs aren't just packets of cholesterol. They are very low in saturated fat and contain many other nutrients that are good for you: protein, some polyunsaturated fats, folic acid and other B vitamins, vitamin D, lutein, and more. So the effect of eggs on heart disease risk can't be predicted by considering only their cholesterol content.

No research has ever shown that people who regularly eat eggs have more heart attacks than people who don't eat eggs. In the late 1990s my colleagues and I looked at the egg-eating habits of almost 120,000 healthy men and women. Those who ate up to an egg a day were no more likely to have developed heart disease or to have had a stroke over many years of follow-up than those who ate less than one egg a week.[16] (A later and larger meta-analysis showed no connection between egg consumption and heart disease or stroke.)[17] Among those with diabetes, though, there did seem to be some connection between eating an egg a day and the development of heart disease.

While these studies, and others like it, don't give the green light for daily three-egg omelets, they should be reassuring to people who enjoy eggs. If your breakfast choices are an egg, a deep-fried doughnut, or a bagel made from refined flour, the egg is the better choice, especially if it is cooked in healthy vegetable oil. If you want to have the healthiest breakfast, though, a combination of oatmeal, nuts, and berries, perhaps with a topping of yogurt, would lower your LDL cholesterol and be better than a "neutral" egg-based breakfast. (This is just one of many examples highlighting that when trying to determine the healthfulness of any food, you always need to ask "Compared to what?")

- lowers the level of harmful LDL without also lowering the level of protective HDL
- prevents an increase in triglycerides, another form of fat circulating in the bloodstream that has been linked with heart disease and that occurs with high-carbohydrate diets

- reduces the development of erratic heartbeats, a main cause of sudden cardiac death
- reduces the formation of potentially artery-blocking blood clots.

Unsaturated fats are so important to good health that they support the foundation of the Healthy Eating Pyramid (see page 16) and are specifically mentioned in the Healthy Eating Plate (see page 19). Both acknowledge that fats and oils make up a substantial chunk of daily calories and can have long-term health benefits. As I describe later in this chapter, not all unsaturated fats are the same, but they share the same beneficial effects.

TRACING THE HEALTH EFFECTS OF DIETARY FATS

Until the middle of the last century, when infectious diseases like tuberculosis and influenza were leading causes of death, calorie-rich diets laden with fat were thought to provide some protection against disease and aid in recovery. As late as the 1950s, a healthy diet meant eggs, bacon, and butter-slathered toast for breakfast and roast beef and mashed potatoes with gravy for dinner.

Our comfortable, almost thoughtless relationship with food was forever changed by separate threads of research that came together after World War II. Large studies in the late 1940s and early 1950s began to focus on diet as a cause of the skyrocketing rates of heart disease. In 1956, a University of Minnesota scientist named Ancel Keys began an international survey called the Seven Countries Study. It suggested a connection between saturated fat and heart disease: in general, the higher the amount of saturated fat in a country's diet, the higher the rate of heart disease. Interestingly, Keys and his colleagues didn't find any connection between the *total* amount of fat in the diet and heart disease. In fact, the area with the lowest rate of heart disease in the study, Crete, had the highest average total fat intake: about 40 percent of calories— mostly due to liberal use of olive oil. At around the same time, the Framingham Heart Study started tracking the health and habits of more than 5,000 men and women living in the town of Framingham, Massachusetts. One of its early findings was that high levels of cholesterol in the bloodstream were often an early signal of impending heart disease. These important studies and others pointed to diet as a key element in the path to heart disease.

Without turning this into a textbook of nutritional epidemiology, I'll briefly describe the consistent evidence from several kinds of studies showing the harmful effects of saturated and trans fats and the benefits that can come from replacing these harmful fats with unsaturated fats.

Cross-Cultural Surveys: More Saturated Fat = More Heart Disease

The country-by-country surveys of Ancel Keys and others showed that heart disease rates varied more than tenfold between Crete and Finland, the Seven Countries Study country with the highest rates. The more saturated fat in a country's average diet, the higher the rates of heart disease. Although the Seven Countries and Framingham studies pointed to saturated fat as a major driver of heart disease, other factors, such as differences in cigarette smoking and amount of physical activity, could have contributed to the large difference in rates.

Metabolic Studies: Good Fats Improve the Cholesterol Profile

In the 1950s and 1960s, dozens of carefully controlled feeding studies among small groups of volunteers showed conclusively that eating saturated fats instead of carbohydrates led to a rise in total cholesterol, and eating polyunsaturated fats instead of carbohydrates led to a reduction in total cholesterol. Thus, for decades we have known that all fats shouldn't be considered equal. Unfortunately, at that time the importance of other blood lipids—protective HDL in particular—wasn't appreciated. So those studies gave an incomplete picture at best.

One of the early and most compelling pieces of evidence to challenge the emphasis on cutting back on all fat and eating more carbohydrates came from an experiment by two Dutch scientists.[18] They recruited forty-eight volunteers for an eight-week study. For the first seventeen days, all of the volunteers ate a typical Western diet with about 40 percent of calories from fat. For the next thirty-six days, half of the volunteers were assigned to a diet in which part of the saturated fat was replaced by olive oil, while the other half followed a diet in which some of the saturated fat was replaced by carbohydrates. In both groups, total cholesterol levels plummeted (see Figure 13).[19] But in the high-carbohydrate group, levels of protective HDL cholesterol also fell, while triglycerides rose—both changes that increase the chances of having a heart attack or developing some other form of heart disease. In the olive oil group, a healthy trend was seen for total cholesterol without the unhealthy changes in HDL and triglycerides. The benefits of cutting back on carbohydrates and adding in more unsaturated fats seen in that study have been confirmed by many research groups.

One of these confirmatory studies, from the University of Washington, documented that these changes weren't fleeting.[20] In this study, 444 men with high cholesterol were asked to follow one of four diets, containing either 30 per-

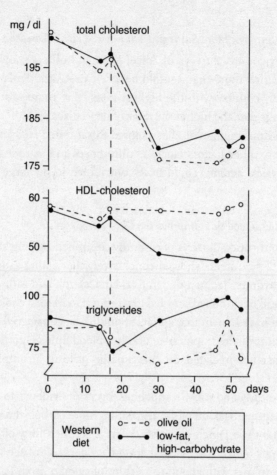

Figure 13. Blood Fat Responses to Olive Oil vs. Carbohydrates. A diet rich in unsaturated fat (olive oil) improved HDL cholesterol and triglyceride levels compared with a diet rich in carbohydrates.

cent, 28 percent, 22 percent, or 18 percent of fat. After a year, all four diets had lowered harmful LDL cholesterol. But the two lowest-fat diets also dropped the level of protective HDL cholesterol and raised the level of triglycerides.

The more we learn about cholesterol in the bloodstream, the more we realize that even though total cholesterol is a decent red flag for heart disease risk, what's really important are the different cholesterol subtypes. The best cholesterol profile is one with a low level of harmful LDL and a high level of protective HDL. This relationship is neatly captured as a ratio of total cholesterol to HDL. Ideally, the ratio should be less than 3.5. The Dutch study, and the many others that have repeated this test, leave no doubt that eating carbohydrates instead of saturated fats—the typical low-fat diet—has little effect on the ratio of LDL to HDL, and that eating unsaturated fats instead of saturated fats improves it.

Cohort Studies: More Good Fats = Less Heart Disease

The connection between dietary fat and heart disease has long been murky, stirred up by many small and short-term studies. To make sense of this important relationship, my colleagues and I completed in 2016 what was the most detailed and comprehensive analysis of dietary fat and health to date.[21] We used information provided by 126,233 initially healthy women and men participating in the Nurses' Health Study and the Health Professionals Follow-Up Study, who were followed for up to thirty-two years. Every two years from the start of the study, we asked the participants about smoking, weight, physical activity, medical diagnoses, medications, and other things that could affect their disease risk. Every four years we asked them to complete detailed questionnaires about their diets. From the diet data we were able to calculate their intakes of various types of fat by using routinely updated databases on the fat composition of thousands of foods.

During the study period, 33,304 of the participants died. We confirmed each cause of death by examining medical records and death certificates. Somewhat to our surprise, participants with the highest intake of total fat (about 42 percent of calories) were 16 percent less likely to have died during the course of the study as those with the lowest total fat intake (25 percent of calories).

My colleagues and I suspect that the lower risk among those with higher-fat diets was due in part to the greatly improved quality of fat in the American diet following the near elimination of partially hydrogenated oils rich in trans fats (see "Trans Fats," page 83) and their replacement by unsaturated oils.

Even more important than the finding for total fat were the strong relationships between specific types of fat and death. When compared to the same number of calories from carbohydrates, trans fats were most strongly associated with increased risk of dying during the study, saturated fats with a slightly higher risk, monounsaturated fats with a moderately lower risk, and polyunsaturated fats with a substantially lower risk. When we looked at types of polyunsaturated fat, omega-6s were strongly linked to a lower risk of dying during the study, while the link with omega-3s was weak.

The findings of this study almost exactly replicate what we had reported nearly twenty years before from a study of heart disease in women.[22]

What was surprising in the 2016 study was that the benefits of unsaturated fats extended to deaths from other causes as well, including cancer, respiratory disease, and neurodegenerative conditions like Alzheimer's disease. The biological basis for some of these findings, especially neurodegenerative disease, is not well understood and is the topic of ongoing investigation.

I must offer a word of caution when interpreting these results. When I say "compared to the same number of calories from carbohydrates," I mean the kinds of carbohydrates actually being consumed by the study participants, which included a large amount of sugar and refined starch. Total fat wouldn't have looked as good, and saturated fat would have looked even worse, if we had compared them to the same number of calories from whole grains. I'll explore these distinctions further in chapter six.

This analysis provides a big picture of the relationship between the amount and type of dietary fat in our diets and health. It isn't an isolated finding but rather stands with findings from many studies of various designs conducted by many investigators around the world. Based on the concordance of this work, I'm confident we can be guided by this overall picture of dietary fat: **Choose foods rich in polyunsaturated and monounsaturated fats, like nuts, salmon, and avocado, over those rich in saturated fats, like red meat. And don't eat those that contain artificial trans fats.**

Clinical Trials: Replacing Saturated Fats with Unsaturated Fats Saves Lives
Clinical trials bear out the overall picture of dietary fats I have been drawing in this book: some fats are good for health and others aren't. Early trials—most of which were done decades ago, were very small, and enrolled people who already had heart disease—showed that eating less total fat, usually by eating more carbohydrate-rich foods like white rice and potatoes, did little for the heart and blood vessels.

In stark contrast to that work, clinical trials in which volunteers were randomly assigned to either a standard Western diet, which is relatively rich in saturated fats, or a diet in which some saturated fats were replaced with polyunsaturated fats have shown benefits such as lower levels of total cholesterol and harmful LDL cholesterol and, more important, reductions in heart disease of one-third or more. (As discussed earlier, "polyunsaturated fats" means both omega-6 and omega-3 fatty acids, which wasn't acknowledged when these trials were conducted.)

One of the most impressive clinical trials was the Lyon Diet Heart Study. Begun in 1988, this French trial set out to test whether a Mediterranean-type

diet could prevent second heart attacks or heart-related deaths among heart attack survivors. Half of the 605 volunteers were asked to follow a low-fat diet. The
other half were asked to follow a Mediterranean-type diet that included olive oil,
whole-grain bread, extra root and green vegetables, fruit every day, more fish
and poultry and less red meat, and a special margarine rich in omega-3 fats.

The trial, which was supposed to run for five years, was stopped after just
two and a half years because the benefits of the Mediterranean-type diet were
so compelling (see Figure 14): a 70 percent reduction in new heart attacks or
deaths from all causes.[23] When the investigators checked in on the participants
a few years later, the benefits of the Mediterranean diet, including a reduced
risk of cancer, were still in evidence. Interestingly, most of those who had been

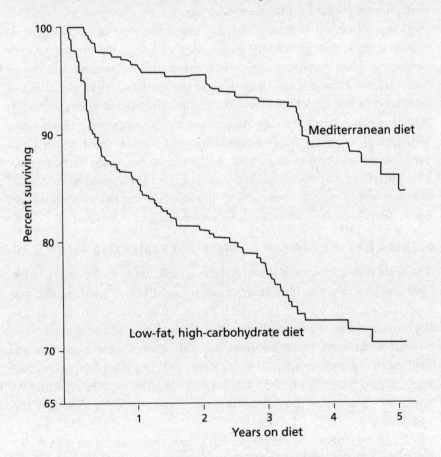

Figure 14. Lyon Diet Heart Study. Heart attack survivors eating a Mediterranean-type diet had fewer second
heart attacks and deaths from heart disease than those on a low-fat, high-carbohydrate diet.

asked to follow the Mediterranean-type diet were still doing so several years after the trial had ended.[24]

A more recent clinical trial shows that a similar type of diet can prevent first heart attacks in relatively healthy people. Researchers recruited nearly 7,500 residents of Spain to take part in the Prevención con Dieta Mediterránea (PREDIMED) trial. All of the volunteers were over age fifty-five. None had ever been diagnosed with heart disease, although all were at high risk for developing it. One-third of the participants were asked to follow a Mediterranean-style diet and were also given a liter of extra-virgin olive oil each week. Another third were asked to follow a Mediterranean-style diet but instead of olive oil were given about seven ounces a week of walnuts, hazelnuts, and almonds. The third group was asked to follow a low-fat diet.

The trial was stopped early, after just under five years of follow-up, when it became clear that participants in the Mediterranean-diet groups were experiencing fewer cardiovascular events—heart attacks, strokes, and deaths from cardiovascular disease—than those in the low-fat diet group, just as had been seen in the Lyon Diet Heart Study. The difference was impressive: 83 cardiovascular events in the Mediterranean diet plus nuts group (8 per 1,000 participants), 96 in the Mediterranean diet plus olive oil group (8 per 1,000 participants), and 106 in the low-fat diet group (11 per 1,000 participants).[25] That difference may not sound like a lot, but if it were applied to the United States, it would translate into tens of thousands fewer hospitalizations and deaths from heart disease each year if everyone shifted to this diet.

PLENTY OF PROOF FOR THE BENEFITS OF UNSATURATED FATS

The popular view of science is that if you assemble the facts, they will give you clear, definite answers. The reality of science usually isn't anything like that, especially when it comes to human nutrition and its connection with disease. We have an ocean of existing facts and a steady deluge of new data, but only a few solid answers. That's because studies are always open to criticism and their results to interpretation. It is standard operating procedure to conclude that "more research is needed," a phrase I have often used in reporting the results of a study or writing an editorial or review on specific aspects of diet and disease.

I don't feel that way at all about what people should be doing with dietary fat. Cutting back on all types of fat and eating more carbs does nothing to protect against heart disease and will ultimately harm some people. Instead, replacing saturated fats with unsaturated fats is a safe, proven, and delicious way to cut the rates of heart disease.

CONFUSING NEWS ABOUT SATURATED FAT

An article published in 2014 set off a maelstrom of misinformation about saturated fat. This *Annals of Internal Medicine* meta-analysis of previously published studies suggested that the prevailing recommendation to eat less saturated fat—abundant in red meat, cheese, and buttery pastries—doesn't lower the risk for heart disease.[26]

The media had a field day with what it called another gigantic flip-flop in dietary advice. Mark Bittman, writing in the *New York Times*, wrote: "Butter is back. Julia Child, goddess of fat, is beaming somewhere." Other headlines were equally effusive. Consumers sighed, blindsided again by confusing and contradictory results from nutrition research.

The media attention was unfortunate, because the analysis was flawed in

The Great Butter Battle

Beginning in the 1970s, many people accepted the demise of butter and gave it up, ruing the loss of its savory flavor but agreeing that the amount of saturated fat it contained might be bad for the heart. They dutifully switched to margarine, as researchers and nutritionists suggested. When later reports highlighted the hazards of margarine, though, many people felt duped.

There never was any good evidence that switching from butter to margarine cut the chances of having a heart attack or developing heart disease. Making the switch was a well-intentioned guess, given that margarine had less saturated fat than butter. But recommendations to switch from butter to margarine overlooked the large amounts of trans fats in many margarines.

Today, the butter-versus-margarine argument doesn't make sense. From the standpoint of heart disease, butter is on the list of foods to use sparingly, mostly because it contains so much of the kind of saturated fat that raises levels of harmful LDL. Many margarines now for sale are low in saturated fat, high in unsaturated fat, and free of trans fats. As long as you don't use too much, you should be fine. (They are still rich in calories.) But before you reach for butter or margarine, think about whether you could use olive oil or another liquid vegetable oil instead.

If you can't do without the taste of butter when sautéing vegetables, scallops, or eggs, melt a small pat of butter and add olive oil.

Good Sources of Essential Fats

Many delicious foods deliver essential unsaturated fats that are good for the heart and the rest of the body. Try to eat at least one source of these every day.

Foods Rich in Omega-3 Fats

- cold-water fish such as salmon, sardines, mackerel, and trout
- canola and soybean oil (as long as they aren't partially hydrogenated)
- flaxseeds and flaxseed oil
- walnuts
- dark green leafy vegetables such as kale, spinach, mustard greens, and collards
- omega-3 enhanced eggs

Foods Rich in Omega-6 Fats

- soybean, safflower, sunflower, corn, and other vegetable oils
- sunflower seeds, walnuts, and pine nuts

many ways. The authors used incorrect numbers from some of the original studies, including the Nurses' Health Study, and omitted important data. Most seriously, the authors did not actually compare the effects of saturated fat with those of polyunsaturated fat; this would have required the original data from the studies that were summarized. These problems called into question a key conclusion of the *Annals of Internal Medicine* study: that replacing saturated fat with polyunsaturated fat does not reduce the risk for heart disease. (In response to the dozens of letters to the journal criticizing this paper, the authors posted several revised versions online. Although some errors were corrected, the most serious limitations could not be addressed.)

A 2016 meta-analysis of butter and heart disease caused a similar ruckus.[27] It concluded that eating a tablespoon or so of butter a day wasn't linked to dying from any cause or having a heart attack or stroke. Although the authors clearly pointed out the benefit of using unsaturated vegetable oils instead of butter, this got lost in the headlines.

Following the publication of those two studies, my team directly compared the effect on risk of heart disease of butter fat compared to other types of foods.

When compared to eating refined grains, eating butter fat was associated with a similar risk of heart disease. When compared to eating whole grains or unsaturated vegetable oils, however, butter was associated with a higher risk.[28]

Here's the key issue: what you choose to eat instead of foods rich in saturated fat makes a huge difference. Eating a bowl of white pasta with a low-fat sauce instead of a juicy, high-fat steak doesn't do much for your health because both choices have harmful effects on risk factors for cardiovascular disease. But swapping that steak for salmon on a bed of greens with an olive oil and vinegar dressing is a very positive switch, because those foods improve risk factors for cardiovascular disease.

OMEGA ADVICE

Given the wide-ranging importance and benefits of omega-3 fatty acids, try to eat at least one good source of them a day. Daily doses of omega-3 fatty acids are especially important for women who are pregnant or hoping to become pregnant. From conception onward, a developing child needs a steady supply of omega-3 fatty acids to form the brain and other parts of the nervous system.

Unfortunately, omega-3 fatty acids aren't as plentiful in the average diet as they once were. Food companies purposely destroy them in vegetable oils to make foods last longer on the shelf without turning rancid. Meat from cows and chickens now contains fewer omega-3 fatty acids. Why? Most animals used for food once foraged on wild plants and seeds, which are rich in omega-3 fatty acids. Today they are fed grains that are low in them.

The best source of omega-3s is fish, especially fatty fish such as salmon, tuna (including canned tuna), mackerel, herring, and sardines. Unfortunately, the relatively high price of fish often puts it beyond the budget of many households. Canned salmon gives the best buy for omega-3 fats and can be used in countless ways.

Eating fish two to three times a week is a good target for almost everyone. Eating more than that adds little extra protection against heart disease. Young children, and women in their childbearing years, should focus on types low in mercury (see "Fish, Mercury, and Fish Oil" on page 147). As research in this area continues to unfold, including in your diet a good source of alpha-linolenic acid (ALA) on most days of the week ensures an adequate intake of omega-3 fats. Good ways to do this include eating walnuts, flaxseeds, or foods made with or cooked in canola or soybean oil.

You don't really need to think about getting more omega-6 fats in your diet because they are found in many common foods. Use plant oils for cooking and you'll get all the omega-6s you need.

DIETARY FAT AND CANCER: A WEAK CONNECTION

The same kind of international comparisons that sparked the dietary fat–heart disease hypothesis have also generated strongly held beliefs about a connection between dietary fat and cancer. Countries with lower average fat intakes—mostly developing or less affluent nations—tend to have lower rates of breast, colon, and prostate cancer than countries with higher average fat intakes. But better, more direct evidence linking diet and cancer has greatly weakened support for this connection.

Breast Cancer

Based on a few retrospective studies, the U.S. National Research Council concluded back in 1982 that reducing the fat content of the diet from 40 to 30 percent of calories would reduce the number of women diagnosed with breast cancer. Two years later, the National Cancer Institute made this the focus of a major health promotion campaign. These efforts have done little to prevent breast cancer.

Since then, larger cohort studies of cancer have not supported a connection between dietary fat and breast cancer. In the Nurses' Health Study, more than 8,000 of the participants have developed breast cancer since 1980. With more than twenty years of follow-up, we didn't see any increase in breast cancer among women with a higher intake of dietary fat. An analysis of all the large cohort studies from around the world also found no connection between dietary fat and breast cancer, except for an unexpected increase among the small number of women with the lowest fat intake.[29] And combining data from the Nurses' Health Study and Nurses' Health Study II, with up to thirty years of follow-up, we looked to see whether the amount of fat in the diet either before or after a diagnosis of breast cancer increased the risk of dying from it. It did not. If anything, higher fat intake before diagnosis was related to a slightly lower risk of dying from breast cancer.[30] (In fact, in the PREDIMED trial described on page 96, women who followed a higher-fat Mediterranean-type diet were less likely to have developed breast cancer over the five-year trial than those following a low-fat diet.[31] Although the number of cases was small, the findings were promising.)

Most studies into the connection between dietary fat and breast cancer have focused on women in midlife or later. That makes sense, because breast cancer is more common in older women. But it can also strike younger women, and breast tissue is particularly vulnerable to carcinogenic influences at younger ages. In the Nurses' Health Study II, which studied women who were ages twenty-six to forty-four in 1989, 714 of the more than 90,000 participants developed breast cancer over an eight-year period. High intake of *animal* fat, especially fat from red meat, increased the chances of having breast cancer. High intake of vegetable fat did not.[32] That finding has persisted through 20 years of follow-up.[33]

As discussed in chapter three, randomized trials are thought to be the best way to test a hypothesis. Because of the strong belief that dietary fat was linked to the development of breast cancer, the Women's Health Initiative was launched in 1991 with dietary fat as a prime focus. It was the most comprehensive and expensive clinical trial ever conducted. More than 48,000 women were randomized to follow either a low-fat diet or their usual diet. After seven years there was no significant difference in rates of breast cancer or, for that matter, heart disease or any other disease.[34] Normally, a finding like that would put an end to the belief that a low-fat diet prevented breast cancer. But questions flew about whether the study had lasted long enough. In a follow-up publication, the authors reported that there were no differences at any time during the trial in blood levels of triglycerides or protective HDL between the two groups of women. We know that on a low-fat diet, triglycerides go up and HDL goes down. The lack of any change in these two indicated there was little if any difference in fat intakes between the study groups.

In another randomized trial conducted in Canada, women at higher risk of breast cancer because of changes in their mammograms were randomly assigned to a low-fat diet or their usual diet for an average of ten years. Levels of protective HDL were lower among women on the low-fat diet, indicating that there was a difference in fat intake between the two groups. Those on the low-fat diet had a 19 percent higher risk of breast cancer. Although this increase was not statistically significant, it was certainly headed in the wrong direction.[35]

The relationship between fat intake and breast cancer risk has been studied intensively over the last three decades. Although it's impossible to prove that dietary fat has absolutely no effect on breast cancer—there could always be a tiny effect too small to detect—we can be confident that low-fat diets don't play an important role in reducing the risk of breast cancer.

There are, however, some hints that replacing fats from animal with those from plants may provide some benefit. The clearest and most consistent finding from both animal and human studies is that too many calories during adulthood, regardless of the foods they come from, are far more important to the development of breast cancer than dietary fat.

Colon Cancer

Early studies suggested a link between dietary fat and colon cancer, the third leading cause of cancer deaths in the United States. But that, too, hasn't been bolstered by more detailed work. There is good evidence that eating a lot of red meat increases the risk of colon cancer. This could stem from the types of fats in red meat or the cancer-causing chemicals generated by cooking red meat at high temperatures. The World Health Organization has warned that regularly eating red meat, especially processed meat, is linked to the development of colorectal cancer.[36] Intake of fats from fish, chicken, and plants has not been associated with risk of colon or rectal cancer.

As is the case for breast cancer, the strongest dietary link with colon cancer is the imbalance between calories consumed and calories burned: people who are overweight are more likely to develop this cancer than people who aren't. Protection from colon cancer comes from getting regular physical activity, not smoking, and getting adequate amounts of folic acid, one of the B vitamins (see chapter eleven).

Prostate Cancer

The situation with prostate cancer is murkier, partly because there have been relatively few studies in this area. International comparisons show that Asian men, who follow relatively low-fat diets, have substantially lower rates of prostate cancer than their Western counterparts. Although Asian men do experience some increases in prostate cancer when they move to the United States, rates in this group always stay lower than among Caucasians, suggesting that some genetic factors play an important role. If there is a connection between dietary fat and prostate cancer, it seems to be mainly related to animal fat or some other component of red meat. That's good news, because it means that olive oil and other unsaturated fats that decrease the risk of heart disease would not increase the risk of prostate cancer.

Research on prostate cancer raises questions about a different kind of balance. Results from the Health Professionals Follow-Up Study and others have shown that men whose diets are rich in omega-3s from seafood—EPA and DHA—are less likely to develop prostate cancer. The connection between omega-3s from plants—alpha-linolenic acid (ALA)—and prostate cancer has been a bit worrisome. Some studies suggest an increase in prostate cancer and advanced prostate cancer among men with high intakes of ALA,[37] although we have not seen this in our most recent follow-up in the Health Professional's Follow-Up Study.

Why might a seemingly healthful oil be implicated in prostate cancer? One possibility is that, until recently, much of the ALA in the American diet was actually a harmful trans fat (see "Trans Fats—A Special Concern" on page 83). For years, oils rich in ALA routinely underwent partial hydrogenation to keep them from spoiling too quickly. But that also added trans fats to them. Partial hydrogenation has been greatly curtailed, which means we will be getting natural, untransformed ALA going forward.

Walnuts offer a clue that this may explain the trend. Walnuts are an important source of ALA. They've never been partially hydrogenated, and consumption of walnuts has never been associated with higher risk of prostate cancer. While scientists will continue to monitor the relationship of ALA with prostate disease, I think men can enjoy walnuts, canola oil, and other foods rich in ALA without worrying about their prostates.

The Bottom Line on Dietary Fats and Cancer

It is impossible to prove that there's no connection between dietary fat and cancer. If fat does influence the development of cancer, though, evidence from large cohort studies with many years of follow-up shows that the effect is small. Given the strong and consistent association that has been observed between type of fat and heart disease, I think it makes sense to focus on dietary fats for their proven impact on heart disease, not for their hypothetical connections with cancers that so far have not been supported by extensive evidence.

SELECTING HEALTHY FATS

The phrase "heart-healthy diet" often conjures up images of steamed rice and vegetables, a platter of baked chicken breasts, pasta—easy on the sauce, please—and only dreams of fried onion rings.

If you believe, as I do, that a low-fat diet isn't the best way to a healthier heart, there's another option. This one requires a bit of cutting back, just as traditional low-fat diets do, but it also means consciously adding some fats to your diet. This takes some practice at first, but the effort will be well worth it, both in taste and health.

Cutting back. Stay away from trans fats and limit your intake of saturated fats. It's gotten easier and easier to avoid trans fats, and it will soon be hard to find them even if you wanted to. When an FDA rule went into effect in 2006 that the amount of trans fat in a food had to be listed on the food label, many companies took that as an "opportunity" to find trans-free replacements (see "Trans Fats—A Special Concern" on page 83).

Limiting your intake of saturated fats means going easy on red meat and whole-fat dairy products, or not eating them at all. It isn't worth making yourself crazy to eliminate all traces of saturated fat from your diet. For one thing, that's almost impossible to do, since foods that are good sources of monounsaturated and polyunsaturated fats also contain some saturated fat. For another, as the Lyon Diet Heart Study, PREDIMED, and others have shown, eating a modest amount of saturated fat along with unsaturated fats is perfectly fine. I don't advise religiously trying to count calories or grams of fat but instead observing a commonly suggested upper limit of 8 percent of calories, or around 17 grams a day of saturated fat. Seven pats of butter, one Pizza Hut pan pizza (personal size), or three glasses of regular milk supply this much.

It isn't necessary to count fat grams or whip out a calculator to compute the percentage of calories from fat. You have better things to do with your time, the payoff is very small, and there's no solid evidence for adopting exact numerical goals for total fat intake. It does make sense to know what is in the foods you eat, or plan to eat, so you can make healthy choices. But I don't recommend keeping precise tallies all day long.

Adding in. Once you have a handle on the saturated and trans fats in your diet, you'll find there are plenty of easy and delicious ways to add in unsaturated fats. The healthiest mix of monounsaturated and polyunsaturated fats hasn't yet been determined. For now, a combination of these is a good strategy and gives you plenty of flexibility in your diet. (See "Percentage of Specific Types of Fat in Common Oils and Fats" on page 105.)

One of the best sources of monounsaturated fats is olive oil, which is every bit as versatile as butter. You can sauté vegetables in it, use it for stir-frying chicken or fish, add it as the base for salad dressings, even dip bread in it at the table instead of using butter, as is done in Spain, Italy, Greece, and my home. Different olive oils have different flavors, giving you a wide range of tastes. Other good sources of monounsaturated fats include canola oil, peanut oil, avocados, almonds, peanuts, and most other nuts.

Percentage of Specific Types of Fat in Common Oils and Fats*

Oils	Saturated	Mono-unsaturated	Poly-unsaturated	Trans	Alpha-linolenic Acid**
Canola	7	58	29	0	12
Safflower	9	12	74	0	0
Sunflower	10	20	66	0	2
Corn	13	24	60	0	1
Olive	13	72	8	0	1
Soybean	16	44	37	0	7
Peanut	17	49	32	0	1
Palm	50	37	10	0	0
Coconut	87	6	2	0	0
Cooking Fat					
Original Crisco	25	36	30	11	2
Lard	39	44	11	1	0
Beef fat	39	49	3	8	3
Chicken fat	27	41	31	0	0
Butter	64	29	6	3	1
Margarines/Spreads					
Imperial Stick	18	2	29	23	4
Fleischmann Tub	19	31	46	6	1
Shedd's Country Crock Tub	21	27	49	5	6
Promise 60% Tub	21	26	51	3	1

*Values expressed as percent of total fat; data are from analyses performed at Harvard School of Public Health Lipid Laboratory and USDA publications.

**Alpha-linolenic acid is also included in polyunsaturated fat.

The main sources of polyunsaturated fats include vegetable oils such as corn and soybean oil, legumes such as soybeans and soy products, and seeds. One easy way to replace saturated fats with unsaturated fats is to use fish, poultry, nuts, and seeds in place of red meat wherever possible. Also, chicken fat is much higher in polyunsaturated fat than beef fat, probably the main reason why substituting chicken for red meat is related to a lower risk of heart disease. (See the recipes in chapter fifteen.)

PUTTING IT INTO PRACTICE

Unsaturated fats are good for you, saturated fats aren't so good, and trans fats are downright harmful. Whenever possible, choose foods that deliver healthy fats.

- Make decisions about dietary fats based on their proven effects on heart disease, not on their weak—if any—connection with cancer.
- Limit the amount of saturated fat in your diet. To do this, cut back on red meat, processed meat, full-fat milk, and other full-fat dairy foods.
- Add in foods that deliver unsaturated fats, such as olive oil, nuts, seeds, and fatty fish.
- Use liquid vegetable oils in cooking and at the table.
- Eat one or more good sources of omega-3 fatty acids every day: fish, walnuts, canola or soybean oil, ground flaxseeds, or flaxseed oil.

Replacing Unhealthy Fats with Healthier Ones

Saturated fats and trans fats are damaging to the heart and to overall health. Make the switch to foods or food ingredients that contain healthful unsaturated fats: monounsaturated fats like olive and canola oils and polyunsaturated fats like soy and corn oil.

Here are several simple substitutions that can help you make this transition:

INSTEAD OF SAUTÉING WITH BUTTER . . .

- Switch to olive, canola, or other healthful oils. The calories are similar but these oils are rich in healthful unsaturated fats and low in saturated fat. Olive oil has only 1.8 grams of saturated fat per tablespoon; butter has 7, which is close to one-half of the daily limit. In fact, each tablespoon of butter gets more than half of its calories from saturated fat.

INSTEAD OF BAKING CAKES, COOKIES, AND QUICK
BREADS WITH SOLID SHORTENING . . .

- Switch to healthful oils whenever possible. The calories are roughly the same but, again, the oils are rich in unsaturated fats. Solid shortenings are now available without unhealthful trans fats, and coconut oil, butter, or lard are options for occasional use when a hard fat is absolutely essential.

INSTEAD OF COOKING PORK LOIN OR FATTIER CUTS OF PORK . . .

- Switch to pork tenderloin. Pork tenderloin is as lean as skinless white meat chicken. A 3-ounce cooked serving contains only 4 grams of fat, just 1.4 grams of it saturated. The same-size serving of cooked pork loin contains nearly 12 grams of fat, 4.5 grams of it saturated. A good rule of thumb is that the leaner the cut of meat, the less saturated fat it contains.

INSTEAD OF COOKING FATTY HAMBURGER MEAT (73 TO 80 PERCENT LEAN) . . .

- Switch to extra-lean ground meat. A 3-ounce portion of a fatty hamburger meat, before it's cooked, can have nearly 23 grams of fat, 9 of it saturated. Lean ground beef, labeled at least 91 percent lean, carries only 8 grams of fat, 3 of it saturated. Cooking, particularly if you broil or grill meat to the well-done stage, can reduce fat—but not dramatically enough to make fatty meat as lean as the extra-lean variety. However, keep in mind that leaner red meat does not necessarily mean lower risk of heart disease or cancer; replacing red meat with alternative protein sources is the best option.

INSTEAD OF USING WHOLE MILK IN SAUCES OR BAKED GOODS . . .

- Switch to skim milk. Eight ounces of whole milk contain close to 8 grams of fat, nearly 5 of it saturated. Eight ounces of skim milk contain about 0.6 grams of fat, of which 0.4 grams are from saturated fat. Better yet, consider using soy milk or almond milk in its place. Although they contain more fat than skim milk, it is mainly unsaturated.

INSTEAD OF ADDING SOUR CREAM TO RECIPES . . .

- Try plain yogurt. A cup of sour cream contains 37 grams of fat, 23 of them saturated, and 136 milligrams of cholesterol. The same amount of full fat yogurt contains about 10 grams of fat and skim milk yogurt carries a mere 0.4 grams of fat and only 5 milligrams of cholesterol.

INSTEAD OF SPREADING SANDWICHES OR CRACKERS
WITH REGULAR PEANUT BUTTER . . .

- Switch to natural-style peanut butter. This doesn't save you any calories, but it does offer a healthful switch in the type of fat. Natural peanut butter

is free of trans fats. Regular peanut butters are usually made with hydrogenated oils that do not contain trans fats but do add more saturated fat.

INSTEAD OF SMOTHERING PIZZA OR SALAD WITH CHEESE . . .

- Use a tiny amount of high-flavored cheeses like Parmesan, blue cheese,
  or extra-sharp cheddar. This adds far less fat, since you're satisfied with a
  smaller amount of cheese. One tablespoon of Parmesan cheese contains
  only 2 grams of fat, 1 gram of it saturated.

Fat Substitutes

The pinnacle of the "All fat is bad" movement may have been the widely hyped introduction
of the fake fat known as olestra. From a scientific standpoint it was a marvel of food engineering. From a public health standpoint, olestra—sold under the misleading trade name
Olean—could have been a disaster had it ever caught on.

Olestra was designed to trigger the same sensations in your taste buds as real fat.
Beyond that, though, it was a completely different compound. The digestive enzymes that
break down fats couldn't attack olestra, so it slid unchanged through the digestive system.
Along the way it picked up vitamins A, D, E, and K, as well as beta-carotene, lycopene, and a
host of other plant pigments and phytochemicals and whisked them out into the stool. This
robbed the body of a host of substances that play roles in preventing heart disease, cancer,
dementia, and other chronic diseases.

Olestra's maker, Procter & Gamble, rolled out chips and other products made with olestra. Fortunately, they were duds in the marketplace.

Many other fat substitutes have been developed. Some, like Simplesse, are made from
milk and egg protein. Some, like Avicel, are made from carbohydrates. Others, like Nutrim, are
made from fiber. This high-fiber product is rich in beta-glucans, a group of soluble fibers that
contribute to the cholesterol-lowering properties of oats and barley.

Fat substitutes like olestra offered health hazards rather than improvements. Those
such as Nutrim could be beneficial if they are used in place of saturated or trans fats. An
equally healthy solution is to use liquid vegetable oils in place of saturated or trans fats.

The bottom line is that we don't need gimmicks or fake foods in order to have healthy
diets. We can do this today in a way that makes eating a pleasure.

CHAPTER SIX

Carbohydrates for Better and Worse

L IKE AN EASY MIDDLE CHILD, carbohydrates were once overlooked. Fats got most of the attention, fruits and vegetables the praise. That's a bit surprising, because carbohydrates make up half of the calories in the American diet and an even higher percentage in many diets around the world. Carbohydrates were thrust into the spotlight with the emergence and incredible popularity of the Atkins and South Beach diets. Carbohydrates—bread, rice, pasta, and the like—plummeted from being the "go-to" foods for healthy eating and weight loss to culinary creeps. The Paleo, Dukan and other carb-bashing diets have kept the pressure on carbs.

As happens with so many fads, the case against carbs began with a kernel of good science that has since been lost in hype and sweeping generalizations. That kernel of good science is this: some sources of carbohydrate, like white bread, white rice, and potatoes, make blood sugar skyrocket. Lost in translation was that other sources, like whole grains, have lower, slower effects on blood sugar; they provide minerals, vitamins, fiber, and phytonutrients that refined grains don't; and they benefit health rather than harm it. Many low-carb faddists have taken another, completely illogical, step: if carbs are bad, then anything else is good for you, such as lots of red meat, sausage, bacon, and butter. And that's just not true.

By wielding control over blood sugar, carbohydrate-rich foods influence the development of diabetes and long-term health. Eating the right types of carbohydrates—meaning grains that are as intact and unprocessed as possible—is an important part of the foundation of a healthy diet.

Before the low-carb diet returned from oblivion, the prevailing attitude was that all so-called complex carbohydrates were good, or at least benign, compared with fats. This idea came from rather simplistic looks at diet and

Fast Fact: Grains Optional

Grains offer an easy way to get the sugars your body needs for energy. But if you aren't partial to grains, don't worry. You can get by just fine if you forgo wheat, rice, and other grains. Your body can make blood sugar from fruits, vegetables, beans, and other foods. Even a very low-carb diet, like the so-called ketogenic diet used to treat epilepsy, can be okay. It forces the body to burn fats rather than carbohydrates. Some people who can't lose weight with standard diets do well with a ketogenic diet, but most find it hard to sustain because food choices are quite limited and, for reasons we don't understand, humans crave carbohydrates when they don't eat them.

If you decide to cut back on carbs, what you eat in their place will make a large difference for long-term health. Foods that deliver healthful protein and unsaturated fats—like fish, nuts, and beans—will be good for your heart and the rest of you too. Foods that deliver a lot of saturated fat—like hamburger, sausage, and other red meats—won't be.

disease in China and other developing countries. Until recently, Chinese people ate mostly carbohydrates, with a sprinkling of protein and fat. They also had low rates of heart disease. Putting one and one together, some dietary experts concluded that the low rates of heart disease in China were the result of the high-carbohydrate, low-fat diet. That idea got transplanted to the West. The "carbohydrates are good" message became a key part of recommendations from the American Heart Association, the American Cancer Society, and the World Health Organization. It also formed the base of the long-standing but misleading Food Guide Pyramid.

This transplant didn't fare so well on foreign soil. Even as Americans tried to cut back on fat and ate more carbohydrates, we got fatter as a nation. The steady decline in rates of death due to heart disease that occurred during the 1970s and early 1980s has slowed in young adults. And the percentage of adult Americans with diabetes skyrocketed, from just under 1 percent in 1960 to more than 8 percent fifty years later.[1] Fortunately, since 2008 there has been a small but steady decline in diabetes, likely due to the large reduction in consumption of trans fat and a 25 percent reduction in consumption of sugar-sweetened beverages.

THE WRONG TYPES OF CARBOHYDRATES DO MORE HARM THAN GOOD

Why isn't a higher-carbohydrate diet paying off for us the same way it used to work for the Chinese? Traditionally the Chinese weighed less and were more physically active than Americans. Weight and exercise matter: high-carbohydrate diets have different effects on metabolism among lean, active people than they do on overweight, sedentary people. So simply eating a high-carbohydrate diet doesn't offer blanket protection against heart disease, cancer, and diabetes. That's something the Chinese are now experiencing. Before 1980, under 1 percent of people in China had diabetes. Today more than 10 percent have it, due mainly to changes in lifestyle that have come with China's rapid economic growth.[2] The problem is worse in Beijing and other urban areas as cars replace bicycles, desk jobs replace manual labor, and carbohydrate intake remains high.

The other problem is that little attention has been paid to the types of carbohydrates we eat. In traditional cultures, grains tend to be eaten whole or lightly refined. But Americans eat mostly highly refined grains. Even in many developing countries, grains have been switched from whole to refined. That means the fibrous bran on the grain's outer surface is stripped away, along with most of the minerals and vitamins. The remaining starch, depleted in nutrients, is quickly digested and absorbed—with damaging consequences. These include higher levels of blood sugar, insulin, and triglycerides, and lower levels of protective HDL cholesterol. In the long run, that means more cardiovascular disease and diabetes.

In the Healthy Eating Pyramid, refined carbohydrates are in the "Use Sparingly" category; the Healthy Eating Plate urges you to limit their use. You will do yourself a double favor by swapping refined carbohydrates for intact, whole-grain carbohydrates. Because whole grains take longer to digest, they help you feel full longer, which means you'll likely end up taking in fewer calories without thinking about it.

Carbohydrates from whole grains, fruits, vegetables, and beans can give you a large share of your daily calories. For optimal health, choose whole grains like brown rice, quinoa, whole oats, and bulgur, and foods made from whole grains like whole wheat bread. Intact grains—those that haven't been ground up or otherwise processed—are best. Not only will whole and intact grains help protect you against a range of chronic diseases, they can also expand the palette of tastes, textures, and colors you can use to please your palate.

NOT JUST SIMPLE VERSUS COMPLEX

Carbohydrates were once divided into two categories: simple and complex. Simple carbohydrates like sugar were portrayed as the bad boys of nutrition, while complex carbohydrates like bread or rice were regarded as the golden children.

That was a gross oversimplification. Not all simple carbohydrates are bad, and not all complex carbohydrates are good. Later in this chapter, I will describe two far more useful ways of categorizing carbohydrates: by their effect on blood sugar (the glycemic index) and by whether they come from refined or whole grains.

Simple carbohydrates are sugars. The simplest simple carbohydrates are glucose (sometimes called dextrose), fructose (also called fruit sugar), and galactose (a part of milk sugar). Table sugar is sucrose, a combination of one molecule of glucose and one of fructose. Milk contains lactose, which is made by joining one molecule of glucose with one of galactose. Simple carbohydrates provide us with energy and little else.

Complex carbohydrates are more . . . well, complex. In essence they are long chains of linked sugars. There are many types of complex carbohydrates in our food. The main one is starch, a long chain of glucose molecules. The human digestive system can rapidly break down starch and other complex carbohydrates into their component sugars. Some complex carbohydrates, like fiber, are quite indigestible and pass largely unchanged through the stomach and the intestines. Although fiber doesn't contribute any energy or molecular building blocks to the body, it is still an important part of our diet. Because the term "complex carbohydrate" includes both starch and fiber, it is a useless and potentially misleading term.

WHY CARBOHYDRATES MATTER

In the average American diet, carbohydrates contribute about half of all calories. In one study from the National Health and Nutrition Examination Survey (NHANES), a staggering half of these "carbohydrate calories" came from just eight sources:[3]

- soft drinks, sodas, and fruit-flavored drinks
- cake, sweet rolls, doughnuts, and pastries
- pizza
- potato chips, corn chips, and popcorn
- rice
- bread, rolls, buns, English muffins, and bagels
- beer
- french fries and frozen potatoes.

Using data from NHANES, my colleagues and I calculated that about 80 percent of the carbohydrates in the U.S. diet come from sugar, refined starch, or potatoes. That means about 40 percent of all the calories we consume come

Fast Fact: Potatoes and Corn—Starches, Not Vegetables

Although the USDA says that potatoes and corn are vegetables, your body treats them more like white rice and other rapidly digested grains than like vegetables (see "The Spud Is a Dud" on page 167). Eating other vegetables instead of potatoes and corn can help control your weight and your health. While corn is technically a whole grain, it has been so intensively bred for high starch content that it is no longer the same nutritious food that Tisquantum (Squanto) gave to the Pilgrims as they tried to eke out a living in North America.

from sugars, highly refined and easily digested grains, or potato starch, all of which are rapidly converted to blood sugar.

When you eat a slice of bread, a potato, or some candy, your body breaks down the digestible carbohydrates it contains. Starch is converted to glucose, which is rapidly absorbed into the bloodstream and swiftly shuttled to the farthest reaches of the circulatory system. Because these simple sugar molecules are a primary fuel for most of the body's tissues, complex mechanisms are in place to make sure that the level of glucose in the bloodstream doesn't shoot too high or drift too low.

The rise in blood glucose is followed quickly by a parallel rise in insulin (see Figure 15). This hormone, produced by special cells in the pancreas,

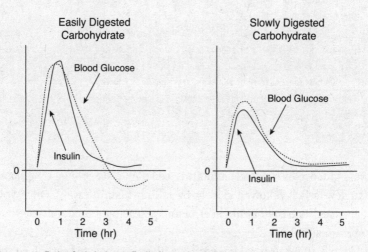

Figure 15. Response to Eating Carbohydrates. Easily digested carbohydrates make blood sugar and insulin rise faster and higher—and fall further—than slowly digested carbohydrates.

Corn Syrup Isn't to Blame

One of the many dramatic changes in the American diet over the past fifty years has been in how we satisfy our craving for sugar. Until the 1970s, we relied almost exclusively on sucrose (table sugar) from sugarcane and sugar beets, with a bit of honey, maple sugar, and molasses thrown in for variety. Today more than half of our sugar comes from corn, much of it in the form of high-fructose corn syrup. It's found in everything from sugared sodas to ketchup and baby food.

Why the change? High-fructose corn syrup tastes a bit sweeter than sucrose. It's easier to blend into beverages. And it costs a few pennies less per pound than sucrose.

High-fructose corn syrup has been cast as one of the villains behind the obesity epidemic for a reason: the jump in its use closely parallels the trajectory of obesity rates.

The body metabolizes fructose differently from glucose. Table sugar contains glucose and fructose in equal proportions (50 percent for both), since sucrose is made of one glucose molecule joined to one fructose molecule. High-fructose corn syrup is pure glucose mixed with pure fructose in almost equal proportions (55 percent fructose and 45 percent glucose). So table sugar and corn sweeteners have much the same physiological impact on blood sugar, insulin, and metabolism.

Some people claim that they've lost weight by cutting high-fructose corn syrup from their diets. That may be so, but it probably isn't because they eliminated corn sweeteners. What likely happened is that by eliminating corn sweeteners they took in fewer added sugars and thus fewer calories.

So far, high-fructose corn sweetener doesn't seem to be a greater dietary disaster than any other kind of added sugar. So swapping a soda made with high-fructose corn sweetener for one made with "natural sugar" won't improve your health. What's important is limiting your intake of all added sugars.

The World Health Organization recommends keeping added sugars under 10 percent of daily calories (roughly 12 teaspoons or 50 grams), and getting under 5 percent of calories from them "would provide additional health benefits."[4]

To help us keep track of added sugars, the FDA is now requiring food companies to list added sugar on their "Nutrition Facts" labels. You may be surprised at how much added sugar some of your favorite foods contain.

ushers glucose into muscle and other cells. As cells sponge up glucose, blood sugar levels fall, followed closely by falling insulin levels. Once your blood sugar nears its baseline, the liver begins releasing stored glucose to maintain a constant supply.

After a snack or meal brimming with easily digested carbohydrates, blood sugar bolts upward. The resulting flood of insulin drives down the blood sugar level, sometimes too fast and too far. If there isn't any more digestible carbohydrate in the stomach or intestines, your gut and brain start sending out hunger signals to make you grab for more food even as the liver starts releasing stored glucose. In contrast, slowly digested whole-grain carbohydrates smooth out this glucose-insulin roller coaster. Because it takes longer for the digestive system to break down whole grains into sugar molecules, blood sugar and insulin levels rise more slowly and peak at lower levels. A more drawn-out process also means it takes longer to get hungry again.

THE PROBLEM OF INSULIN RESISTANCE

In a growing number of people, the body's tissues don't respond to insulin as they should. Instead, they resist its "Open up for sugar" signal. This resistance to insulin keeps the amount of sugar in the bloodstream at high levels for longer periods and forces the pancreas to produce extra insulin in order to jam glucose into cells. Like an overworked, undermaintained pump, insulin-making cells in the pancreas may wear out and eventually stop producing enough insulin to keep blood sugar under control. Insulin resistance and faltering insulin production are early signs of type 2 diabetes, which was once called non-insulin-dependent diabetes and adult-onset diabetes.

Several things contribute to insulin resistance. Here are four key factors:

Obesity is at the top of the list. The further you get above a healthy weight (see page 40), the more your body has trouble handling glucose.

Inactivity comes next. The less active you are, the lower the ratio of muscle to fat you have, even if your weight is perfectly fine. Fat cells don't handle glucose as efficiently as muscle cells, especially regularly exercised muscle cells. The less muscle you have, the harder it is to clear glucose from the bloodstream. Working your muscles with daily physical activity improves their ability to remove glucose from the blood, even when you are resting or sleeping.

Dietary fats play a modest role in insulin resistance, with low intake of polyunsaturated fat and high intake of trans fats leading to greater resistance.

Genes also play a part. Insulin resistance is more common among Native Americans, Pacific Islanders, and people of Asian heritage than it is among those of European descent. But, like everyone else, people with a genetic predisposition to insulin resistance can beat the condition by staying lean, being physically active, and eating the right diet.

Insulin resistance isn't just a blood sugar issue. It has also been linked with a variety of other problems, including high blood pressure, high levels of triglycerides, low protective HDL cholesterol, heart disease, and possibly some cancers.

HIGH-CARBOHYDRATE DIETS ARE ESPECIALLY BAD FOR PEOPLE WHO ARE OVERWEIGHT

People who are overweight fare worse on high-carbohydrate diets than do lean people. In the Nurses' Health Study, for example, eating a lot of easily digested carbohydrates is most strongly connected to increased odds of having a heart attack among women who are overweight. What's more, experiments in which volunteers were asked to follow high-carbohydrate, low-fat diets ended up with heart-unhealthy changes in levels of HDL and triglycerides, not to mention higher levels of blood sugar and insulin.[5] These adverse changes are the most pronounced in overweight people.

Put more plainly, a low-fat, high-carbohydrate diet may be a terrible eating strategy for individuals who are overweight and not physically active. They fare better with a diet that includes fewer refined carbohydrates, more whole and intact grains, more healthy protein, and more good fats. Whether or not you are overweight, the switch from refined to whole grains will be good for you because of the increased intake of micronutrients.

THE GLYCEMIC INDEX: HOW CARBOHYDRATES AFFECT YOUR BODY SUGAR

Some carbohydrate-rich foods make blood sugar spike in a flash. Others yield their sugars more slowly, acting like those sustained-release cold capsules you may have seen advertised on television.

Not long ago, the rule of thumb was that sugars triggered rapid rises in blood sugar and insulin, while complex carbohydrates caused more delayed responses. But nutrition researcher David Jenkins and his colleagues at the University of Toronto overturned this conventional wisdom by systematically testing the impact of different foods on blood sugar levels (see "Measuring the Glycemic Index and Glycemic Load" on page 121). The carbohydrate ranking they developed, called the glycemic index (GI), counters the notion that all complex carbohydrates are good and all simple ones are bad.[6] The higher a food's glycemic index, the faster and stronger it affects blood sugar and insulin levels. As a reference point, pure glucose—the rapidly digested essence of blood sugar—is assigned a score of 100. On this scale, anything below 55 or so is considered a low-glycemic-index food.

Some of the glycemic index rankings are exactly what you might expect.

Low Glycemic Foods and Prevention of Diabetes: the Building Blocks of Evidence

Over time, high blood sugar levels and a high demand for insulin will damage insulin-secreting cells in the pancreas and lead to type 2 diabetes. That's good reason to suspect that diets with a high glycemic index will increase the risk of this disease. And there's evidence for it: in large cohort studies, my research team and others have found that people consuming diets with a high glycemic index have a greater risk of developing type 2 diabetes. This was borne out in an updated analysis of data from the Nurses' Health Study and Health Professionals Follow-Up Study.[7] Among more than 175,000 women and men followed for up to twenty-four years, 15,027 developed type 2 diabetes. In all three cohorts, participants who consumed diets with the highest glycemic index were 33 percent more likely to have developed diabetes than those consuming diets with the lowest glycemic index.[8]

A large study using a drug, not diet, adds to what I think is conclusive evidence that there's a cause-and-effect relationship between the glycemic index and the development of diabetes. The drug, called acarbose (brand name Precose), has long been used to treat diabetes. It specifically inhibits the body's ability to chop up starch molecules into glucose molecules. In effect, it converts a high glycemic food into a low glycemic food without affecting its content of fiber or micronutrients. In a large randomized trial that compared acarbose with placebo, those taking the drug had a 25 percent lower risk of diabetes, as well as a similar reduction in risk for cardiovascular disease and high blood pressure.[9]

An apple has a glycemic index of 38. A serving of old-fashioned (not instant) oatmeal has a glycemic index of 58. Jelly beans have a glycemic index of 78. Other rankings come as a surprise. Cornflakes, surely a complex carbohydrate, are in the 80s, while ice cream and a Snickers bar—which most people would assign to the simple carbohydrate camp—have lower glycemic index rankings than white bread, a classic complex carbohydrate. Perhaps surprisingly, whole-grain bread can have just as high a glycemic index value as white bread if the flour is finely ground. However, its higher content of fiber and other nutrients sets it apart as a healthier choice.

Foods with a high glycemic index offer a fast energy boost by quickly increasing blood sugar levels. (That's one reason some people who use insulin to treat diabetes are urged to carry glucose tablets when they travel or exercise.) But such foods also promote equally swift drops in blood sugar that may trigger the early return of hunger. In contrast, the steadier, more sustained release of glucose from low-glycemic-index foods can stave off hunger for longer periods. There is

Glycemic Index and Glycemic Load Values for Commonly Eaten Foods (Relative to Glucose)

The glycemic index and glycemic load offer information about how a food affects blood sugar and insulin. The lower the glycemic index or glycemic load, the less the food affects blood sugar and insulin levels. A glycemic index below 55 and a glycemic load below 10 are considered low.

Foods	Serving Size	Glycemic index (%)	Carbohydrate (grams)	Glycemic Load*
Pancake	2 six-inch	83	56	46
Cornflakes	1 cup	81	48	38
Total	1 cup	76	40	31
Grape-Nuts	½ cup	71	41	29
Coca-Cola	12 ounces	63	39	25
Cranberry juice	1 cup	68	36	24
White rice	5 ounces	64	36	23
Jelly beans	1 ounce	78	28	22
Snickers bar	1 bar (2 ounces)	68	32	22
Raisin Bran	1 cup	61	35	21
Pasta	1 cup	42	47	20
Shredded Wheat	2 biscuits	75	20	15
Potatoes, mashed	1 cup	74	20	15
Cheerios	1 cup	74	20	15
Oatmeal (rolled oats)	1 cup	58	22	13
Banana (ripe)	1 medium	51	25	13
Orange juice	1 cup	52	23	12
White bread	1 slice	70	14	10
Strawberry jam	1 tbsp	51	20	10
Pizza Hut Super Supreme Pizza	2 slices	36	24	9
Whole wheat bread	1 slice	71	13	9
English muffin	1 muffin	77	11	8
Ice cream	½ cup	61	13	8
All-Bran	½ cup	42	21	8
Sugar, table	1 tsp	68	10	7
Baked beans	1 cup	48	15	7
Apple	1 medium	38	15	6
Pumpernickel (dark rye bread)	1 slice	41	12	5
Milk, skim	1 cup	32	13	4
Carrots	½ cup	47	6	3

* The glycemic load is calculated by multiplying the grams of carbohydrate by the glycemic index.

Source: Foster-Powell K., Holt, S. H., and Brand-Miller, J. C. "International Tables of Glycemic Index and Glycemic-Load-Values." American Journal of Clinical Nutrition 62 (2002): 5–56. The entire list is available for free at http://ajcn.nutrition.org/content/76/1/5.full. The University of Sydney (Australia) maintains a free searchable database of glycemic index and glycemic load values at www.glycemicindex.com.

Fast Fact: Comparing Carbs, Fats, and Protein

Whole grains and other carbohydrate-rich foods low on the glycemic index are better for you than refined carbs. Compared to healthy unsaturated fats and protein, though, all carbohydrate-rich foods, regardless of the glycemic index, boost blood triglycerides and blood pressure and lower protective HDL cholesterol.[10] Swapping refined grains for whole grains is a smart move. Swapping some of them for unsaturated fat or protein may be even better.

also now strong evidence that eating foods lower on the glycemic index will help keep diabetes at bay (see "Whole Grains Protect Against Diabetes" on page 124).

GLYCEMIC LOAD: THE AMOUNT OF CARBOHYDRATE MATTERS TOO

Although the glycemic index of a food is helpful information, it is only part of the story. The full effect of a food on blood glucose and insulin levels depends on both its glycemic index and the amount of carbohydrate consumed (protein and fat have small effects on blood sugar).

For this reason, my colleagues and I developed the concept of "glycemic

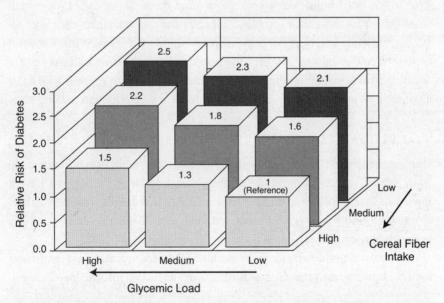

Figure 16. Combined Danger of Low Fiber and High Glycemic Load. In the Nurses' Health Study, women whose diets were low in cereal fiber and high in glycemic load were twice as likely to develop diabetes.

load." This is the amount of carbohydrate in a food multiplied by its glycemic index. As with the glycemic index, lower numbers are better. Good choices include foods with a glycemic load of 10 or less per serving, such as beans, fiber-rich fruits and vegetables, and edamame (soybeans still in the pod) and foods made from soybeans. Moderate choices such as oatmeal, sweet potatoes, and some whole-grain crackers have glycemic loads of 11 to 19. Foods with high glycemic loads (20 and above) include sugar-sweetened soda and fruit juice, white rice, french fries and baked potatoes, and pizza.

Glycemic load better reflects a food's effect on your body's biochemistry than either the amount of carbohydrate or the glycemic index alone. This is important: Some popular diet books warn against eating carrots because they were initially found to have a high glycemic index. Even if they do, carrots are mostly water, with only a small amount of carbohydrate. Finally, it's important to consider the other nutrients in a food. For example, the glycemic load of most commercial whole wheat bread is only slightly lower than for white bread because the starch is pulverized into fine particles in both products. But the whole wheat bread is a better choice because it delivers fiber and other nutrients that are removed from the white bread. Best of all would be a coarsely ground whole-grain bread that would also have a lower glycemic index.

While the glycemic index and glycemic load are useful tools for deciding what to eat, don't build your whole diet around them. Some carbohydrate-rich foods deliver far more than just blood sugar. Fruits and vegetables offer fiber, vitamins, minerals, and plenty of active phytochemicals. The same is true for intact or slightly processed grains. The biggest value of the glycemic load may be for deciding among various options. When picking a snack or meal, foods with a low glycemic load are likely to be better for your heart and your insulin-making cells.

WHAT DETERMINES A FOOD'S GLYCEMIC INDEX AND GLYCEMIC LOAD?

One general trend you can see in the glycemic index table is that foods made from refined grains—things like white bread, bagels, and crackers—have a rapid and strong influence on blood sugar. Those that are less refined, such as coarsely ground whole-grain breads, oatmeal, and brown rice, have relatively lower glycemic index values, as do beans, vegetables, and fruits.

Several things determine how rapidly the carbohydrates in a particular food are broken down and the resulting glucose absorbed into the bloodstream:

- *How swollen (gelatinized) the starch grains are.* Starch grains swollen to the bursting point with water or heat, such as those in a boiled or baked potato,

Measuring the Glycemic Index and Glycemic Load

Building the library of glycemic index values for foods has been a relatively slow, painstaking effort. That's because each food must be tested on a number of volunteers, and each volunteer must be tested several times. The basic steps are the same. A healthy volunteer fasts overnight. The next morning, he or she drinks a glass of water in which 50 grams of glucose have been dissolved (or, alternately, eats 50 grams of white bread). Over the next two hours, blood samples are taken at regular intervals to measure the rise and fall of glucose. On another day, the same volunteer eats enough of the test food—cooked potato, whole-grain bread, kiwi fruit, ice cream, and so on—to consume 50 grams of carbohydrates and sits through another two hours of blood sampling. The glycemic index for that food for that individual is calculated by dividing his or her blood sugar response to the test food by the response to pure glucose or white bread. The numbers in the tables, then, represent percentages. For example, black beans have a glycemic index of 30. This means that they boost blood sugar only 30 percent as much as pure glucose.

Because everyone processes food and responds to glucose a little differently, the glycemic index published in tables is usually the average of eight to ten volunteers.

Once a food's glycemic index is in hand, calculating the glycemic load is easy. It involves multiplying the glycemic index by the amount of carbohydrate actually consumed. One-quarter of a cantaloupe, then, with a glycemic index value of 65 and 5.6 grams of carbohydrate, would have a glycemic load of about 3.7 (65 percent times 5.6). A serving of mashed potato, with a glycemic index of 74 and 20 grams of carbohydrate, would have a glycemic load of 15.

are more easily digested than the relatively unswollen starch grains found in brown rice.

- *How much the food has been processed.* Grinding wheat into superfine flour dramatically increases the attack rate of digestive enzymes. Not only does flour have greater surface area than coarsely ground wheat grains, it has been stripped of the protective, hard-to-digest, fibrous outer coat that temporarily fends off enzymes from digesting the starch inside. Regular oatmeal, which is made of smashed oat grains, has a higher glycemic index than oats that are intact or sliced, usually sold as steel-cut oats. Instant oatmeal has an even higher glycemic index.
- *How much fiber it contains.* As indigestible fiber passes through the intestine, it carries along partly digested food, shielding it from immediate digestion. This spreads out the release of glucose into the blood.
- *How much fat the food contains.* Fats tend to increase the time it takes for

food to leave the stomach and enter the intestine. So a food that contains fat may temper the rise in blood sugar.

- *What else is consumed.* Something acidic, like vinegar or lemon juice, can slow the conversion of starch to sugar, as do oils and fats. That means the glycemic index of a whole meal is influenced by the combination of foods that are eaten together. That said, eating a low glycemic food instead of a high glycemic food will lower the impact of the overall meal on blood sugar.

INTACT GRAINS, WHOLE GRAINS, AND REFINED GRAINS

Various terms are used to describe grain. Here are the key terms that I use. *Intact grains* are those that have barely been processed, if they've been processed at all. They look much the same as they did when they were harvested. *Whole grains* include intact grains and also grains that have been processed—ground, chopped, steamed, or the like—but nothing has been removed. (If you aren't familiar with intact and whole grains, check out the "Directory of Whole or Intact Grains" on page 272.)

Webster's defines the word "refined" as "free from impurities." That certainly applies to refined grains. Unfortunately, the "impurities" removed by refining include fiber, vitamins, minerals, and a variety of other beneficial micronutrients and phytochemicals.

Let's look at wheat as an example. Wheat is a gigantic relative of the grass that grows in yards and parks all across America. The hollow stem supports a seed head that's tightly packed with many individual grains. Our ancestors often used these grains as they came from the plant, and many people still use these "wheat berries" with meals or in breakfast porridges. Today, though, most wheat is processed and refined. The milling process first cracks the wheat grains. The starchy, carbohydrate-rich center, called endosperm, is separated from both the dark, fibrous bran and the wheat embryo, called the wheat germ. The endosperm is then pulverized with a series of rollers to make white, powdery flour. If the wheat grain is milled into fine flour without removing the bran and germ, this is technically a whole-grain product, since all the original parts are still present. But it is no longer an intact whole grain.

At each stage of milling, something is lost. Removing the germ pulls out unsaturated fats and fat-soluble vitamins. Whacking away the branny outer layer removes fiber, magnesium, and more vitamins. By the time wheat grains

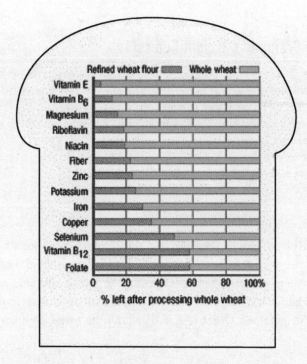

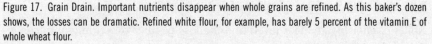

Figure 17. Grain Drain. Important nutrients disappear when whole grains are refined. As this baker's dozen shows, the losses can be dramatic. Refined white flour, for example, has barely 5 percent of the vitamin E of whole wheat flour.

have been turned into white flour, the final product is a pale shadow of the original, literally and nutritionally (see Figure 17 above).

If intact grains are so healthy, why did we stop eating them and shift to highly refined grains? It's partly a function of perception. Once it became possible to refine wheat, white flour was marketed as being purer than whole-grain flour. At first, white flour was a novelty for the upper classes. The bread and pastries it made were lighter and airier than their whole-grain cousins. In time, buying white flour became a symbol of moving up in the world. The shift was also driven by the reality of storage: white flour, with almost none of the healthy oils found in whole-grain flour, keeps longer. Whole-grain flours must be used more quickly and/or refrigerated.

For the past four decades, my colleagues and I have been studying the health effects of refined and whole-grain foods with the dedicated help of more than 200,000 women and men participating in the Nurses' Health

Whole Grains and Weight Control

The slower, gentler effects of whole grains on blood sugar and insulin, and the feeling of fullness after eating provided by greater fiber intake, translates into better weight control. My colleagues and I looked at the effects of whole grains in three long-term cohorts of nearly 173,000 men and women. Those who ate several servings of whole grains a day were less likely to have gained weight, or gained less weight, over twenty-four years' follow-up than those who rarely ate whole grains.[11] By helping you feel full longer after a meal or snack, whole grains can help you eat less.

Study, the Nurses' Health Study II, and the Health Professionals Follow-Up Study. The result of this work is compelling: eating whole grains and foods made from them is clearly better for sustained good health and offers more protection against a variety of chronic diseases than a diet high in refined carbohydrates or potatoes. Other research around the world points to the same conclusion.

WHOLE GRAINS PROTECT AGAINST DIABETES

Roller-coaster blood sugar levels and the loss of fiber-containing bran can affect more than just how fast you get hungry after a meal or snack. They can also influence the development of diabetes.

My colleagues and I studied all participants in the Nurses' Health Study and the Health Professionals Follow-Up Study who were free of diabetes when we first collected data on diet in the 1980s. During twenty-plus years of follow-up, more than 15,000 of the participants developed type 2 diabetes. Those whose diets scored highest on the glycemic index were 33 percent more likely to have developed diabetes than those with low glycemic index diets.[12] Participants with high glycemic index diets and low-fiber diets were 60 percent more likely to have developed type 2 diabetes. In these studies, eating high-fiber cold breakfast cereal seemed to help reduce the risk of developing diabetes, while consuming soft drinks, white bread, white rice, french fries, and cooked potatoes were all associated with increased risk of diabetes.

Developing healthy dietary habits as early as possible, ideally during childhood, is best for long-term health. The good news about preventing diabetes is that no matter how old you are, if you have managed to escape diabetes so far, adopting a healthy diet and physical activity program today will lower your risk starting tomorrow. That's a terrific immediate return on investment. Other benefits, such as reduced risks of heart disease and cancer, will follow but some may take years to show up.

WHOLE GRAINS MEAN LESS HEART DISEASE

Refined grains pose other problems in addition to diabetes. They are also linked to heart disease and stroke.

In the Nurses' Health Study, women who reported eating the most intact grain foods, an average of 2.5 servings a day, were 30 percent less likely to develop heart disease than women eating the fewest, about 1 serving a week.[13] Most of their whole grains came from whole-grain breakfast cereals, brown rice, and whole-grain bread. We estimated that eating a bowl of cold breakfast cereal that supplies about 5 grams of fiber cuts the chance of developing heart disease by about one-third compared with a fiber-free breakfast. The apparent benefit was larger in overweight women than it was in lean women. These benefits have also been seen consistently in other long-term studies of heart disease. Systematic reviews and meta-analyses of long-term cohort studies have linked high glycemic index and high glycemic load diets to increased risk of heart attack, stroke, and heart-related deaths.[14]

WHOLE GRAINS IMPROVE GI HEALTH TOO

Constipation is the number one gastrointestinal complaint in the United States. It affects more than 60 million Americans, accounting for more than 4 million physician visits and three-quarters of a million trips to emergency departments a year.[15] We spend more than $1 billion a year on over-the-counter laxatives. But there's a dietary remedy to this problem: foods rich in fiber. By keeping the stool soft and bulky, the fiber in intact grains helps prevent this troubling problem.

Two other common GI problems are diverticulosis, the development of tiny, easily irritated pouches inside the colon, and diverticulitis, the often painful inflammation of these pouches. Fiber from grains, as well as from fruits and vegetables, adds bulk to the stool and softens it. Together, these actions decrease pressure inside the intestinal tract and help prevent diverticular disease.

UNCERTAIN EFFECTS ON CANCER

Although a number of early studies suggested that higher consumption of whole grains or fiber reduced the odds of developing mouth, stomach, colon, gallbladder, and ovarian cancer, later and larger studies haven't consistently borne this out. Analyses from the Nurses' Health Study, the Health Professionals Follow-Up Study, and a compilation of large cohort studies from around the world showed that men and women with the highest fiber intake did not have lower risks of colorectal cancer.[16]

The timing of fiber intake, however, may be important. Among the middle-aged participants of the Nurses' Health Study, we saw no relation between fiber intake and risk of breast cancer. In the Nurses' Health Study II, which was established to look at diet earlier in life, we found that higher fiber intake during adolescence predicted a lower risk of breast cancer later in life.[17]

Even if whole-grain, high-fiber foods have no effect on cancer, their impact on heart disease and diabetes is reason enough to eat grains in this form instead of their stripped-down counterparts.

WHAT MAKES INTACT AND WHOLE GRAINS BETTER?

It may be almost impossible to isolate the ingredient or ingredients in whole grains that reduce the risks of heart disease and diabetes. However, a few contenders have been identified. The fiber in whole grains delays absorption of glucose into the bloodstream and eases the workload for insulin-making cells in the pancreas. Fiber helps lower cholesterol levels in the blood. It may also rev up some of the body's natural anticoagulants and help prevent the formation of small blood clots that trigger heart attacks or strokes. Antioxidants like vitamin E in whole grains prevent cholesterol-containing low-density lipids from reacting with oxygen, a key early step toward the formation of cholesterol-clogged arteries. Phytoestrogens, or plant estrogens, may protect against some cancers. The bran layer of many grains contains essential minerals such as magnesium, selenium, copper, and manganese that may be important in reducing the risk of heart disease and diabetes.

SEPARATING THE WHEAT FROM THE CHAFF

What exactly is a whole-grain food? This shouldn't be a trick question, but it is. Part of the problem is our lack of knowledge about the foods we eat. The other is that food makers, eager to promote any health benefits that might sell their products, jumped on the fiber/whole-grain bandwagon and haven't gotten off. Stroll the aisles of your favorite grocery store and you'll see what I mean. General Mills Total is a whole-grain breakfast cereal; Quaker Puffed

Wheat isn't. Nabisco Triscuit and Wheat Thins are whole-grain crackers, while Keebler Toasteds Harvest Wheat crackers are mostly refined wheat.

Some choices are easy. Brown rice is whole grain, white rice isn't. Most of the time, though, it takes a savvy shopper to separate the whole grain from the refined. You have to read food labels with the discriminating eye of a food critic, alert for subtle nuances that spell the difference between whole grain and refined grain. If the label says "made with wheat flour," it may be a whole-grain product—or it may just be an advertising gimmick and made with entirely refined wheat flour. The silkiest, most refined white cake flour is "made with wheat flour." True whole-grain products should list as the main ingredient whole wheat, whole oats, whole rye, or some other whole grain. To be 100 percent whole grain, no other type of grain should be on the list. The FDA isn't helpful here: a product can be labeled as whole grain if 51 percent of the grain is whole grain; the rest can be refined starch.

Low-Carb Claims

When the Atkins diet took the country by storm, food companies and entrepreneurs rushed to introduce new products. Even today you can buy low-carb bread, bagels, cereal, pasta, ice cream, chocolate bars, and beer. Books, monthly magazines, and online sources offered advice on following a low-carb lifestyle. You can even take a low-carb cruise!

Although the low-carb market peaked in the mid-2000s, Americans still buy millions of dollars' worth of branded, low-carb products per year. And that's without the blessing of the FDA, which hasn't been keen on allowing food companies to use the term "low carb" on food labels because it hasn't been precisely defined. This hasn't stopped savvy marketers, who bypass this roadblock with terms like "carb smart," "carb friendly," and "net carbs."

Some so-called low-carb products are ones we have been eating for years that are naturally low in carbohydrates, such as salad dressings and peanut butter, dressed up with new labels. Others have been engineered or reformulated to carry fewer digestible carbohydrates. Companies do this in several ways. They can replace refined wheat flour with fiber, soy protein, or lower-carbohydrate, higher-protein soy flour; replace sugar with less digestible sugar alcohols, such as sorbitol; or add more fat.

These changes aren't necessarily bad, but they can be misleading. Many consumers erroneously equate "low-carb" with "low-calorie." In fact, many low-carb products deliver just as many calories as their normal-carb counterparts, and sometimes more. They also cost more: following a low-carb diet can nearly double what you pay for food. So it's questionable whether you are getting the best nutritional bang for your buck.

Bran cereals and wheat germ aren't technically whole-grain foods. Bran cereals lack the vitamin- and oil-rich germ, while wheat germ lacks the fiber-rich bran. Both are missing the starchy endosperm. If your diet is high in refined grains, adding bran and wheat germ makes sense. But this strategy doesn't give you the full benefits of eating intact grains, such as a protective shield that slows down the absorption of the starch inside the grain.

The Healthy Eating Pyramid and Healthy Eating Plate emphasize the importance of including whole grains in your daily diet.

PUTTING IT INTO PRACTICE

Given the myriad health benefits of eating whole grains, why do most Americans eat less than one and a half servings a day?

For one thing, we aren't used to eating whole grains. For another, they haven't always been that easy to buy. Until fairly recently, you could only find products such as whole-grain pasta, whole-grain couscous, and bulgur in health food stores, co-ops, and organic-type grocery stores. Finding them in restaurants or cafeterias was even harder. A third barrier has traditionally been time: many intact grains take longer to cook than their refined counterparts. Brown rice, for example, takes twice as long to cook as white rice.

Carb-to-Fiber Ratio

Although "whole grain" has become a healthy eating buzz phrase, not everything that bears this label is worth eating. Kellogg's, for example, can tout sugary Froot Loops as a whole-grain food. To find healthful, whole-grain foods, the *Dietary Guidelines for Americans* recommends choosing grain products that have the word "whole" before any grain in the ingredient list and that contain few or no added sugars. With its 10 grams of added sugar and whole grain oat flour as the fourth ingredient, Froot Loops certainly doesn't qualify as a true whole-grain food. You can also look for the Whole Grain Council's Whole Grain Stamp, which a company can place on its packaging if the product contains at least 8 grams of whole grains per serving.

Or here's another way: Make sure that a whole-grain food has at least 1 gram of fiber for every 10 grams of carbohydrate (1 to 5 is even better).[18] Why 1:10? That's about the ratio of fiber to carbohydrate in a genuine whole grain—unprocessed wheat. If the fiber is a fake one, like inulin or other artificially added fiber, all bets are off.

Beware of Added Sugar

Our bodies don't need lots of carbohydrates each day, and they certainly don't need any of them from added sugar. Yet the average American consumes more than 20 teaspoons of added sugar a day, which amounts to more than 300 calories. Most of this comes from processed and prepared foods, with breakfast cereals and sugar-sweetened beverages such as soda and juice leading the pack. Post Golden Crisp Cereal, for example, has 14 grams of sugar, which account for more than half the calories in a serving. A single can of cola has 10 teaspoons of added sugar.

The 2015 *Dietary Guidelines for Americans* recommends getting no more than 10 percent of your daily calories from added sugar—about 13 teaspoons. The American Heart Association recommends even less: no more than 100 calories worth a day (about 6 teaspoons or 24 grams of sugar) for most women and no more than 150 calories a day (about 9 teaspoons or 36 grams of sugar) for most men.

It hasn't always been easy knowing if prepared or packaged foods contained added sugar, since the FDA required companies to list only total sugar on the "Nutrition Facts" label. Figuring out the added sugar content was made even more difficult by the plethora of ingredients that add sugar to a food. Here are just a few of them: agave nectar, brown sugar, cane sugar, corn sweetener, corn syrup, dextrose, evaporated cane juice, fructose, fruit juice concentrates, glucose, high-fructose corn syrup, honey, inverted sugar, malt syrup, maltose, maple syrup, molasses, raw sugar, sucrose, and syrup.

Spotting added sugar is now easier, thanks to a rule the FDA made in 2016 that food companies must list added sugars in addition to total sugars on the "Nutrition Facts" label.

The food industry, always on the lookout for new markets and marketing ideas, is helping to break down the last two barriers. More and more mainstream grocery stores now carry a fair selection of whole-grain products. You can now get quick-cooking brown rice—although it comes with a higher glycemic index—that's ready in the same twenty minutes as white rice. Better yet, make the old-fashioned, slow-cooking kind of brown rice a day or more in advance and microwave as needed.

Gluten in Grains: A Danger for Some

Gluten-free foods have become the latest health food fad. Supermarket aisles abound with products proudly labeled "Gluten-free," and many restaurants now offer gluten-free options.

Gluten is a mixture of proteins found in mainly in wheat, rye, and barley. It helps dough rise and keep its shape.

People with celiac disease can't tolerate gluten, not even small amounts. Their bodies mistakenly mount an immune response to the protein. This attack on gluten damages the lining of the small intestine. Just 50 milligrams of gluten—about the amount in a few crumbs of bread—is enough to cause trouble. The resulting immune response interferes with the absorption of nutrients from food. It also causes a host of symptoms, such as gas, bloating, abdominal cramps, diarrhea, weight loss, and skin rashes. Over time it may lead to problems such as osteoporosis, infertility, nerve damage, and seizures.

People with celiac disease must do everything they can so they don't eat foods that contain gluten. Although the influx of gluten-free foods is making this easier, gluten can lurk in unexpected foods, such as soy sauce, french fries, processed meats, prepared soups and sauces, and herbal supplements.

A related condition, called gluten sensitivity or non-celiac gluten sensitivity, can generate symptoms similar to celiac disease but without the intestinal damage. Many people erroneously believe that gluten is harmful to health even among people who don't have celiac disease or evidence of antibodies to gluten. So far, though, there's no evidence from the Nurses' Health Study, the Health Professionals Follow-Up Study, or other large cohorts that link high intake of gluten with poorer health.

If you and your health care provider think that gluten is causing you problems, it's a good idea to have a simple blood test to check for antibodies that are a giveaway for celiac disease. Do this *before* cutting gluten from your diet. If you've been off gluten for a while, it becomes very difficult to determine whether you have celiac disease or gluten sensitivity. That's because the tests look for your body's reaction to gluten. If you haven't been eating gluten, they can't do this.

If you decide to go gluten free, keep in mind that you'll need to take steps to get the nutrients you need. Breads and cereals are important sources of folic acid and other B vitamins in the United States. Many gluten-free breads and cereals aren't fortified with vitamins. Not getting enough B vitamins can be a problem for anyone, but it's especially worrisome for women who are pregnant or may become pregnant, who need a steady supply of folic acid (an important B vitamin) to help prevent the development of the birth defect known as spina bifida. If you're planning to adopt a gluten-free diet, take a multivitamin-multimineral supplement to make sure you are getting the vitamins and minerals you need.

"Fake" Fiber: Give It a Pass

To boost the fiber content of generally fiber-free foods—yogurt, cookies, ice cream, diet drinks, and the like—food companies are turning to fiber additives such as cellulose, guar gum, pectin, locust bean gum, hydroxypropyl methylcellulose, inulin, maltodextrin, and polydextrose. Don't be fooled. These additives don't offer the same health benefits as foods that are naturally rich in fiber.

These faux fibers don't come with the vitamins, minerals, and other micronutrients that food-based fiber delivers. And they likely don't slow the absorption of glucose from the digestive system as does fiber from whole grains that partially encapsulates carbohydrates.

Food companies are allowed to list synthetic and isolated (purified) fiber on the "Nutrition Facts" label as plain old fiber. Beginning in 2018, the Food and Drug Administration will require companies to send it documentation that these additives have at least one health benefit, such as a laxative effect, but there may be none of the other benefits that come from eating real fiber from real foods.

Take a minute to check the ingredient list to see where the fiber in a food is coming from. If it includes the fake fibers listed above, think about choosing a food with real fiber instead.

Here are a few suggestions for adding more intact grains to your diet (see page 272 for more ideas and details). Start slowly and add new grains or products as your appetite grows for these tasty foods:

Eat whole grains for breakfast. Make a habit of starting the day with a bowl of whole-grain cereal. If you're partial to hot cereals, try old-fashioned or steel cut oats. Quick and instant oatmeals are better than many choices, but they have a higher glycemic index than less processed oats. If you'd rather have cold cereal, look for one that lists something whole—wheat, oats, barley, or other grain—first on the ingredient list. A few possibilities are Wheaties, Great Grains, Wheat Chex, Grape-Nuts, shredded wheat, and Kashi cereals.

Discover whole-grain breads. Choose breads made from whole grains instead of from refined grains. Again, check the label to make sure the first ingredient includes the word "whole." You can now buy whole-grain pita bread and sandwich rolls.

Forget the spuds. Instead of potatoes, cook up some brown rice to accompany a meal. Or get really adventurous and try some "newer" grains, like

Fast Fact: Grams of Sugar

Keep this in mind when reading nutrition labels:

4 grams of sugar = 1 teaspoon = 15 calories

kasha, bulgur, oat groats, wheat berries or cracked wheat, millet, quinoa, or hulled barley.

Whole wheat pasta can be a delicious alternative. Look for whole wheat pasta in your grocery store. If it's a bit too chewy for you, Eden, Prince, Barilla, and other companies make pasta that is half whole wheat flour and half white flour.

Bake with whole wheat flour. Try substituting whole wheat flour for white flour. Start with a mixture that's one part whole wheat to three parts white flour. If you like the results, try increasing the ratio of whole wheat to white flour. Some companies sell a "white wheat" whole-grain flour that has a milder taste and texture than traditional whole wheat flour, although it also tends to have less fiber. Precooked whole wheat pizza shells are also showing up in grocery stores.

CHAPTER SEVEN

Choose Healthier Sources of Protein

W E KNOW LESS ABOUT PROTEIN in the diet and the role it plays in health than we do about fats and carbohydrates. This is not because protein is unimportant—quite the contrary: it's extremely important—but because it has been studied far less intensively than the other main components of food in relation to long-term health and disease. Much of the focus to date has been on the minimum amount of protein that children need for healthy development and that adults need to keep from slowly breaking down their own tissues. Far less attention has been paid to other important questions, like how much protein is best, if it matters whether your protein comes from animals or plants, and whether a high-protein diet is better for losing or controlling weight than a low-fat, high-carbohydrate diet. Intriguing research on soy and weight loss has kindled new interest in protein that is yielding better information.

As we wait for better answers, eating more protein from plant sources like beans and nuts, or from fish and chicken, and getting less from red meat and dairy foods is a key healthy eating strategy. It is also a good choice for the health of the planet (see chapter twelve).

WHAT IS PROTEIN?

Your hair and skin are mostly protein. Ditto your muscles, the oxygen-carrying hemoglobin in your blood, and the multitude of enzymes that keep you alive and active. In fact, your body is home to at least 10,000 different proteins. Together they make up about 15 percent of your weight.

On the molecular level, proteins are long, intricate chains fashioned from just twenty or so basic building blocks called amino acids. Because our bodies are constantly making new proteins, and because we don't store amino acids, we need a near daily supply of protein.

Some proteins in food are complete, or "high quality." That means they contain all of the twenty-plus types of amino acids needed to make new protein. Others are incomplete, lacking one or more *essential* amino acids; those are the ones we can't make from scratch or from other amino acids. Meat, poultry, fish, eggs, and dairy foods tend to be good sources of complete proteins, while proteins from plants are often incomplete. That's why vegetarians need to eat combinations that complement each other, such as rice and beans, peanut butter and bread, and tofu and brown rice.

High-Quality Protein: Is Too Much a Bad Thing?

The human body can make most of the amino acids it needs from scratch. The nine it can't manufacture—histidine, isoleucine, leucine, lysine, methionine, phenylalanine, threonine, tryptophan, and valine—must come from food.

High-quality or complete protein contains all of the amino acids the body needs to make new proteins. This complete combination of amino acids stimulates growth far better than protein that is missing one or more essential amino acids. Complete protein is perfect for developing babies, children, burn victims, and others who need an extra developmental or growth push. But large amounts of high-quality protein during adulthood may not be needed and may even be harmful.

Three essential amino acids—leucine, isoleucine, and valine, the so-called branched-chain amino acids—in high-quality protein turn up production of insulin-like growth factor 1 (IGF-1). This hormone does what its name suggests: stimulates growth. Too much of it, though, increases the risks of developing breast, prostate, and probably other cancers.

Milk and dairy foods are excellent sources of high-quality protein. That's why they are so good for young children. But drinking too much milk throughout life may overstimulate growth. For example, milk consumption among children and adolescents is an important driver of height. (A dramatic increase in milk consumption has contributed to the rapid increase in height among Japanese boys and girls.) Socially, being taller may be a good thing. But it has been linked to increased risks of several types of cancer, including lymphoma and breast, prostate, colon, and ovarian cancers.[1]

Later in life, many people lose muscle, which increases the risk of falling and breaking a bone. This happens partly due to lack of exercise and partly due to the falloff in growth hormone production. A growth-promoting boost from high-quality protein at this stage in life may be helpful.

HOW MUCH PROTEIN DO YOU NEED?

The National Academy of Medicine (formerly known as the Institute of Medicine) set the recommended daily allowance (RDA) for protein at 0.8 grams per kilogram of body weight, or just over 7 grams per 20 pounds. Translated to real body weights, that means 50 grams of protein a day for a 140-pound person and 70 grams for a 200-pound person. (Calculate your daily protein needs here: fnic.nal.usda.gov/fnic/interactiveDRI.)

You can hit this goal almost without thinking, given the abundance of protein-containing foods (see "Dietary Sources of Protein" on page 136). For example, a serving of yogurt at breakfast, a peanut butter and jelly sandwich for lunch, and a serving of chicken plus rice and beans for dinner adds up to about 85 grams of protein. Because it is so easy for us to get protein, it's uncommon for healthy adults in this country to have a protein deficiency.

Aside from the minimum amount of protein needed to keep the body running, there's little guidance on the ideal amount of dietary protein or the healthiest proportion of calories contributed by protein. Country-to-country comparisons of protein intake and health aren't much help because diets around the world tend to have similar amounts of protein. In the average American diet, which we tend to think of as meat-centered, about 15 percent of calories come from protein. In the largely vegetarian, rice-based diets that are common throughout Asia, about 12 percent of calories come from protein. (Rice, which we think of as a carbohydrate, is about 8 percent protein.) Other types of human studies haven't paid that much attention to protein. Diet fads further confuse the issue, with competing claims for high-protein, low-carbohydrate diets and low-protein, high-carbohydrate diets.

Until there's a good reason to change, getting 7 to 8 grams of protein per 20 pounds of body weight is a good guide for most people, but I don't recommend that you count and track your daily grams of protein.

PROTEIN AND HUMAN HEALTH

The amount and type of protein in the diet has been linked at one time or another with chronic diseases such as cancer and heart disease. It may also influence diabetes in children, obesity, and gastrointestinal disorders. Specific proteins in food, the air, and elsewhere are responsible for a variety of allergies, although this book doesn't cover that topic in detail.

Dietary Sources of Protein

Food	Serving Size	Calories	Protein (grams)	Protein % Daily Value*
Beef, top sirloin, broiled	3 ounces	155	26	52
Chicken, roasted	3 ounces	162	25	50
Salmon, fillet, cooked	3 ounces	130	21	42
Hamburger patty, 90% lean	3 ounces	178	21	42
Yogurt, Greek, low-fat	7-ounce container	146	20	40
Tuna, water-packed	3 ounces	73	17	34
Soy milk	1 cup	140	11	22
Soybeans, cooked	½ cup	127	11	22
Peanuts, dry-roasted	1½ ounces	242	10.5	21
Cottage cheese, low-fat	3 ounces	69	9	18
Lentils, cooked	½ cup	115	9	18
Cheese pizza	1 slice	181	8	16
Milk, skim	1 cup	102	8	16
Black beans	½ cup	114	8	16
Whole milk	1 cup	149	8	16
Almonds	1½ ounces	254	8	16
Whole wheat bread	2 slices	161	8	16
Tofu, firm	3 ounces	65	7.5	15
Cheddar cheese	1 ounce	115	7	14
Macaroni, cooked	1 cup	190	7	14
Egg	1 large	90	6	12
Walnuts	1½ ounces	270	6	12
Brown rice, cooked	1 cup	248	5	10
Baked potato, flesh and skin	1 medium	161	4	8
Corn, cooked	1 medium ear	99	4	8
Broccoli, cooked	½ cup chopped	27	2	4

*Based on a daily value of 50 grams of protein per a 2,000-calorie daily diet

Source: USDA National Nutrient Database for Standard Reference, Release 28, 2016. ndb.nal.usda.gov/ndb/foods.

Protein and cancer. There's no good evidence that eating a little or a lot of protein influences the risk of cancer in humans. You may have heard about low cancer rates in China or Japan, where the average diet contains a bit less protein—and certainly less animal protein—than the average American diet. In reality, though, total cancer rates in these countries have traditionally been about the same as they are in the United States, although the *types* of cancers that are the most common in each country are different.

Among more than 130,000 men and women in the Harvard Nurses' Study and Health Professionals Follow-Up Study who were followed for up to thirty-two years, protein intake wasn't linked to total deaths from cancer.[2]

The *source* of protein may make a difference. The International Agency for Research on Cancer, part of the World Health Organization, has concluded that processed meat is "carcinogenic to humans," while red meat is "probably carcinogenic."[3] The link between processed meat consumption and cancer is mainly with colorectal cancer, but connections were also seen between consumption of processed and red meat and pancreatic and prostate cancer.

Age may also make a difference. Most studies have looked at diet during adulthood. It is possible that the seeds of cancer may be planted earlier. Recent analyses in the Nurses' Health Study have found that higher intake of red meat during adolescence was associated with an increased risk of premenopausal breast cancer, while higher intakes of poultry, nuts, and legumes were associated with lower risks.[4]

Protein and heart disease. Country-to-country surveys of protein consumption and heart disease hint that the more plant protein in the diet, the less heart disease, and the more animal protein, the more heart disease. But different dietary and lifestyle habits in each of these countries—things like consumption of saturated fat, smoking rates, and amount of physical activity—make such surveys difficult to interpret. In the relatively few prospective studies of protein and heart disease, the source of protein makes a difference. In an analysis my colleagues and I did among more than 43,000 men, intake of total protein was minimally associated with heart disease risk, while intake of protein from meat was associated with higher risk.[5] A slightly lower risk of heart disease was inconsistent: getting more protein from plants, or from poultry and fish, is linked to lower risk of heart disease, while getting more protein from meat, especially red meat, is related to higher risk.

Protein and diabetes. The source of dietary protein has important implications for type 2 diabetes too. Eating more red meat increases the risk of developing this chronic condition, while eating more nuts, legumes, and poultry is related to lower risk.

One or more proteins found in cow's milk may—and I stress the "may"—play a role in the development of type 1 diabetes in children, one reason why infants should consume mother's breast milk rather than cow's milk if possible.

Premature death. In a large analysis of the dietary habits of women and men in the Harvard cohorts led by my colleague Mingyang Song, eating more protein from meat was linked with a modestly higher risk of premature death, while eating more protein from plant sources was associated with a lower risk. Similar findings were seen in a prospective study of women living in Iowa.[6]

Protein and other chronic diseases. The medical literature is full of reports linking allergic responses to specific protein sources with conditions ranging from arthritis and breathing problems to chronic digestive disorders. Eggs, fish, milk, peanuts, tree nuts, and soybeans cause allergic reactions in some people. A startling and well-documented report published in the *New England Journal of Medicine*, for example, showed that something in cow's milk causes an allergic response leading to severe chronic constipation in some young children.[7] In a group of sixty-five toddlers with chronic constipation, two weeks' worth of soy milk in place of cow's milk cleared up the problem in two-thirds of the children. A return to cow's milk led to the return of constipation. What's more, the "responders" were also more likely to have had constant runny noses, bronchospasm, and skin inflammation when drinking cow's milk. This may be a sentinel report pointing the way to other links between specific proteins and chronic disease.

Gluten, a mixture of proteins found mainly in wheat, rye, and barley, triggers a mistaken immune response in people with celiac disease (see "Gluten in Grains: A Danger for Some" on page 130). For some reason the immune response recognizes gluten as a foreign invader and attacks it. This attack damages the lining of the small intestine. People with celiac disease can't tolerate *any* gluten. Even a little bit of it, say from a few crumbs of bread, is enough to cause problems.

Protein and weight control. As I described in chapter six, a diet higher in fat and protein and lower in carbohydrates tends to work better than a low-fat, high-carbohydrate diet for helping people shed pounds quickly. There are two reasons for this: First, chicken, beef, fish, beans, and other high-protein foods slow the movement of nutrients from the stomach to the small intestine. Slower stomach emptying means you feel full for longer. Second, protein's rather gentle, steady effect on blood sugar avoids the quick, steep rise and fall in blood sugar caused by a carbohydrate like white bread or baked potato.

Once again, the protein *package* matters. In a detailed analysis of long-term weight change among the participants of the Harvard Nurses' Health Study and Health Professionals Follow-Up Study cohorts, eating red meat, chicken with skin, and regular cheese was associated with greater weight gain, while eating yogurt, peanut butter, walnuts and other nuts, chicken without skin, low-fat cheese, and seafood was associated with less weight gain.[8]

Protein and bone health. Early research raised the theoretical problem that eating a lot of protein could be bad for bones. The digestion of protein releases acids into the bloodstream. At normal levels of protein intake, calcium and other agents in the blood neutralize these acids. With a high-protein diet, however, extra calcium is needed to neutralize these acids. Some experts worried that this neutralizing calcium would be pulled from bone. According to a systematic review of sixty-one studies, that doesn't appear to happen.[9]

PAY ATTENTION TO THE PACKAGE

Pure protein from meat probably has about the same effect on your health as pure protein from beans or nuts. As I have mentioned before, it's the protein *package*—what comes along with the protein, like healthful or harmful fats, beneficial fiber, or hidden salt—that makes a substantial difference in health.

Beef is a good source of complete animal protein. But it also delivers a lot of saturated fat. The same is true for whole milk or dairy foods made from whole milk, such as butter, ice cream, and cheese. Poultry and nuts are good sources of protein, but unlike red meat or beef they also deliver healthy unsaturated fats.

There's more to the protein package than fats. People who regularly eat hot dogs, bologna, bacon, and other processed meats are more likely to develop type 2 diabetes and colon cancer than those who don't. That may be due to the salt, nitrates, and other additives these products contain. Men whose diets include a lot of dairy foods seem to be more likely to develop prostate cancer,

Go Nuts

The next time you're racking your brain over what to have for a snack or to make for dinner, think about using nuts as part of the main dish or as a garnish. Your taste buds and your heart will thank you.

Some people think that nuts are "junk food." Nothing could be further from the truth. They're a great source of protein and other beneficial nutrients. An ounce of almonds, walnuts, peanuts, or pistachios gives you about 8 grams of protein, the same as a glass of milk. It's true that nuts contain quite a bit of fat, but this is mostly healthy unsaturated fat that reduces harmful LDL cholesterol and keeps protective HDL cholesterol high.

People who regularly eat nuts are less likely to have heart attacks or die from heart disease than those who rarely eat them. Several large cohort studies, including the Adventist Health Studies, the Iowa Women's Health Study, and the Nurses' Health Study, have shown a consistent 30 to 50 percent lower risk of heart attack or heart disease associated with eating nuts several times a week. Regularly including nuts in the diet also seems to help prevent type 2 diabetes and gallstones.

The value of eating nuts was documented in the PREDIMED trial (see page 96). In this five-year trial, participants who were asked to eat an ounce of nuts each day in addition to a Mediterranean diet had lower risk of heart disease than those who followed a low-fat diet.[10] Notably, the nut eaters did not gain more weight than those on the low-fat diet.

The evidence for the health benefits of nuts is strong enough that the FDA let food companies claim on nutrition labels that "eating 1.5 ounces per day of most nuts as part of a diet low in saturated fat and cholesterol may reduce the risk of heart disease."

How do nuts benefit the heart? There are plenty of possibilities. Their unsaturated fats help lower harmful LDL cholesterol and boost protective HDL cholesterol. One type of unsaturated fat found in walnuts, the omega-3 fatty acid known as alpha-linolenic acid (ALA), seems to help prevent blood clots and potentially deadly erratic heartbeats (see "Omega-3 Fats: A Special Benefit" on pages 80–83). Nuts are also rich in arginine, an amino acid needed to make a tiny but important molecule called nitric oxide. Nitric oxide helps relax blood vessels and ease blood flow. It also makes blood platelets (tiny blood particles that are involved in clotting) less sticky and less likely to form clots in the bloodstream. Vitamin E, folic acid, potassium, fiber, and other phytonutrients found in nuts may also contribute to their heart-health benefits.

Whatever the mechanism, the message is the same: Nuts are good for your heart and the rest of you—*if* you eat them the right way.

Here's the wrong way: eating nuts on top of your usual snacks and meals. At 160 calories an ounce, having a handful of almonds a day without cutting back on anything else could translate into adding 10 to 20 pounds over the course of a year. This extra weight would cancel out any benefit from nuts and tip the scales toward, not away from, heart disease.

Here's the right way: eating nuts instead of chips or a candy bar as a snack. They'll take the edge off hunger every bit as well as junk food, they taste as good as or better than junk food, and they give you healthy nutrients to boot.

Better yet, use nuts instead of meat in main dishes. Mediterranean and other traditional cuisines use nuts this way in all sorts of delicious dishes and sauces. For example, check out the delicious Roasted Walnut and Brown Rice Loaf on page 339.

Comparing protein packages

Food	Protein (grams)	Saturated fat (grams)	Monoun-saturated fat (grams)	Polyun-saturated fat (grams	ALA* (grams)	Marine** Omega-3 fats (grams)	Fiber (grams)	Sodium (milligrams)
Sirloin steak, broiled (4 oz)	33	4.6	4.9	0.4	0.4	0.	0	66
Sockeye salmon, grilled (4 oz)	30	1.1	2.1	1.5	0.3	1.0	0	104
Chicken, thigh, no skin (4-oz)	28	2.7	3.9	2.0	0.1	0.1	0	120
Ham steak (4 oz)	22	1.6	2.2	.5	.5	0	0	1,439
Lentils (1 cup cooked)	18	0.1	0.1	0.3	0.3	0	4	4
Milk (8 ounces)	8	3.1	1.4	0.2	0.3	0	0	115
Peanut butter (2 tbl)	7	3.3	8.3	4.0	0	0	1.6	136
Almonds, dry roasted, unsalted (1 oz)	6	1.2	9.4	3.4	0	0	3.1	1

* Alpha-linoleic acid. Small amounts of other 18:3 omega-3 fatty acids are included.

** Mainly EPA and DHA.

Source: USDA National Nutrient Database for Standard Reference Release 28, 2016. ndb.nal.usda.gov/ndb/foods

especially quickly spreading (metastatic) prostate cancer, than men who don't often eat dairy foods.[11] Dairy foods increase the blood level of insulin-like growth factor 1, which in turn is related to higher risk of prostate cancer.

How meat is prepared may also contribute to its effects on health. Frying and grilling meat, poultry, and fish to a well-done degree causes some of the protein to turn into a group of chemicals called heterocyclic amines that cause cancer in animals. How much this increases cancer risk in humans hasn't been clearly determined.

Antibiotic Resistance: A New Dietary Hazard

For years, doctors were able to turn to a multitude of antibiotics that could stop virtually any type of bacterial infection. No longer. Several strains of bacteria have emerged that are resistant to the antibiotics we currently have. These so-called superbugs have appeared around the world, including in the United States.

The use of antibiotics in food production has contributed to the emergence of these superbugs.[12] Antibiotics are often given to healthy animals to help them grow faster. That's a recipe for creating antibiotic resistance. By allowing more opportunity for random mutations, giving healthy animals antibiotics for a long time allows bacteria that become resistant to the antibiotic mutations to thrive. This is truly evolution at work. Recognizing this problem, the FDA announced in 2016 a voluntary program to limit such routine use of antibiotics in food production.[13] The major poultry producers have indicated they will stop routinely using antibiotics, and some quickly began to use this as a selling point to consumers, touting that their products were raised without antibiotics. Beef and pork producers are finding it harder to do the same thing, because cows and pigs live longer than poultry and they are raised in less sanitary conditions.

As a consumer, eating less meat will reduce the likelihood of your taking in antibiotic-resistant microbes. If you do plan on eating meat, try to find products without antibiotics. Some companies say that on the packaging; others don't.

THE SCOOP ON SOY

At the turn of the twenty-first century, several research groups turned their attention to soybeans and soy protein. The media routinely churned out articles with provocative headlines like this one from the *Washington Post*—"Touting the Joys of Soy: Studies of the Protein-Rich Bean's Positive Effects on Cholesterol May Be Only the Beginning"—trumpeting the "power" of soy to lower cholesterol, prevent heart disease, ease hot flashes and other menopause-related problems, preserve memory, and protect against breast, prostate, and other cancers. That work didn't hold up.

- *Soy and heart disease.* Based largely on an analysis published in the *New England Journal of Medicine* that eating soy in place of red meat can reduce the level of harmful LDL cholesterol,[14] the FDA approved a health claim for soy in 1999. Foods that contain at least 6.25 grams of soy per serving can claim on the label that "diets low in saturated fat and choles-

Fats in 1½ Ounces of Various Nuts and Seeds

Types (# pieces/1½ ounces)	Calories	Total Fat (grams)	Saturated Fat (grams)	Mono-unsaturated Fat (grams)	Poly-unsaturated Fat (grams)	Ratio of Un-saturated to Satu-rated Fats
Hazelnuts (27–30)	275	26.5	1.9	19.8	3.6	12.3
Almonds (30–36)	246	22	1.7	14.1	5.5	11.5
Pine nuts	286	29.1	2.1	8	14.5	10.7
Flaxseeds	224	17.7	1.5	3.2	12.1	10.2
Pecans (27–30 halves)	293	31.6	2.7	18.7	8.7	10.1
Walnuts (12–16)	270	25.5	2.3	3.5	18.6	9.6
Pistachios (73–77)	243	19.5	2.4	10.4	5.7	6.7
Sesame butter (tahini, 2 tbsp.)	178	16.1	2.3	6.1	7.1	5.7
Sesame seeds	240	20.4	2.9	7.7	8.9	5.7
Mixed nuts (30–36)	258	22.7	3.4	14.7	4.2	5.6
Macadamia nuts (15-18)	32.3	32.2	5.1	25.2	0.6	5.1
Peanuts (42–45)	250	21.1	3.3	11.1	4.2	4.6
Cashews (24–28)	244	19.7	3.9	11.6	3.2	3.8
Peanut butter (smooth, 2 tbsp.)	191	16.4	3.3	8.3	4	3.7
Brazil nuts (9–12)	280	28.5	6.9	10.1	10.4	3.0

Source: USDA National Nutrient Database for Standard Reference, Release 28, 2016.
ndb.nal.usda.gov/ndb/foods.

terol that include 25 grams of soy protein a day may reduce the risk of heart disease."

Keep in mind that you would need to drink four 8-ounce glasses of soy milk (which would deliver a whopping 600 calories) or eat almost a pound of tofu to get 25 grams of soy protein a day. Soy alone can't counteract a diet that's high in calories and saturated fat, or for lack of exercise. And later studies don't fully back this health claim for soy, with some trials showing that soy protein has little or no effect on cholesterol levels.

One problem with the soy research is that in nutrition, the issue of substitution—what you choose to eat instead of something you prefer not to eat—is vitally important. If you eat a soy food instead of red meat in an entrée, say, this will reduce the risk of heart disease, in part because of the much healthier mix of fatty acids in soy than in red meat.

Soy and breast cancer. Biologically speaking, there's a good reason why soybeans and soy products may act against cancer. Soybeans are rich in compounds called phytoestrogens, literally plant estrogens. There are two main types of phytoestrogen, isoflavones and lignans. They act a bit like human estrogen, sometimes erroneously called the "female hormone." Yet exactly what phytoestrogens do depends on the amount of them and where they are acting. In some tissues phytoestrogens mimic the action of estrogen, while in other tissues they block it. Estrogen stimulates the growth and multiplication of breast and breast cancer cells. So the estrogen-blocking effects of soy estrogens *could* protect against breast cancer.

Support for this idea comes from a 2009 cohort study in Shanghai, where soy intake has traditionally been much higher than in the United States.[15] In Shanghai, women who ate more soy foods during both childhood and early adult life were less likely to develop breast cancer during their premenopausal years, when natural estrogens are high; no relation was seen for postmenopausal breast cancer. Women with the highest soy protein intakes throughout adolescence and early adulthood had nearly a 60 percent lower risk of premenopausal breast cancer than women with the lowest intakes.

In Western populations, little relation has been seen between soy consumption and breast cancer risk, possibly because the amounts of soy eaten by those groups are relatively low.

Soy and hot flashes. Menopause is a time of dwindling estrogen production. If the phytoestrogens that are thought to block the effects of estrogen in breast tissue can mimic the effects of estrogen elsewhere in the body, they could provide a natural way to cool hot flashes and ease other problems that plague many women during menopause. A recent meta-analysis of clinical trials of soy foods showed that eating these foods appeared to help reduce the frequency of hot flashes and may ease vaginal dryness but had no effect on night sweats.[16] Yet the studies included in the analysis had significant limitations, so it is hard to tell whether or not women in menopause should eat extra soy.

Soy and prostate cancer. Soy foods have also been promoted as a way to prevent prostate cancer by inhibiting the hormones that help this disease grow. A few prospective studies support this idea.[17] However, more research is needed, since most of the studies have been small. We know little about how much soy would be needed to prevent prostate cancer and when in life one should start eating it for the biggest payoff.

Soy and the brain. Can soy keep your memory sharp as you get older? It's an interesting idea. Naturally falling estrogen levels in both women and men have been suggested as one possible cause of aging-related memory loss and cognitive problems. A few studies, mostly using isoflavone supplements, suggest that getting more soy may preserve memory and thinking skills. Others say that more soy won't make any difference.[18]

SOY MAY HAVE A DARK SIDE

The flip-flopping research on soy and health wouldn't be a huge concern if eating soy protein was completely and totally safe and free of side effects. We don't know if that's the case. Two disconcerting reports suggest that, in some situations, overdoing soy protein could do more harm than good.

One showed that women with a suspicious breast lump who took a soy supplement containing 45 milligrams of isoflavones a day for the fourteen days until a scheduled breast biopsy had biopsies showing more cell growth and division than biopsies from women not taking soy.[19] While this might suggest a possible link between soy and risk of breast cancer, the large study from Shanghai that I described earlier, as well as other prospective studies from Asia, provide reassurance that soy does not promote breast cancer.

The other, done among older individuals of Japanese ancestry living in Hawaii, showed that those who continued to eat a traditional soy-based diet were more likely to have memory loss and other cognitive problems than those who had made the switch to a more Western diet.[20] Similar increases in cognitive problems have been seen in two other reports from Asia, but studies from the United States have generally shown no problems, and even possible benefits, from eating soy foods for maintaining memory.

These conflicting findings point out the absolutely critical need to learn more about how soy foods affect different tissues at different life stages. The estrogen-blocking activity of phytoestrogens may be beneficial for young women, whose breast, ovarian, and other tissues are bombarded by more human estrogens that may promote the development of cancer. But it would be a shame to make blanket recommendations for eating more soy as a way to prevent breast cancer if phytoestrogens also cause problems with memory later in life, when the natural output of estrogen is dwindling.

One thing we know for certain about soy is that the phytoestrogens it contains are potent biological agents. Whether they trigger, suppress, or have no effect on breast cancer, prostate cancer, or memory is unfortunately an open question. That's why you should treat concentrated soy supplements or isoflavone pills with the same caution you would a totally untested new drug.

These findings don't mean to steer you completely clear of soy. Instead, eat it now and then rather than several times a day.

PUTTING IT INTO PRACTICE

Protein is a key part of any diet. The average person needs about 7 grams of protein a day for every 20 pounds of body weight. Many people can get that amount without any trouble. What's probably more important for health is the foods you turn to for protein. Red meat, poultry, eggs, fish, milk and dairy foods, and other animal sources can provide plenty of protein. So can beans, soy, nuts, seeds, and other plant sources.

There's no need to go overboard on protein and eat it to the exclusion of everything else. By shunning fruits, vegetables, and whole grains, you would miss out on fiber, vitamins, minerals, and other phytonutrients you can't get from protein. Supplements can add back some of the main phytonutrients, but they leave out hundreds of others that may be equally important for long-term health. You also need to pay attention to what's coming along with your protein. A serving of salmon gives you 19 grams of protein plus 2 grams of unhealthy saturated fat and 7.4 grams of healthy unsaturated fats. A standard hamburger delivers the same amount of protein but with more than double the saturated fat (4.5 grams) and only 5 grams of unsaturated fat. Choosing high-protein foods low in saturated fat will help your heart even as it helps your waistline.

Here are suggestions for shaping your diet with the best protein choices:

- *Get your protein from plants when possible.* Eating beans, nuts, whole grains, and other plant sources of protein is good for your health and the health of the planet. If you enjoy milk and other dairy foods, do so in moderation. If you enjoy red meat, eat it in small amounts or on special occasions, as is done with traditional Mediterranean diets. Chicken, turkey, and fish are better options than red meat.
- *Mix up your proteins.* If most of your protein comes from plants, make sure you eat a mix of beans, nuts, whole grains, and vegetables to be sure that no essential components of protein are missing.
- *Balance carbohydrates and protein.* Eating more protein and cutting back on carbohydrates, especially refined carbohydrates, improves blood pressure,

Fish, Mercury, and Fish Oil

If you like to eat seafood, or think you should eat more of it, you may feel you're caught between the devil and the deep blue sea. Fish is a great choice for many reasons: it tastes good, it's a healthier source of protein than red meat, and the omega-3 fats in most types of seafood help the heart. Yet some species contain mercury, polychlorinated biphenyls (PCBs), and other contaminants. Should you stop eating fish? Cut back? Hold the line?

The answer depends on who you are.

Mercury and PCBs are definitely dangerous at the high doses you'd see in an industrial accident. In the small amounts found in fish, their effects aren't as clear-cut.

Young children and women who are pregnant, who might become pregnant, or who are breastfeeding need to be the most careful about mercury. This metal, which comes from natural sources, industrial emissions, and coal-burning electricity plants, can harm the developing brain and nervous system. At the same time, getting enough omega-3 fats from fish and other foods is important during pregnancy and when breastfeeding, because they are essential building blocks for a developing child's nervous system.

What about PCBs, which were banned in the 1970s but are still present in the environment? High doses kill fish and cause cancer in laboratory rats. Low doses may cause subtle developmental problems in babies. Studies in adults haven't linked PCBs to cancer or other diseases.

To be on the safe side, children and women of childbearing age should stay away from high-mercury fish like shark, swordfish, king mackerel, and tilefish (sometimes called golden snapper or golden bass). It's also wise to avoid eating fish caught near industrial areas, where PCBs are likely to be most abundant. Safe choices include cod, haddock, salmon, sardines, shrimp, and tilapia. The EPA's and FDA's "Advice About Eating Fish" sheet (www.fda.gov /downloads/Food/FoodborneIllnessContaminants/Metals/UCM536321.pdf) offers information about choosing healthy sources of seafood during pregnancy.

But that doesn't mean avoiding seafood altogether. Instead, it's best to eat up to twelve ounces (two average meals) a week of a variety of lower-mercury fish and shellfish such as salmon, pollock, catfish, and shrimp to get the omega-3s you need.

Canned tuna warrants special attention because it is easy and inexpensive, making it something that people tend to eat often. Unfortunately, it also contains intermediate amounts of mercury. To be prudent, eat canned *light* tuna, which has less mercury than canned *white* (albacore) tuna.

What about men and older women? If you're old enough to worry about heart disease, the definite benefits from eating seafood greatly outweigh the possible (and possibly minuscule) risks from mercury and PCBs. It's prudent to limit your seafood choices to species known to carry high levels of mercury to once a month, and you might not want to eat fish—even ones low in mercury—every single day.

(*continued on next page*)

The benefits of eating fish extend beyond the heart and arteries. It's also good for your brain. The overall benefit of fish for brain health was vividly illustrated in a 2016 study by Martha Claire Morris at Rush University in Chicago. She autopsied brains from participants in her long-term study of diet and brain function who had died. Higher consumption of fish before death was associated with fewer of the harmful changes of Alzheimer's disease. Fish consumption was also correlated to the amount of mercury in the brain, but it wasn't linked to harmful changes.[21]

If you don't like to eat fish or are worried about contamination, fish oil supplements are an alternative. They deliver plenty of two essential omega-3 fats, EPA and DHA, without the mercury; several chemical analyses of fish oil supplements show negligible amounts of the metal. However, they don't deliver the same benefit as fish as a replacement for a less healthy source of protein such as steak. And you might consider talking with your doctor about taking a fish oil supplement that contains 600 to 800 milligrams of EPA plus DHA if you:

- have angina (chest pain), have had a heart attack, or are at high risk for one. (You can calculate your risk of having a heart attack using an online calculator provided by the Harvard T.H. Chan School of Public Health, www.diseaseriskindex.harvard.edu.)

- engage in high-intensity sports or activities. Even though the overall risk of heart disease is generally low among people who exercise hard, fatal heart rhythms can appear during and shortly after intense activity. Formal studies haven't yet been done on the effect of fish oil supplements in this group. Even so, it's prudent to have plenty of omega-3 fats aboard if you exercise or play hard.

blood triglycerides, and protective HDL, all of which may reduce your odds of having a heart attack, stroke, or other form of cardiovascular disease. However, if that extra protein comes from red meat and dairy foods, you are likely to be increasing, not decreasing, your risks of cardiovascular disease and diabetes.

- *Eat soy in moderation.* Soybeans, tofu, and other soy foods can be a good alternative to red meat. Just don't overdo it. Aim for a few servings a week, not a few a day. For women in the midst of menopause or beyond who are plagued by hot flashes or other problems related to estrogen loss, boosting soy intake for a while probably won't do any harm and can be worth a try. At the same time, it probably isn't much more effective than the tincture of time. For women living with breast cancer, moderation makes sense. No one should take pills that deliver concentrated soy protein or pure isoflavones unless there is a clear medical reason to do so.

Fast Fact: Be Wary of Protein Supplements

Athletes, bodybuilders, and others take protein supplements, such as whey protein, to build muscle. Taking protein supplements without exercising has only a small effect on adding muscle and is no replacement for exercise. It's an expensive strategy that isn't any better than a high-protein diet. In addition, trying to rev up muscle growth with protein supplements might be accompanied by a revving up of cancer cells that lurk around for years and don't show up until far down the road (see "High Quality Protein: Is Too Much A Bad Thing?" on page 134).

CHAPTER EIGHT

Eat Plenty of Fruits and Vegetables

A S A CHILD, YOU HATED to hear it. As a teenager, you promised your-self you'd never say it to your own children. Yet as an adult, it—"Eat your vegetables; they're good for you!"—springs out of the mouth un-bidden, like wisdom that must be passed from generation to generation.

That's actually a good description. "Eat plenty of fruits and vegetables" is timeless advice that science is only now catching up to. It is a simple, easy-to-remember, and tasty morsel of dietary advice that ranks high on the list of smart and healthy nutritional habits.

With apologies to Elizabeth Barrett Browning, how do fruits and vegeta-bles help thee? Let me count the ways. A diet rich in fruits and vegetables can:

- decrease the chances of having a heart attack or stroke or developing dia-betes
- lower blood pressure
- help you avoid constipation and the painful intestinal ailment called diver-ticulitis
- guard against two common aging-related eye diseases: cataract, the grad-ual clouding of the eye's lens; and macular degeneration, the major causes of vision loss among people over age sixty-five
- delay or prevent memory loss and a decline in thinking skills
- help you feel full with fewer calories and so control your weight and waist-line
- add variety to your diet and enliven your palate.

Notice that I keep saying "fruits and vegetables." Pills that contain one or two or ten substances made by plants just won't do. Why not? Plants make a seemingly endless cornucopia of compounds that have biological activity in

Why Supplements Are Not a Substitute for Fruits and Vegetables

So far, no one has found a magic bullet that works as well as fruits and vegetables against heart disease, cancer, and a host of other chronic diseases. In theory, one could cram all of the good things that plants make—essential elements, fiber, vitamins, antioxidants, plant hormones, and so on—into a pill. But it would have to be a very large pill, and scientists honestly can't say they know exactly what should go into it. Or in what proportions.

Take the antioxidant pigments known as carotenoids. When you eat a tomato or carrot, the different carotenoids it contains eventually work their way into different types of cells and different parts of each cell. This offers antioxidant protection throughout the cell and to a wide variety of cell types. When eaten in the proportions usually found in foods, carotenoids and other phytochemicals benefit cells by working together in ways we don't yet completely understand. But when delivered in unnatural proportions or missing some essential components—say, via a poorly designed supplement pill—an oversupply of one carotenoid or phytochemical could block the activity of others.

This isn't to say that vitamin and mineral supplements are worthless. As described in chapter eleven, vitamin supplements are excellent insurance. But they aren't a substitute for a healthy diet.

Health issues aside, the biggest drawback is that a pill would always taste like a pill. It can't give you the earthy smell and taste of a fresh ear of corn, the sweetness of a juicy tomato still warm from the afternoon sun, the crunch of an apple, the festive green of a snap pea or broccoli floret, or the smooth, nutty taste of an avocado. Stick with real fruits and vegetables: they contain a bounty of phytochemicals that do not come in capsules, and they taste better too.

the human body. So far, only a tiny minority have been flagged as agents that may be responsible for the health benefits of fruits and vegetables, sometimes on the basis of surprisingly little solid evidence. The vast majority of phytochemicals have yet to be discovered, named, chemically characterized, and biologically evaluated. The odds are high that the benefits I listed for fruits and vegetables emanate from many different substances found in plants and quite possibly from the interactions among them.

BUT FIRST, EXACTLY WHAT ARE FRUITS AND VEGETABLES?

To a botanist, a fruit is any plant part that contains seeds. By the process of elimination, a vegetable is everything else: leaves, stems, flowers, roots, and bulbs. Things get hazy in the kitchen, though, because many of what are com-

Fruit or Vegetable?

The argument over whether certain foods are fruits or vegetables has been around for years. Back in 1893, the U.S. Supreme Court ruled that tomatoes were a vegetable, and they've remained so ever since. Why was the highest court in the land asked to make a legal and somewhat unscientific rule like that? Fruit importers John, George, and Frank Nix sued New York's collector of customs taxes, Edward Hedden, to recover taxes he had levied on a shipment of tomatoes the Nixes had imported from the West Indies. Back then, imported fruits weren't taxed, while vegetables were. In its decision, the Court acknowledged that tomatoes were technically fruits. But "in the common language of the people" the Court determined that tomatoes, as well as cucumbers, squashes, beans, and peas, "are vegetables which are grown in kitchen gardens" and are usually served at dinner with the main part of the meal and not as dessert.[1]

monly called vegetables are technically fruits: Think of the seeds in avocados, cucumbers, eggplants, squashes, and tomatoes, to name just a few. In this book, I will stick with the culinary concept of fruits as sweet, dessert- or even snack-like foods, and vegetables as savory, salad- or dinner-type foods.

I am not including potatoes and corn in the vegetable category, even though they are among the most popular "vegetables" in America (see "The Spud Is a Dud" on page 167). In your digestive system they act more like carbohydrates.

FAMILY NUTRITION

When studying the connection between fruits, vegetables, and health, it helps to talk about groups of plants. One of the most common classification schemes is by plant "family." Those you usually find in the market or on the table include the following:

- The crucifer family (Cruciferae) gets its name from the tiny cross you can see if you look at a recently sprouted seed. It includes a number of those vegetables that children (and some adults) instinctively but unwisely avoid—broccoli, Brussels sprouts, cabbage, cauliflower, collard greens, kale, kohlrabi, mustard greens, radishes, rutabaga, turnips, and watercress. Some members of the crucifer family are excellent sources of isothiocyanates, indoles, thiocyanates, and nitriles. These chemicals may protect against breast and some other types of cancer.

- The melon/squash family (Cucurbitaceae) includes cucumbers, summer squashes such as pumpkin and zucchini, winter squashes such as acorn and butternut, cantaloupes, and honeydew melons.
- The heath or heather family (Ericaceae) gives us cranberries, blueberries, lingonberries, and more. These fruits are particularly high in a flavonoid called anthocyanin, which may be linked to the prevention of diabetes, heart disease, and dementia.
- The legume family (Leguminosae) includes alfalfa sprouts, beans, peas, and soybeans. Legumes have plenty of fiber, folate, and substances called protease inhibitors, all of which may offer some protection against heart disease and cancer.
- The lily family (Liliaceae) includes asparagus, chives, garlic, leeks, onions, and shallots. These vegetables contain a number of sulfur-containing compounds, especially allicin and diallyl sulfate, that may fight cancer.
- The rose family (Rosaceae) includes almonds, apples, apricots, cherries, peaches, pears, plums, raspberries, and strawberries.
- The citrus family (Rutaceae) encompasses grapefruits, lemons, limes, oranges, and tangerines. Citrus fruits are high in vitamin C and the carotenoid beta-cryptoxanthin and also contain the compounds limonene and coumarin, which have been shown to have anticancer properties in laboratory animals.
- The solanum family (Solanaceae) is a diverse group that includes eggplant, peppers, potatoes, and tomatoes. Tomatoes contain high amounts of lycopene, a type of antioxidant that may play a key role in preventing prostate and other cancers.
- The umbels (Umbelliferae) include carrots, celeriac, celery, parsley, and parsnips. Carrots are an excellent source of beta-carotene, which the body uses to make vitamin A. Strong evidence supports a benefit of beta-carotene and possibly the related compounds called carotenoids in maintaining memory into old age. Other studies suggest a possible role in preventing some cancers.

While any one fruit or vegetable contains dozens, maybe hundreds, of different compounds that your body uses for something besides energy, no single fruit or vegetable contains all of the substances you need. That's why it's a good idea to get a few servings a week from each of these major groups.

CHOOSE A RAINBOW OF FOODS

It's a good idea to eat for color variety as well. Painting your diet with the bold colors of ripe red tomatoes, crisp orange carrots, creamy yellow squash, emerald-green spinach, juicy blueberries, indigo plums, violet eggplants, and all shades in between not only makes meals more appealing but also ensures that you get a variety of beneficial phytonutrients.

INADEQUATE GUIDANCE FROM THE USDA AND OTHERS

Back in 1991, the National Cancer Institute launched its 5 A Day public health campaign. Through grocery store banners, labels on fruits and vegetables, public service announcements in the media, and educational materials for schoolchildren, it urged us to eat five or more servings of fruits and vegetables a day. This campaign was incorporated into early *Dietary Guidelines for Americans* as well as into guidelines from the American Heart Association, the American Cancer Society, the World Health Organization, and others. In 2007 it was replaced by a new campaign called Fruits & Veggies—More Matters.

The name of the new campaign, More Matters, gets to the heart of fruit and vegetable guidance. One thing it lacks is clear definitions about what qualifies in meeting the "More." Two glasses of orange juice, an apple, an order of

Presidential Passion for Olive Oil and Vegetables

Olive oil drizzled over roasted eggplant or grilled peppers conjures up images of Mediterranean cooking. Yet the use of olive oil is as all-American as the founding fathers. Here's what Thomas Jefferson had to say about the olive tree and olive oil in a letter to William Drayton, a South Carolina lawyer, congressman, and planter: "The olive is a tree the least known in America, and yet the most worthy of being known. Of all the gifts of heaven to man, it is next to the most precious, if it be not the most precious. Perhaps it may claim a preference even to bread, because there is such an infinitude of vegetables which it renders a proper and comfortable nourishment."

Our third president knew something that cooks and chefs have rediscovered—that olive oil can perk up vegetables and other foods. Jefferson, a curious naturalist and ardent horticulturalist, repeatedly tried to cultivate olive trees in South Carolina and Georgia, but with little success. He ultimately had to rely on imported olive oil for his table. Little did he know that Spanish priests had brought olives to California in the late 1700s and that they would become a native source of olive oil for the country.

french fries at lunch, and a potato with dinner puts you well on the road to meeting its recommendation. While that's better than no fruits and vegetables at all, it doesn't offer the full dose of health benefits I describe here.

The 2015–2020 *Dietary Guidelines for Americans* recommend eating a variety of vegetables from all of the subgroups: dark green, red and orange, and legumes (beans and peas). But they include potatoes and corn as vegetables, when the body recognizes them as starchy carbohydrates.

NOT MEASURING UP

Few of us take advantage of the incredible bounty of fruits and vegetables grown in this country and elsewhere. The average American relies on roughly a dozen fruits and vegetables. Daily consumption is just as limited, hovering around four servings a day, and that figure is vastly inflated by potatoes. A recent national survey showed that only 1 in 9 Americans gets the minimum recommended daily "dose" of five servings of fruits and vegetables a day.[2] That limited consumption is a pity, given the clear-cut benefits of eating fruits and vegetables.

FRUITS AND VEGETABLES PREVENT CARDIOVASCULAR DISEASE . . .

A diet that includes plenty of fruits and vegetables can help control or even prevent high blood pressure and high cholesterol, two of the main precursors of heart disease and stroke. Even better, investing in a plant-rich diet pays off in terms of lower chances of developing several forms of heart disease and stroke.

High blood pressure often sets the stage for stroke, heart attack, and other kinds of circulatory problems. High blood pressure, formally known as hypertension, affects more than 70 million Americans and a staggering 1 billion people worldwide.[3] It's increasingly common with age: under 10 percent of U.S. adults between the ages of twenty and thirty-four have high blood pressure, compared to more than 75 percent of those over age seventy-five. Up to 90 percent of Americans develop high blood pressure over their lifetimes. Sometimes called the silent killer, high blood pressure causes no real symptoms. That's one reason at least one-third of people with it don't know they have it. Of those who are well aware they have high blood pressure, many have a hard time keeping it under control.

The effect on blood pressure of adding more fruits and vegetables to your diet, while not quite as huge as comes from exercise, is well worth the small effort. Among more than 185,000 men and women participating in the Nurses' Health Studies and the Health Professionals Follow-Up Study, those who reported eating four or more servings of fruits and vegetables a day were about 7 percent less likely to have developed high blood pressure over a fifteen-year period than participants who reported eating four or fewer servings a week.[4] Foods that appeared to be especially helpful included broccoli, carrots, tofu or soybeans, raisins, and apples.

Other reviews and meta-analyses have shown that eating about thirty servings of fruits and vegetables a week (or just under five a day) was associated with a 30 percent lower risk of the most common type of stroke (ischemic stroke), the kind caused by a blood clot blocking an artery in, or to, the brain.[5] My colleagues and I calculated that eating one extra serving of fruits or vegetables a day decreases the chances of having an ischemic stroke by about 6 percent. In that study, most of the benefit seemed to come from eating broccoli, spinach, kale, romaine lettuce, and citrus fruit or juice. Many nutrients in these foods contribute to the lower risk of stroke. One of them is folate, the plant form of folic acid (the terms are derived from the word "foliage"). Folic acid has been shown to reduce the risk of stroke when taken as a supplement too.[6]

An innovative study called DASH, short for Dietary Approaches to Stop Hypertension, clearly showed that eating more fruits and vegetables can substantially lower blood pressure, especially as part of a diet low in animal fat.[7] DASH wasn't your garden-variety nutrition study but a full-blown clinical trial, much like those done to test a new drug. All 457 of the DASH participants—some with high blood pressure, some without—were randomly assigned to one of three diets: a control diet that mirrored the typical American diet (about three servings of fruits and vegetables a day, nearly 40 percent of calories from fat, and one dairy food daily); a fruit-and-vegetable diet similar to the control diet but with eight servings of fruits and vegetables a day; and a combination diet that included nine servings of fruits and vegetables a day plus three servings of low-fat dairy foods. The beauty of the DASH method was that all of the volunteers' meals during the study were specially prepared in hospital kitchens, a strategy that minimized variation from person to person.

After eight weeks, the combination diet (fruits and vegetables plus three servings of dairy) substantially lowered blood pressure among the volunteers who had high blood pressure. So did the fruit-and-vegetable diet, though not quite as much. For both experimental diets, the reductions were about as large as what drug therapy can do for mild high blood pressure. Both the combination diet and the fruit-and-vegetable diet also lowered blood pressure in people without hypertension, suggesting that this may be an easy, side effect–free way to prevent this condition. A second DASH trial showed that a low-salt version of the DASH diet can subtract a few extra points from blood pressure (see chapter eleven).

Many components of the DASH diet contribute to its ability to lower blood pressure. A follow-up study showed that the single most important factor is the extra potassium provided by the fruits and vegetables.

Cholesterol levels also seem to respond to a diet with plenty of fruits and vegetables. This may be one of the ways that fruits and vegetables reduce the risk of heart disease and stroke. No one knows for sure how fruits and vegetables lower cholesterol. Since eating more plant foods often means eating less meat and dairy products, lower cholesterol levels may come from eating less saturated fat. They could also be due to the ability of soluble fiber to block the absorption of cholesterol from food. In spite of what food companies are claiming, though, soluble fiber's effect on cholesterol is relatively small.

. . . AND EYE DISEASES . . .

Eating plenty of fruits and vegetables helps keep those portals to your soul healthy, clear, and focused. This goes way beyond the common admonition to eat carrots for better vision (actually better night vision). People who regularly eat dark green leafy vegetables like spinach and collard greens are less likely to develop two common aging-related eye diseases, cataract and macular degeneration. Together, these two afflict millions of Americans over age sixty-five. A cataract is the gradual clouding of the eye's lens, a disk of protein that focuses light on the light-sensitive retina. Like clear floor wax that turns dull and cloudy from the pounding and scuffling of feet, decades of "insults" damage and cloud the lens. Macular degeneration, the leading cause of blindness among older people, is caused by cumulative damage to the macula, the center of the retina. It starts as a blurred spot in the center of what you see. As the degeneration spreads, vision shrinks.

In both diseases, free radicals are believed to be responsible for causing much of the damage. Free radicals are highly reactive and out-of-control substances generated inside the eye by bright sunlight, cigarette smoke, air pollution, and infection. Dark green leafy vegetables contain two pigments, lutein and zeaxanthin, that accumulate in the eye. These two, along with phytochemicals called carotenoids, can snuff out free radicals before they can harm the eye's sensitive tissues.[8] Getting lutein and zeaxanthin from fruits and vegetables is probably better than taking them as pills. Good sources include dark green lettuce, kale, turnip greens, collards, spinach, and broccoli.

. . . AND BOWEL TROUBLE . . .

What you can't digest of fruits and vegetables is as healthful as what you can. As I describe later (see "Fiber: Praise for the Indigestible," page 161), fiber, or what some call roughage, is essential for healthy bowel function. Without enough indigestible material in the diet, stools can become hard and difficult to pass. Fiber sops up water like a sponge and expands as it moves through the digestive system. This can calm the irritable bowel. By prompting regular bowel movements, fiber can relieve or prevent constipation. The bulking and softening actions of fiber also decrease pressure inside the intestinal tract and so may help prevent diverticulosis (the development of tiny, easily irritated pouches inside the colon) and diverticulitis (the often painful inflammation of these pouches). Almost twenty years ago, my colleagues and I found that men who ate more fiber were less likely to develop symptoms of diverticular disease.[9] This was recently confirmed in a six-year study of nearly 700,000 women in the United Kingdom.[10]

. . . AND CONTROL WEIGHT

Adding more fruits and vegetables to your diet won't necessarily help you lose weight, or even maintain it, *unless* you cut back on something else. As I described earlier, ideally that something else would be highly refined carbohydrates (like breads, crackers, and other foods made from white flour, or sugar-sweetened beverages) and red meat (see "A Low-Carb Diet May Help," page 53). That said, data from the Nurses' Health Studies and the Health Professionals Follow-Up Study show that women and men who increased their intakes of fruits and vegetables over a twenty-four-year period were more likely to have lost weight than those whose fruit and vegetable consumption remained steady or decreased.[11] An interesting pattern appeared: increased intake of berries, apples, pears, soy, and cauliflower were all linked to weight loss or control, while increased intake of starchy vegetables such as potatoes, corn, and peas was linked to weight *gain*.

BUT DO THEY PROTECT AGAINST CANCER?

Three decades ago, two eminent epidemiologists estimated that "dietary factors"—not enough of something or too much of something else—accounted for 35 percent of cancer deaths in the United States, or roughly the same percentage that was chalked up to smoking at the time. Major reports from the U.S. National Academy of Sciences (*Diet and Health: Implications for Reducing*

Fast Fact: A Shout Out for Blueberries

In our analyses of connections between specific fruits and vegetables and disease risk, one group of foods kept rising to the top: berries. Several studies have linked eating these tasty fruits, especially blueberries, to lower risks of heart disease, memory loss, diabetes, estrogen-receptor negative breast cancer, Parkinson's disease, and more. Berries are no miracle food, mind you, and eating them can't undo the harms caused by less-than-healthful food choices. But sprinkled on cereal, added to a fruit salad, munched as a snack, and turned into low-sugar desserts, berries can be a terrific addition to your diet.

Chronic Disease Risk) and the World Cancer Research Fund and the American Institute for Cancer Research (*Food, Nutrition, Physical Activity, and the Prevention of Cancer: A Global Perspective*), among others, have echoed this conclusion. While 35 percent may be overly optimistic, the basic message that better diets—heavy on the plant foods, please—can help guard against a variety of cancers is perfectly sound.

So far, several hundred studies have looked at the connection between diets high (or low) in fruits and vegetables and the development of cancer. Initially, they estimated a 50 percent reduction in most major cancers if everyone got at least five servings of fruits and vegetables a day. That was the basis of the National Cancer Institute's ongoing 5 A Day program.

Most of the early studies were case-control studies (see page 32). In a nutshell, these involve comparing differences in diet, habits, and other possible causes of cancer between a group of people with a particular cancer and a group without it. Such comparisons aren't always fair or without bias. People with cancer, for example, tend to seek reasons why they were stricken and may be more apt to find fault with their diets than those without the disease. The consistency of results from case-control studies created a deceptively strong idea that eating plenty of fruits and vegetables helped ward off cancer.

Cohort studies, in which information on diet and other lifestyle factors are collected before cancer, heart disease, and other conditions occur, tend to give more reliable and durable results. More than a decade ago, my team at the Harvard School of Public Health combined information on fruits and vegetables and cancer from our two large cohort studies, the Nurses' Health Studies and Health Professionals Follow-Up Study, after the 110,000 participants had been followed for almost twenty years. During this time, 9,100 had developed some type of cancer. Those who averaged eight or more servings of fruits and vegetables a day developed cancer at about the same rate as those who ate fewer than one and a half servings a day.[12] Also, in two randomized trials in which fiber supplements and a high-fiber, low-fat diet were compared with control groups, higher fiber intake didn't reduce the recurrence of new polyps.[13] The lack of a strong relation with overall cancer incidence was confirmed in a large prospective study in Europe.[14]

Does this mean that eating fruits and vegetables has no impact whatsoever on cancer? No. Although they don't have a blanket anticancer effect, some specific fruits and vegetables may work against specific cancers. Drill down a bit into the data and there's some evidence that certain types of fruits or vegetables work against specific cancers. Examples include the following:

- *Bladder cancer.* Eating cruciferous vegetables like broccoli has been linked with lower rates of bladder cancer.

- *Breast cancer.* One problem with studying breast cancer is that it isn't a single disease. It is several different diseases, each with its own risk factors. One type, estrogen-receptor-negative breast cancer, is particularly aggressive and more likely to be deadly. By combining data from cohort studies around the world, my team was able to examine breast cancers by their estrogen receptor status and found that consuming more vegetables was linked to a lower risk of developing estrogen-receptor-negative breast cancer.[15] Eating broccoli and other cruciferous vegetables has been linked to lower risk of developing breast cancer.[16]

- *Colon and rectal cancer.* There is strong evidence that the vitamin folate (also called folic acid) helps protect against colon and rectal cancer. Vegetables such as spinach and beets are good sources of folic acid and so can help fight these cancers. Today, though, with so many foods fortified with folic acid (see chapter eleven), the contribution of this vitamin from fruits and vegetables to protection against colon and rectal cancer may be dwindling.

- *Prostate cancer.* Lycopene from tomatoes and cooked or processed tomato products, such as tomato sauce and ketchup, seems to be involved in the prevention of prostate cancer. In the Health Professionals Follow-Up Study, for example, men who consumed several servings of tomatoes, tomato sauce, or tomato juice a week were less likely to develop advanced prostate cancer than those who ate one to two servings a week.[17] This finding has been supported by studies that look at blood levels of lycopene and other carotenoids.

Although the anticancer effects of fruits and vegetables aren't quite what they were thought to be a few years ago, every little bit helps. It is also possible that the benefits of fruits and vegetables may be underestimated, because almost all studies so far have examined intakes during midlife and later, while the critical time period for preventing cancer may be in childhood, adolescence, or young adulthood. For example, in one of the few studies to examine diet during adolescence, we have seen that consumption of fruits and vegetables was more strongly related to lower risk of breast cancer than was diet in midlife.[18]

The genes you inherited from your parents play a role in determining whether or not you will get cancer. So do habits like smoking cigarettes, drinking too much alcohol, getting too much sun, and not exercising. Your occupation may also play a role. Still, a nutritious diet—and that includes plenty of fruits and vegetables—is an important part of any stay-healthy strategy.

FIBER: PRAISE FOR THE INDIGESTIBLE

From a health standpoint, one of the wonderful things about eating fruits and vegetables is that they contain much you can't digest. Many of the substances that give plants their strength and flexibility aren't broken down by the acids and enzymes in the human stomach or intestines. These substances, generically called fiber, include cellulose, pectin, and gums. There are two classes of fiber, soluble and insoluble. Both pass through the digestive system largely untouched. The big difference is that soluble fiber dissolves in the intestinal fluid, while insoluble fiber doesn't.

Soluble fiber is plentiful in peas, apples, and citrus fruits, as well as in oats and other grains and seeds. It forms a sticky, gooey, Jell-O–like mass as it passes through the intestines. This gummy substance traps cholesterol-rich bile acids and carries them out of the body in the stool. The more cholesterol you excrete, the less is available for transfer into the blood and the more your cholesterol will be lowered. The lower your cholesterol, the lower your risk of heart disease and other circulatory problems.

Insoluble fiber comes from the cell walls of plants. The main component is cellulose, a long string of glucose molecules linked in a way the human digestive system can't separate and that can't dissolve in the intestines' fluids. Several decades ago, research among the Bantu people of South Africa suggested that their high-fiber diet was responsible for their low rate of colon cancer. As insoluble fiber passes unchanged through the intestine, so the thinking went, it carries along partly digested food, and by speeding the passage of food through the digestive system, it may reduce the intestine's exposure to toxic or cancer-causing substances found in food. After a few small studies showed much the same thing, the fiber craze was on. Media reports prompted many of us to start crunching through bran flakes or bran muffins for breakfast, and food manufacturers began adding fiber to cereals, breads, and pastries. In reality, though, most studies did not show lower colon cancer risks among persons who ate higher amounts of fiber from grain products. In a combined analysis of thirteen studies from around the world that included more than 725,000 men and women, fiber intake was not related to risk of colon cancer.[19] Earlier analyses had failed to find a link between dietary fiber and colon polyps, the tiny growths from which most cancers arise. Also, in two randomized trials in which fiber supplements and a high-fiber, low-fat diet were compared with control groups, higher fiber intake didn't reduce the recurrence of new polyps. Taking these findings together, high-fiber diets don't appear to be an effective way to prevent colon cancer.

Despite the disappointments for colon cancer, don't throw out the All-Bran and stock up on Wonder Bread. By dragging partly digested food through the intestines, insoluble fiber delays the absorption of sugars and starch. This helps blunt the spikes in blood sugar and insulin that occur after eating foods that are easily converted into glucose and a similar spike in triglycerides, particles that ferry fat from the intestines to the tissues. Consistently high levels of insulin and triglycerides in the blood increase the chances of having a heart attack, and the repeated demand for large amounts of insulin can increase the risk of developing type 2 diabetes. Not surprisingly, many studies have shown that eating more fiber can lower the risks of having a heart attack or developing diabetes, providing more reason to consume an abundance of fruits, vegetables, and whole grains.

The vast community of microbes that live in your digestive system, called your gut microbiome, helps digest food as it passes through your intestines. It also makes certain vitamins, breaks down toxins, and trains your immune system. Your microbiome plays an important role in keeping you healthy or making you sick, and may help control your weight or nudge you toward gaining weight. A powerful way to keep your microbiome in shape is to feed it plenty of fiber, a preferred food of gut microbes. This promotes what is believed to be the healthiest mix of microbes.

Over the past decade or so, research in animals has shown that adding more fiber to the diet can change the community of microbes from one that promotes weight gain to one that is linked to a leaner physique. Fiber-starved microbes in the gut can start to feed on the protective mucus that lines the gut, which may trigger inflammation and disease. How well this applies to humans is a hot area of research.

PHYTONUTRIENTS AT WORK

How fruits and vegetables protect us from certain cancers, heart disease, gastrointestinal problems like diverticulitis, age-related eye diseases, and other ailments is still something of a mystery. Although we've been eating plants for eons and seriously studying them for decades, what we know today is the proverbial tip of the iceberg.

Identifying the benefits of fruits and vegetables has been a challenging job, especially since plants have tremendous nutritional variability. A single type of plant—say, a Macoun apple—isn't a stable, well-defined entity. Instead its chemical composition varies with the season, the soil in which it grew, the amount of water it got, what pests it had to withstand, how ripe it was when picked and eaten, and under what conditions it was stored. What's more, the nutrients it delivers depend on how it is processed or cooked.

It will be decades before we have identified all of the complex compounds in food and even longer before we truly understand how they interact with one another and what they do in our bodies. Even so, scientists have isolated a number of substances that plants make or store that may play critical roles in keeping us healthy. These include the following:

Vitamins. The first set of phytochemicals discovered were what we today call vitamins. By definition, vitamins are carbon-containing compounds the body needs in small amounts to maintain tissue and keep metabolism humming. Vitamins have traditionally been defined by studying diseases of deficiency, things like rickets (too little vitamin D), pellagra (not enough niacin), and beriberi (not enough thiamine). More and more it looks as though cancer, heart disease, stroke, diabetes, osteoporosis, and other chronic diseases are, in part, diseases of deficiency. Exactly what the deficiencies are is the focus of intense research. Inadequate intake of folic acid is a likely risk factor for cardiovascular disease and some cancers. Low consumption of a special class of vitamins known as antioxidants, which capture and neutralize free radicals, appears to be involved in the early stages of heart disease, cancer, aging-related eye disease, dementia, and possibly aging itself (see chapter eleven). Perhaps some of the known or yet-to-be-discovered phytochemicals will earn vitamin status for preventing these diseases. You could think of whole fruits and vegetables as vitamins, given their already proven ability to prevent these new diseases of deficiency, but they are much more.

Essential elements. Plants are excellent sources of potassium, magnesium, and other elements the body needs for a host of critical tasks. Magnesium and potassium help control blood pressure and may reduce the risk of fatal rhythm disturbances of the heart.

Plant hormones. The Food and Drug Administration has given food manufacturers the go-ahead to claim in ads and on packages that eating protein from soybeans lowers the risk of heart disease. One group of compounds found in soy, the isoflavones, can mimic or inhibit the hormone estrogen (see chapter seven). Another group, the phytosterols, can influence the absorption and metabolism of cholesterol.

Carotenoids. These pigments give plants their orange or reddish colors. Some of them, such as beta-carotene and alpha-carotene, can be converted to vitamin A and so are considered to be vitamins. Others, like lutein and beta-cryptoxanthin, don't contribute to vitamin A, but the evidence is strong that they play important roles in maintaining vision and memory, probably by acting as antioxidants.

Because the chemical makeup of fruits and vegetables can vary so widely—what does a carrot have in common with a blueberry?—we should not expect that they would all have the same effects on health. Until recently, however, nutrition recommendations have just lumped them together as "fruits," "vegetables," or "fruits and vegetables." There are now a few studies, including the Nurses' Health Studies and Health Professionals Follow-Up Study, that are large enough to look at specific fruits and vegetables. For example, in an analysis combining these cohorts, with more than 185,000 men and women followed for up to twenty-four years, we examined consumption of specific fruits in relation to risk of diabetes. Total fruit consumption was related to lower risk of diabetes. Consumption of blueberries, grapes, raisins, and prunes seemed particularly beneficial for preventing diabetes, while oranges, strawberries, and cantaloupe were not.[20] Drinking fruit juice was linked to a *higher* risk of diabetes, probably because of the large amount of rapidly absorbed sugar.

OUR HEALTH DEPENDS ON PLANTS

The diet we eat today doesn't look a thing like the diet our hunter-gatherer ancestors ate over hundreds of thousands of years. They probably relied on a wide variety of fruits and vegetables, scrabbling to pick and eat whatever edible morsels they could find. It is likely that, over time, humans became metabolically dependent on hundreds of compounds made by plants. These phytochemicals help detoxify the harmful substances found in plants; help some of our enzymes fight cancer, infection, and other cellular disruption; and work with others to repair damage to cells. So far, only a small number of these compounds have been labeled essential nutrients.

"Vegetables and fruits contain the anticarcinogenic cocktail to which we are adapted," noted cancer researcher John Potter once wrote. "We abandon it at our peril."

TOO MUCH OF A GOOD THING

Could eating too much of some kinds of fruits or vegetables be *bad* for you? The answer is yes.

Almost all essential nutrients can be toxic if you take in too much of them. That cautionary note likely applies to fruits and vegetables as well. Legendary biochemist Bruce Ames once pointed out that plants evolved to make chemicals that are toxic to insects and other animals that might eat them, or to ward off infections by bacteria, yeast, and other organisms.[21] Many of these chemicals are natural carcinogens when tested, but, as Ames pointed out, we have evolved multiple detoxification mechanisms to protect us. It is possible that some of these plant-made agents will slip through our defenses. And we have also altered the chemical content of the foods we eat, especially fruits and vegetables, by selective breeding for many characteristics, such as sweetness, that could increase the natural carcinogens.

Here are a few examples of potential harms:

Too much spinach. This green leafy vegetable is a healthful, versatile plant. You can eat it raw in salads, use it as a bed for salmon, or sauté it as a side dish. But spinach is quite high in oxalates. The kidneys can turn these naturally occurring acids into kidney stones. The more oxalates consumed, the greater the risk of developing these painful stones.[22] This doesn't mean you should avoid spinach. But if you have had a kidney stone, it would make sense to limit spinach to a few times a week and rely on a wider variety of greens, most of which are lower in oxalates. You might also eat cheese or some other dairy food along with spinach, because these foods reduce the absorption of oxalates.

Grapefruit juice. This popular juice contains potent compounds that alter the metabolism of many drugs. Depending on the drug, these changes can lead to too much or too little of the drug in the bloodstream (see "Juice" on page 174). If you take medications and you like to drink grapefruit juice or eat grapefruit, talk with your health care provider about possible interactions.

Brussels sprouts. Many people like the edgy bitterness of this cruciferous vegetable. But this bitterness is sometimes a signal of potentially cancer-causing chemicals. In a pooled analysis of cohort studies, my colleagues and I saw a modest increase in pancreatic cancer among people consuming Brussels sprouts three times a week.[23] In a separate analysis, high consumption of Brussels sprouts was also linked to a higher risk of developing high blood pressure.[24] If you think about the unusual shape of the Brussels sprout, the tight packages of leaves that we eat emerge from the stalk, which would normally be covered with bark or spines for protection. The fragile sprouts don't have anything like that, and so turn to a different defense mechanism: chemical warfare. Given what we've found, it makes sense to eat this vegetable not more than once a week while we wait for more data.

As we dig more deeply into the roles of specific fruits and vegetables, I expect to see more of the unexpected. Plants may seem like simple organisms compared to animals, but their biology is complicated!

PUTTING IT INTO PRACTICE

There isn't any magic daily number or combination of fruits and vegetables for optimal health. Instead, I offer two words of advice: "five" and "variety." Keep in mind that potatoes and corn don't count for the five-plus servings a day, and that you should count juice as only one fruit serving, even if you drink it two or three times a day.

Aim for five. The five servings a day used as the goal for national programs turns out to have been a good choice. When it comes to cardiovascular disease and premature death, a large meta-analysis linked higher consumption of fruit and vegetables to a lower risk of dying from any cause. The biggest benefit came from hitting five servings a day.[25] Eating more than five servings of vegetables and fruits a day is perfectly fine, but you don't need to put that high on your priority list.

In the DASH study described on page 156, the target of nine servings a day was definitely beneficial. But there's no way to know if five or six or seven servings a day would have done the same thing.

Eat for variety and for color. Getting five servings of fruits and vegetables a day is important, but variety matters too. On most days try to get at least one serving from each of the following fruit and vegetable categories:[26]

- dark green, leafy vegetables
- yellow or orange fruits and vegetables
- red fruits and vegetables
- legumes (beans) and peas
- citrus fruits.

Cook your tomatoes. Treat yourself to tomatoes: processed tomatoes or tomato products cooked in oil on most days. Tomatoes are rich in lycopene, a powerful antioxidant that has been linked with lower rates of prostate cancer and memory loss. Because lycopene is tightly bound inside cell walls, your body has a hard time extracting it from raw tomatoes. Cooking breaks down cell walls, and oil dissolves lycopene and helps shuttle it into the bloodstream.

Fresh is best. Eat several servings of fresh, uncooked fruits and vegetables each week because cooking damages or destroys some important phytochemicals. Vitamin C and folic acid, for example, are sensitive to heat. Otherwise, the physical state of the fruits and vegetables you eat doesn't much matter. Frozen fruits and vegetables are nearly as good as fresh ones and may even be more nutritious than "fresh" fruits and vegetables that have been stored for weeks or months under conditions that prevent ripening. Canned fruits and vegetables are usually fine, although many come loaded with salt and added sugar.

THE SPUD IS A DUD

As I have said earlier, potatoes and corn don't deserve to be called vegetables in the nutritional sense. Sure, they meet the minimum requirements—they are plants, after all—but the resemblance ends there. When it comes to healthy

Fresh Fruits and Vegetables

The freshest produce is what you grow yourself and pick just before you eat it. You don't need a farm plot or a big suburban backyard to do this. My backyard is only about 40 feet by 20 feet. Yet in that space, not far from busy Harvard Square, my wife and I have a peach tree that yields several bushels of fruit a year, a pear tree, raspberries that bear fruit in both June and October, blueberries, four varieties of grapes, and herbs. We used to grow tomatoes, cucumbers, and greens, but the fruit trees have made the space too shady, so we visit farmers' markets for these vegetables. Our garden gives us something fresh, tasty, and healthy for at least four months of the year.

eating, it's best to think of potatoes and corn as starches like rice and pasta, since they deliver mostly easily digested starch.

The average American consumes more than 100 pounds of potatoes a year,[27] making the spud the most popular "vegetable" in America. (Compare that with about 10 pounds of carrots and 8 pounds of broccoli per person.) Because potatoes are such a huge commodity, they have received special treatment from the USDA and from politicians.

The potato is one of several starchy vegetables mentioned by name in the *Dietary Guidelines for Americans*. The USDA has said that batter-coated frozen potatoes—the ones used to make french fries—can be classified as a fresh vegetable.

Congress even promoted potatoes a few years back when senators from Maine, Idaho, and other potato-growing states, backed by the National Potato Council, added potatoes to the list of vegetables that could be bought with vouchers from the federal Special Supplemental Nutrition Program for Women, Infants, and Children (WIC). The 2014 omnibus appropriations bill directed the USDA to allow all varieties of fresh, whole, or cut vegetables to be part of the WIC program, which included white potatoes and french fries. That's just one more example of promoting agribusiness over health.

More than two hundred studies have shown that people who eat plenty of fruits and vegetables decrease their odds of having heart attacks or strokes, of developing a variety of cancers, or of suffering from constipation or other digestive problems. Yet the same body of evidence shows that potatoes don't contribute to this benefit and may even contribute to poor health. Here are just two examples:

In the analysis of long-term weight that I described on page 158, eating fruits in general and vegetables with high fiber and low glycemic load was related to low weight gain over a twenty-four-year period. Eating starchy vegetables such as potatoes, corn, and peas was linked to greater weight gain.

High blood pressure afflicts millions of Americans, putting them at risk of having a stroke and developing cardiovascular disease. Potatoes are a good source of potassium, which can help reduce blood pressure. They also have a high glycemic load (see page 118), which can boost blood pressure and increase the risk of diabetes. We have shown that higher consumption of potatoes is linked to the development of type 2 diabetes, especially when compared with the same number of servings from whole grains.[28]

Juice and Smoothies: No Recipe for Health

Eating fruits and vegetables is unquestionably good for health. Pulverizing them into juices and smoothies isn't, for two key reasons:

You will consume extra calories. Ordinary servings of fruits and vegetables tend to be relatively low in calories. Turning them, especially fruits, into juice or smoothies almost always adds calories. Take orange juice as an example. Eating a medium-size navel orange gives you about 12 grams of sugar. A cup of orange juice gives you more than twice that amount of sugar, because you end up drinking the juice from more oranges than you would eat. We also tend to absorb calories more quickly from juice than from whole fruits, because the sugar is locked up inside of cells, which slows down their release into the bloodstream.

You can overdo it. Kale became a miracle food, lionized by celebrities such as Gwyneth Paltrow, Kevin Bacon, and Bette Midler. This green, leafy vegetable is rich in vitamins K, A, and C, delivers fiber, and more. It is great in salads and soups, and when sautéed makes a wonderful side dish. If a little bit is good, more is better, right? Sadly, no. As a member of the Cruciferae family, kale contains chemicals that can block the formation of thyroid hormone, which helps regulate an individual's metabolism. Consuming too much kale—hard to do when eating the vegetable but easy to do when drinking kale smoothies—can cause the thyroid gland to slow its production of thyroid hormone. This condition, known as hypothyroidism, can cause symptoms that range from fatigue and increased sensitivity to cold to weight gain, muscle aches and stiffness, thinning hair, depression, and memory loss.

It's best to eat fruits and vegetables the way they grow, not concentrated into juice and smoothies.

To directly evaluate the overall impact of eating potatoes on blood pressure in a contemporary population of Americans, we turned to data from the Nurses' Health Studies and the Health Professionals Follow-Up Study. Participants on the higher end of the potato-consumption spectrum—baked, boiled, and mashed, and fried—were more likely to have developed high blood pressure.[29]

The trade-off of risks and benefits for potatoes, corn, and other starchy vegetables depends on other aspects of diet and lifestyle, especially physical activity. My grandfather was a dairy farmer in Michigan. He was active from sunup to sundown and was as lean as the rails that bordered his fields. He ate potatoes and ate them often. But he was able to tolerate their glycemic load in a way most sedentary Americans can't today.

I'm invoking solid evidence when I recommend that most people not eat potatoes often and turn instead to nonstarchy vegetables like carrots, broccoli, and spinach.

CHAPTER NINE

You Are What You Drink

"TO YOUR HEALTH." THAT TRADITIONAL toast captures an essential nugget of nutrition information: what and how much you drink is just as important to your health as what and how much you eat.

More than half of your body weight is made up of a briny fluid that is similar to the oceans that nurtured primordial life. This fluid bathes, cushions, and lubricates your cells, tissues, and organs. It gives cells their shape and provides their substance. And it forms the watery highways that transport nutrients, wastes, hormones, and other substances throughout your body.

When it comes to fluids, the constant struggle for survival can be reduced to this: you dry, you die. Your skin, kidneys, nasal passages, and several hormones work together to keep the fluid part of you from drifting off into the air. But preventing water loss isn't enough. You need to take in enough fluid to carry out a variety of critical metabolic tasks—things like making urine to flush away toxic by-products of digestion and metabolism, maintaining blood volume, and preventing body salts from getting too concentrated, as well as replenishing whatever water you lose.

The average person uses about a milliliter of fluid for every calorie burned. That's about 64 ounces for a 2,000-calorie-a-day diet. Exactly how much fluid you need to take in each day depends on you. Your needs are partly genetically programmed and largely determined by diet, the environment, and activity.

- *Diet.* If you eat lots of fruits and vegetables, which are mostly water, you may not need to drink as much as someone who eats a lot of meat, bread, or salt. In western Tanzania, people drink much less water than elsewhere in the world because they satisfy much of their daily fluid needs by eating water-rich cooked bananas, which make up a large part of the diet.
- *Environment/weather.* When the temperature is perfectly comfortable, you lose about 64 ounces of water a day through your skin, the moist air you

Do You Need to Drink Eight 8-Ounce Glasses of Water a Day?

You may have heard or read that you need to drink eight 8-ounce glasses of water a day. That's a medical myth, one of those "facts" that is repeated so often it gains the ring of truth.[1] Where it came from no one really knows. One possible source is the physiological requirement that burning 2,000 calories' worth of food a day requires about 64 ounces of water. Another is a 1945 report by the National Food and Nutrition Board (under the National Academies of Sciences, Engineering, and Medicine) that included this recommendation: "A suitable allowance of water for adults is 2.5 liters daily in most instances."[2] Two point five liters is a little more than eight 8-ounce glasses. If that's the source, the next sentence in the report—"Most of this quantity is contained in prepared foods"—has been overlooked or ignored. Recommendations from the same board in 2004 raised the bar to about fifteen 8-ounce glasses of water for men and eleven for women, with more needed during strenuous activity.[3]

Some of the fluid your body needs comes from your food. If you eat a lot of fruits, vegetables, and soups, you don't need to drink as much as someone who eats "drier" foods. The rest comes from what you drink. Water is your best bet, but coffee, tea, juice, soda, sports drinks, beer, and other water-based beverages can also resupply the water you lose.

exhale, and urine. When it's "too darn hot," as Ella Fitzgerald croons, you lose even more. You can also lose extra fluid in the winter, when the relative humidity plummets and the dry air draws water out of your skin.

- *Activity.* The more active you are, the more fluid you need. When your muscles burn glucose, they generate heat. As you sit and read these words, some of that heat helps keep your body temperature near 98.6°F. Start scraping old wallpaper off a wall or running around a track and you quickly make more heat than you need. This extra heat must be vented or you literally risk cooking the temperature-sensitive proteins that make you you. That's what sweat does. As sweat forms on your skin and evaporates, it carries heat away from your body. When you are giving your body a real workout, you can lose up to a quart (32 ounces) of fluid an hour.

Because your body doesn't have an easy-to-read gauge that tells you when your fluid level is low, several rules of thumb are often offered: Drink when you are thirsty. Drink before you are thirsty. Drink enough so your urine is consistently clear or pale yellow rather than bright or dark yellow. None of these are great guides.

By the time you feel thirsty, your fluid level can already be low. That's especially true when you are working or playing hard and losing water quickly. Aging tends to uncouple the sense of thirst from the body's fluid level, and many older people become dehydrated without realizing it. Urine color is influenced by what you eat and some vitamin supplements.

The consequences of not taking in enough fluid each day range from the merely irritating to the life-threatening. Minor dehydration can make you feel grumpy and tired. Chronic minor dehydration is a cause of constipation, especially among older people. It can also contribute to the development of kidney stones and bladder cancer. Extreme dehydration, though relatively uncommon, can be deadly. It occurs mostly among children and older people during very hot weather, and among endurance athletes.

Overhydration can be a problem too. Drinking too much water, sports drink, or any other beverage can throw off the body's balance of water and minerals. It has led to the deaths of runners in the Boston and other marathons, several high school football players, and other athletes. One way to prevent overhydration, which can lead to a deadly condition known as hyponatremia, is to consume a balanced mix of water and minerals, such as Gatorade, when you are engaged in prolonged, intense activity.

Think of hydration as a day-long process. Drink at least one glass of your beverage of choice soon after arising, with each meal, and in between meals. Drink before and after exercising. And drink if you are feeling thirsty.

So far I have been deliberately general in talking about *fluid* intake rather than specifying any specific beverage. Plenty of beverages qualify for the task, including water, juice, soda, milk, coffee, tea, and alcohol. Some are better than others, especially as routine thirst quenchers. Let's take a look at each one. The "healthy" list may surprise you.

WATER

For plain old topping off your tank, water is hard to beat. It has 100 percent of what you need—pure H_2O—and no calories or additives. And when it comes from the tap, water costs a fraction of a penny per glass.

In most cities across the United States, tap water is pure and healthy. In others, tap water contains lead, chromium, pesticides or herbicides, and other potentially dangerous chemicals that leach into water supplies from leaking underground storage tanks, factories and other businesses, landfills and garbage dumps, aging water pipes, and a variety of other sources. The possibility exists that the chlorine-based chemicals used to rid tap water of disease-causing bacteria can react with organic matter to create potentially cancer-causing compounds. So far, the available evidence doesn't support that as serious health threat. To be on the safe side, though, we need to invest in public water treatment facilities that minimize the levels of these compounds.

Many people believe that bottled water is safer than tap water. That's not necessarily true. In fact, some bottled water actually comes from the tap, not from the pristine mountain springs conjured up by their names or the images on their labels. Bottled water doesn't have to meet standards set by the federal Environmental Protection Agency that require regular testing for bacterial and chemical contamination. Tap water from public supplies, by comparison, must meet those standards and the reports must be made public.

There's also a widespread belief that bottled water tastes better than tap water. In blind taste tests, though, tap water often comes out on top. There are certainly exceptions, as some water systems have chlorine levels that give the water an "off" taste.

In terms of cost, tap water is the clear winner. In Boston, it costs about $1.25 a year to drink eight glasses of tap water a day. Getting that much from bottled water would cost two hundred times more (about $225) if it's from large home-delivery bottles or four hundred times more ($500) if it comes from individual bottles.

There are also environmental considerations. It takes as much water to make disposable, individual-size water bottles as the bottle contains. Transporting bottled water uses fossil fuels and contributes to global warming. And many of the billions of bottles consumed each year in the United States end up in landfills or incinerators.

The bottom line is that our public water supplies are generally very safe and that chlorination has saved countless lives by blocking the spread of infectious diseases. If there are risks to drinking tap water, they are generally very low compared with other "hazardous" habits. That said, some city water can be a health hazard, as we've sadly seen in Flint, Michigan. In such cases, drinking bottled water is an inexpensive and healthy alternative to drinking soda, juice, or other beverages in place of tap water.

JUICE

A glass of real fruit juice or vegetable juice tastes delightful. It also gives you water plus vitamins, minerals, and maybe some fiber. As a morning eye-opener or as a small part of your total fluid requirement, real juice (as opposed to juice-flavored sugar water) can be part of a healthy diet. In fact, scurvy, a disabling condition caused by a deficiency of vitamin C, was eliminated in the United States after World War II in part by the tradition of having a small glass of orange juice with breakfast. Orange juice also happens to be a good source of beta-cryptoxanthin, a healthful carotenoid that would otherwise be low in our diet.

As a regular beverage, though, fruit juice can add a hefty daily dose of calories (see "Beware of liquid calories" on page 65). A 12-ounce serving of orange juice, for example, gives you 150 calories or so, or the equivalent of three chocolate-chip cookies or a can of sugar-sweetened soda. That's an awful lot of calories if you just need something to quench your thirst.

The fundamental problem with drinking juice is that it is just too easy to consume a large amount of fruit—and its accompanying sugar—in a few moments. Think of squeezing your own oranges to make a glass of juice. This would require about three oranges, depending on their size. Almost no one would eat three whole oranges at a sitting; spacing them out over a day would have a very gentle effect on your blood glucose. As juice, though, three oranges go down the hatch quite quickly, and you can do that several times a day if you aren't careful.

If you enjoy drinking juice, try diluting it with regular or sparkling water. Start with two parts juice to one part water and gradually work your way to one part juice to three or four parts water. Another trick for putting some zest into plain water is adding a squeeze of fresh lemon or lime. Vegetable juices tend to have fewer calories than fruit juices, but check the labels to be sure and look at the sodium content: some vegetable juices deliver nearly a day's dose of sodium in a single serving.

"Infused" Water: A Detox Myth

Can you flush "toxins" from your body by drinking water that's been infused with a few slices of cucumbers, some grapefruit, and a few sprigs of mint? Media personalities like Dr. Oz, trainer Jillian Michaels, and celebrity Khloé Kardashian have touted the health benefits of "detox water," which is made by letting water sit for a few hours with vegetables and fruits.

What makes this detox water so magical? Nothing. For starters, no one can explain exactly what toxins this special water helps people eliminate. Any benefits—if there are any—come from drinking extra water. Adding grapefruit, cucumbers, or mint gives the water a pleasant taste but no detoxification power.

The biggest problem with drinking fruit juice instead of water is that many people don't eat less to adjust for the extra calories. That's a surefire recipe for gradual weight gain.

Among the many types of juices, grapefruit juice needs a special mention because it changes the way some people absorb and metabolize certain drugs. Grapefruit juice can reduce the absorption of the allergy medication fexofenadine (Allegra); digoxin, used to treat congestive heart failure; losartan (Cozaar), used to control blood pressure; and the anticancer drug vinblastine. Grapefruit juice can also boost the blood levels of other drugs, sometimes to dangerous heights. Drugs in this category include calcium channel blockers such as felodipine (Plendil), nifedipine (Procardia), and nisoldipine (Sular), which are used to control high blood pressure; carbamazepine (Carbatrol, Tegretol), used to control epilepsy; some widely used cholesterol-lowering medications such as lovastatin (Mevacor), atorvastatin (Lipitor), and simvastatin (Zocor); cyclosporine, an immunosuppressant taken mainly by people who have had an organ transplant; and buspirone (BuSpar), used to fight alcohol abuse, depression, panic disorder, and a variety of other problems.

SODA AND OTHER SUGAR-SWEETENED BEVERAGES

Imagine dumping seven to nine teaspoons of sugar onto a bowl of cereal. Too sweet to eat? That's how much sugar is in a 12-ounce can of Coca-Cola, Pepsi, Orange Crush, or most other sugared soft drinks. We drink the stuff by the gallon—nearly five hundred 12-ounce servings of soda, pop, tonic, or whatever you call it per person each year, most of it the full-sugar variety. Keep in mind that this is the average, and many people consume several times that amount. That's an awful lot of a beverage that has absolutely no nutritionally redeeming value.

I say this because soda delivers pure calories completely divorced from the healthful nutrients you might get from real fruit juices—things such as vitamins, minerals, other phytochemicals, and maybe some fiber. That's a problem on several levels.

Most Americans already take in too many calories and struggle to lose weight. One 12-ounce serving of soda a day doesn't seem like a big deal, especially if you manage to cut back on food calories. If you don't, though, an extra 150 calories a day can translate into a 15-pound weight gain over a year! The danger of drinking sugared sodas and juices instead of water is that many people treat "liquid calories" as somehow different from "food calories" and often don't make up for the calories in soda or juice by eating less.

The simple sugars in soda trigger rapid and intense increases in blood sugar, which causes the pancreas to pump out more and more insulin. When this happens several times a day on top of the rises in blood sugar and insulin that occur after eating, it can increase the risk of type 2 diabetes, especially for people who are growing more and more resistant to insulin's ability to ferry glucose inside cells. In a meta-analysis that included nearly 500,000 men and women followed for an average of twenty-two years, the risk of developing type 2 diabetes went up by 13 percent for each daily serving of sugar-sweetened soda or juice.[4] Given the rate of soda consumption in the United States, that would translate into 1.8 million new cases of type 2 diabetes over a ten-year period. Notably, this increase in risk was on top of the contribution of soda to weight gain, which itself is a powerful risk factor for diabetes. Taking in lots of easily digested carbohydrates—like those found in soda—raises the blood level of triglycerides, a kind of fat-carrying particle, and depresses the level of HDL cholesterol. Both of these changes would tilt the scales in the direction of heart disease. Not surprisingly, that is exactly what we found when studying soda consumption in the Nurses' Health Studies.[5]

Drinking a fair amount of sugar-sweetened soda also appears to boost the odds of developing painful kidney stones. In the Nurses' Health Study and the Health Professionals Follow-Up Study, participants who drank one or more sugar-sweetened sodas a day were 33 percent more likely to have developed kidney stones over an eight-year period than those who drank less than one serving a week.[6]

What about calorie-free sodas, often called diet sodas? The FDA has approved six sugar substitutes for use in foods and beverages—advantame (no brand name yet), aspartame (Equal and NutraSweet), acesulfame potassium (Sweet One), neotame (Newtame), saccharin (Sweet'N Low), and sucralose (Splenda). Two other so-called nonnutritive sweeteners, Stevia and extracts of the Swingle or monk fruit, are derived from plants, so they aren't "artificial." Instead, they fall into the FDA's "generally recognized as safe" category.[7]

As a beverage, diet sodas are better than the sugared versions, although they're an expensive way to get water. As a weight-loss gambit, don't count on this approach all by itself. Artificial sweeteners may affect the body's ability to gauge how many calories are coming in.[8] Our brains respond to sweetness with signals to eat more. By providing a sweet taste without any calories, artificial sweeteners may cause us to crave more sweet foods and drinks, which can add up to extra calories. The relation between diet soda and obesity is complicated to study because many people who are overweight switch to diet soda with the hope of losing weight, making it difficult to determine cause and effect—a simple analysis done at one point in time may show that consumption of diet soda is associated with overweight and obesity. My colleagues and I have looked at this carefully over time. Men and women who consumed diet soda gained less weight than those who consumed sugar-sweetened soda.[9] A similar trend was seen in a randomized trial conducted among adolescents that compared sugared and diet sodas.[10] In the same way, after taking into account the tendency of overweight people to select diet soda, consumption of this beverage does not appear to increase the risk of diabetes.

Despite what you might read on the Internet or hear in the popular press, nonnutritive sweeteners probably don't pose a health hazard for adults. However, the reality is that most of these have not been examined adequately in long-term human studies. No one knows how they affect children, who may consume large amounts of them over a lifetime.

Why bother with the uncertainty when plain water or water with a twist of lemon or a dash of juice is a healthier option? My bottom line: Think of diet soda as you might a nicotine patch for smoking. It may help wean you from drinking sugar-sweetened soda, but you don't want to rely on it for the long haul.

MILK

Milk from cows, sheep, goats, and other species is a brew of high-quality proteins, minerals such as calcium and phosphorous, hormones, and other nutrients that make baby animals—including humans—grow fast. For very young children, it's a good but second-best alternative to breast milk. For older children, it can help promote growth. Milk and dairy foods may be good for elderly individuals who need extra protein and other nutrients. But for adolescents and most adults, there is potential harm in drinking too much milk. That's why I believe that you should think of milk and other dairy foods as optional parts of your diet to be consumed in modest amounts, not something you need to drink or eat two or three times a day.

The *Dietary Guidelines for Americans* have long recommended that most Americans get three servings of milk or other dairy foods a day. That recommendation was enshrined in the old Food Guide Pyramid and resurrected in MyPlate. The 2015–2020 *Dietary Guidelines for Americans* say that a healthy eating plan includes fat-free or low-fat dairy, including milk, yogurt, cheese, and/or fortified soy beverages, and still set three servings a day as the target for most people.

The main rationale is that milk and other dairy foods give us the calcium we need to strengthen bones. Milk has also been touted as a weight-loss food.

But as I point out in chapter ten, we don't need two to three servings of dairy foods a day to prevent osteoporosis and fractures, and many Americans may be getting too much calcium. The evidence doesn't support the link between drinking milk and long-term body weight, although eating yogurt may help control weight.[11]

You may be thinking, *If I'm not getting enough calcium every day, why not play it safe and drink three glasses of milk a day?* Here are several good reasons: lactose intolerance, extra saturated fat, extra calories, unneeded hormones, possible increased risks of heart disease or cancer, and environmental problems.

Lactose intolerance. All babies are born with the ability to digest milk. Some, especially those of northern European ancestry, keep this trait for life. Most children, though, gradually lose it as their bodies stop making an enzyme called lactase that breaks down milk sugar (lactose). In fact, only about a quarter of the world's adults can fully digest milk. In the United States, as many as 50 million Americans aren't equipped to digest milk. Half of Hispanic Americans, 75 percent of African Americans, and more than 90 percent of Asian Americans can't tolerate much lactose. For them, drinking a glass of milk can have unpleasant consequences, such as nausea, bloating, cramps, and diarrhea.

A lot of effort has gone into helping lactose-intolerant people drink milk or eat cheese or ice cream. The Agriculture Research Service (part of the USDA) touts its development of the lactose-modified milk known as Lactaid as one of its top accomplishments in the last fifty years. A variety of lactose-digesting powders or tablets that can be added to milk or taken before eating dairy products are available over the counter. And dairy proponents point to a number of studies showing that people who have trouble digesting lactose can tolerate small amounts throughout the day, especially when consumed with other food. But because there are easier ways to get enough calcium, I don't believe that people who have trouble digesting lactose need to spend the extra money or time drinking milk or eating dairy products. It is perfectly fine if you want to do that, but you shouldn't force yourself to do it or feel guilty if you don't. After all, you're in good company with three-quarters of the world's adults.

Saturated fat. An 8-ounce glass of whole milk contains almost 5 grams of saturated fat. Drinking three glasses a day would be the equivalent of eating twelve strips of bacon or a Big Mac and an order of fries. That's a substantial amount of saturated fat. Cheese can also deliver a lot of saturated fat. A 1-ounce serving of American cheese made from whole milk delivers about as much calcium as a glass of milk and the same amount of saturated fat.

Despite confusion in both the scientific and general media, saturated fat is a real health concern. As discussed in chapter five, saturated fat was once over-vilified as uniquely harmful and the primary cause of heart disease. We now know that trans fat has a more harmful effect on the cardiovascular system, and saturated fat is about the same, calorie for calorie, as refined starch and sugar. If you are aiming to optimize your health, replacing butter and other sources of dairy fat with unsaturated plant oils is a good step in that direction.

That isn't to say that you should entirely eliminate milk, cheese, and ice cream. If you really like them, eat them in modest amounts, buy the best quality you can afford, and enjoy them.

You might think that if enough people made the switch to low-fat or skim milk, lower rates of heart disease would follow. But that won't happen, at least not at the population level. That's because once a cow is milked, the fat from that milk is in the food supply, and someone ends up drinking or eating it. Much of the fat skimmed from milk resurfaces as butter and cream, which are used to make premium ice cream, buttery pastries, and high-fat snack foods such as cookies and candy bars. Many of the same people who have switched to skim milk have a bowl of high-fat Ben & Jerry's or Häagen-Dazs ice cream before going to bed, and people who drink whole milk or don't drink milk at all—often poorer, less educated, or less health-savvy people—are eating more and more high-fat products made with milk fat.

Extra calories. Three glasses of whole milk a day add 450 calories to your diet—nearly one-quarter of the average person's recommended daily intake. Low-fat milk, at 330 calories, adds a bit fewer, but that is still a lot of calories if the main goal is just to get more calcium.

Extra hormones. Cows make most of the same hormones that humans make. Before farming turned into agribusiness, the hormone levels in milk weren't an issue. Today, though, they may well be a cause for concern.

Over the years, dairy cattle have been bred to produce more milk. Since 1960, American Holstein cows' genetic potential for milk production has increased nearly 7,000 pounds after each birth. Cows today are routinely milked while they are pregnant, which also keeps milk production high. This is great for cattle farmers and milk producers, and it helps keep the price of milk relatively low. But it also means that today's milk contains a more concentrated mix of hormones than it did years ago. Naturally occurring hormones in milk include estrogens and progestins (so-called female hormones), testosterone and other androgens (so-called male hormones), and insulin-like growth factor, to name just a few. Estrogens and progestins can stimulate breast cancer, testosterone and androgens can promote prostate cancer, and elevated levels of insulin-like growth factor have been linked with breast, prostate, and colon cancer.

Twenty years ago, my colleagues and I started the Growing Up Today Study. It enrolled more than 25,000 volunteers, all children of women in the Nurses' Health Study. The participants complete questionnaires on diet, exercise, lifestyle factors, and health, much as their mothers do. In this group, teenage acne, a largely hormone-driven condition, is more common among milk drinkers.[12] This is important, because it suggests that the hormones in milk are strong enough or abundant enough to stimulate glandular tissue such as the sebaceous glands in the skin—and possibly mammary glands in the breast. Low-fat and skim milk were more strongly associated with acne than whole milk. That's probably because removing fat from milk also removes fat-soluble female hormones (estrogens), which tend to counter the acne-driving effects of water-soluble male hormones (androgens), which are left behind.

Cardiovascular disease. There's no clear overall connection between consuming milk or other dairy foods and cardiovascular disease. That's largely because what individuals choose to drink in place of milk influences their overall health. Swapping milk for soda would tip you toward worse health. Swapping it for water, coffee, tea, or water with a splash of fruit juice would benefit your heart and blood vessels by helping cut calories. Eating a peanut butter sandwich instead of a cheese sandwich, or sprinkling nuts on a salad instead of cheese, would reduce your risk of heart disease.

Prostate cancer. A diet high in milk or dairy foods has been implicated as a risk factor for prostate cancer. In a meta-analysis of thirty-two cohort studies, total dairy foods, milk, low-fat milk, and cheese were all significantly associated with a higher risk of prostate cancer.[13] In the most detailed of these studies, the Health Professionals Follow-Up Study, men who drank two or more glasses of milk a day were almost twice as likely to develop advanced or metastatic (spreading) prostate cancer as those who didn't drink milk at all.

What's the connection? Drinking milk increases blood levels of insulin-like growth factor 1, which has been linked to higher risk of prostate cancer. This growth factor is what's partly responsible for helping children and teens grow taller. It continues to rev up cell multiplication throughout life. But it also stimulates the growth of cancer cells. It's possible that calcium contributes to the excess risk of prostate cancer too. In the Health Professionals Follow-Up Study, men who took in more than 2,000 milligrams of calcium a day from food and supplements combined were almost three times as likely to develop advanced prostate cancer and more than four times as likely to develop metastatic prostate cancer as men who got less than 500 milligrams a day. Inside the prostate (and elsewhere), the active form of vitamin D may act like a brake on the growth and division of cancer cells. Too much calcium slows or even stops the conversion of inactive vitamin D to its biologically active form and so may rob the body of a natural anticancer mechanism.

Uterine cancer. Endometrial cancer, the glandular form of cancer affecting the uterus, is strongly promoted by higher estrogen levels, whether they are naturally produced or result from medication. Because of concerns about the naturally occurring hormone levels in milk, we examined milk consumption and risk of this cancer in the Nurses' Health Study. Overall, there was a modest increase in risk with greater milk consumption. But among postmenopausal women not taking hormone medications, there was a 60 percent higher risk when the women consumed three or more servings of dairy foods per day.[14] This finding adds to evidence that the hormone levels in milk are high enough to be biologically important.

Other cancers. Overall, there is little connection between drinking milk during midlife or later and breast cancer.[15] Milk consumption during this period is related to lower risk of colorectal cancer, almost certainly due to its calcium content, but it's probably better to get calcium from other sources without the extra calories or saturated fat. Drinking milk during childhood and adolescence, however, may be a different story. Children and adolescents who drink a lot of milk tend to be taller than those who don't drink much milk, and greater height has been linked to an increased risk of cancers of the breast, colon, and other sites.[16] Today we have limited data directly relating consumption of milk during childhood and adolescence to risk of cancers during adulthood, but the potential for increases in risk suggest caution over high dairy consumption during these formative years.

Fractures. As noted in chapter ten, the observation that rates of hip fractures are highest in countries with the greatest milk consumption has been a long-standing paradox. Because of the provocative finding that being tall is associated with increased risks of many cancers, we explored our data on diet during adolescence in the Growing Up Today Study to identify the aspects of diet that were most strongly predictive of gain in height and ultimately attained height. The answer was simple and clear: milk.[17] Even the same amount of protein from red meat wasn't related to gain in height. This shouldn't be surprising, because milk is beautifully designed to promote the growth of young mammals, including humans. But we are the only mammal to continue to drink milk after we are weaned from our mothers' milk.

Twenty years ago my research team published a paper showing that greater height is a strong risk factor for hip fracture, probably because of simple physics: a long stick is easier to break than a shorter stick.[18] I hypothesized that high milk consumption during adolescence might actually *increase* fracture risks later in life by promoting greater height. Fortunately, we had the data to test this idea, because we had asked participants in our adult cohort studies about their milk consumption during high school. As expected, their reported milk consumption during high school correlated with their adult height and in men also predicted higher risk of hip fracture later in life. The risk increased by 9 percent for each additional glass of milk per day.[19] Among women, we didn't see an increase or a decrease in hip fractures with milk consumption, possibly because height is determined earlier in girls than in boys. While these relationships need further examination, the international correlation between milk consumption and fracture risk is a bit less paradoxical than it seems.

- *Environmental issues.* As practiced in the United States, it takes a lot of water and energy to make milk. Dairy farming and milk production make significant contributions to the greenhouse gases we generate each year.[20] The average American currently consumes about one and a half glasses of milk or equivalent amounts of other dairy foods a day. Getting us up to three a day would appreciably increase the already substantial environmental impact of dairy farming and milk production—from water use and water pollution to the release of greenhouse gases.

COFFEE

Here's something you may not have been expecting to read in a book about food and health: coffee is a remarkably safe and healthy beverage. Its dubious reputation, which stretches back hundreds of years, is more image than substance.

Over the years, hundreds of studies have been done on the health effects of coffee. Some early ones linked the bitter brew with breast cancer, pancreatic cancer, and heart disease. Many of these studies had a major flaw: they didn't take into account a key habit—cigarette smoking—that once went hand in hand with coffee drinking. More carefully controlled studies eventually showed that it was the smoking, not the coffee drinking, that accounted for health problems.

In fact, a growing body of research shows that coffee may actually be good for a few things that ail us.

I don't mean to imply that coffee is as innocuous as water. It isn't. The caffeine in coffee—and tea, many sodas, and chocolate—has definite drug-like activity. The pep and mild euphoria that caffeine offers is probably why most people drink coffee and other caffeine-containing beverages. As with any drug, there are downsides to caffeine. Too much of it can give you the shakes, make you irritable, and keep you from sleeping. Many people don't connect their caffeine consumption with trouble sleeping; for some people, consuming any caffeine after lunch can do this. It's also mildly addictive. Regular caffeine consumers tend to get nasty headaches if they miss their morning dose. Drinking espresso, French press, or other coffee that doesn't drip through a paper filter can increase your cholesterol a few points. However, when drunk in moderation, coffee is low on the totem pole of health risks and even has a number of benefits. In addition to the gentle pick-me-up, these include the following:

Lower chance of developing kidney stones. Few afflictions are as painful as kidney stones. These nuggets of calcium, oxalate, and phosphate plague hundreds of thousands of adults each year in the United States alone. Stones form for a variety of reasons: not drinking enough water, chronic urinary tract infections, diseases such as gout, and as a side effect of some medications. Among the men and women of the Health Professionals Follow-Up Study and the Nurses' Health Study, coffee drinkers were less likely to develop these stones than non–coffee drinkers.[21] While we aren't certain why this is so, caffeine's activity as a diuretic—a substance that stimulates the body to excrete more water—may help flush out the plumbing and make urine that is too dilute to form kidney stones.

Lower chance of developing gallstones. Each year, about 1 million Americans are diagnosed with gallstones. These solidified chunks of cholesterol or bile salts can be as small as a grain of sand or as large as a golf ball. People who drink coffee aren't as prone to gallstones as those who don't partake of the bean. Exactly how coffee does this isn't exactly clear. It stimulates the gallbladder to contract regularly, and this churning may stir things up enough to prevent stone formation. Caffeine also interferes with cholesterol crystallization, a key step in stone formation. Some of this reduction in risk may come from the same metabolic benefits of coffee consumption that are related to lower risk of diabetes; gallstone formation has long been known to be part of the metabolic disorder that includes type 2 diabetes.

Lower risk of type 2 diabetes. Coffee drinking has been associated with lower risk of type 2 diabetes with remarkable consistency. A meta-analysis of twenty-eight studies that included more than 1 million men and women who were followed for an average of eleven years showed a clear connection between coffee drinking and diabetes—and the more coffee, the better.[22] Compared with non–coffee drinkers, those who drank a cup a day had an 8 percent lower risk of developing type 2 diabetes, while those drinking six cups a day had a 33 percent lower risk. Similar benefits were seen for both caffeinated and decaffeinated coffee. It is possible that the many potent antioxidants in coffee beans may be responsible.

Fewer suicides. Coffee and other caffeinated beverages act like mild antidepressants. Findings from the Nurses' Health Study, the Health Professionals Follow-Up Study, and other cohorts have shown that suicide rates are as much as 50 percent lower among coffee drinkers than they are among non–coffee drinkers.[23]

Less Parkinson's disease. Connections between coffee consumption and protection against Parkinson's disease, a debilitating neurodegenerative disorder, were first suggested at least fifty years ago. In one of the latest analyses, coffee drinkers were about 25 percent less likely to have developed Parkinson's disease.[24] The benefit peaked at about three cups of coffee a day.

Lower risk of liver cancer. Drinking more coffee has been consistently connected with lower risk of liver cancer. Substantially lower risks have been seen in Asia, Europe, and the U.S.[25] Although this is a relatively rare type of cancer in the U.S., it is more common in other parts of the world.

Hidden Calories in Coffee Drinks

All by itself, coffee is a *very* low calorie drink: an 8-ounce cup contains just 2 calories. Adding a spoonful of sugar and a tablespoon of cream turns that into a 50-calorie beverage. Drinking that three times a day is like drinking one sugar-sweetened soda. Without cutting back on calories elsewhere, that could translate into packing on 15 extra pounds over the course of a year.

The real caloric danger comes from specialty mochas, lattes, and blended coffee drinks. These are often supersized and can contain 500 calories or more. If you like such sweet coffee-based beverages, enjoy them as a treat or dessert, and stick with plain, minimally sweetened coffee for your day-to-day drink.

Lower overall mortality. Adding up all of these benefits, including a modestly lower risk of heart disease, the overall risk of dying prematurely seems to be slightly lower among those who drink three or more cups of coffee per day—caffeinated or decaffeinated—compared to those who drink little coffee.[26]

Bottom line: Given the massive body of research on coffee, it's safe to say that there aren't any major health hazards lurking in the murky depths of your cup. In short, when drunk in moderation, coffee is no threat to your health and there are, in fact, some important benefits. Some of these are due to the caffeine, but decaffeinated coffee also appears to contribute to lower risks of type 2 diabetes.

TEA

According to Chinese mythology, Emperor Shen Nung discovered how to make tea in 2737 B.C. using the leaves of the plant known today as *Camellia sinensis.* Nearly 5,000 years later, tea is right up there with coffee as one of the most consumed beverages in the world behind water. The health-promoting properties long ascribed to tea are only now receiving the careful scientific scrutiny they deserve.

Some of the benefits attributable to coffee also apply to tea, such as a gentle mental and physical pick-me-up and lower risk of kidney stones and gallstones. Some studies have suggested that drinking tea may protect against specific types of cancers, but a massive review found no clear evidence for reductions of common cancers.[27] Substances in tea called flavonoids may reduce the risk of cardiovascular disease. In the laboratory, tea and/or flavonoids improve cholesterol levels and artery function, but in real life the evidence is mixed and often contradictory.

Flavonoids aren't limited to tea. Other good sources include berries, apples, tomatoes, broccoli, carrots, and onions. It may be necessary to look at all their contributions simultaneously to determine whether or not the current enthusiasm for flavonoids is warranted.

Bottom line: For now, don't count on tea to bring any special benefits besides a reduced risk of kidney stones and a pleasant way to begin, enjoy, or end the day.

ALCOHOL

Public health campaigns have traditionally urged people to cut back on their drinking or to avoid alcohol altogether. Concerns about alcohol are definitely justified. Alcohol is implicated in about one-third of all deadly traffic accidents. Heavy drinking is a major cause of preventable deaths in the United States. It contributes to liver disease, a variety of cancers, high blood pressure, so-called bleeding strokes, and a progressive weakening of the heart and other muscles. Too much alcohol can dissolve the best of intentions and the closest relationships.

Alcohol in moderation, though, can have benefits. A drink before a meal can improve digestion or offer a soothing respite at the end of a stressful day, and the occasional drink with friends can be a social tonic. These physical and psychic effects may improve health and well-being. Well-documented benefits exist for most adults who are middle-aged or older.

Drinking alcohol helps raise levels of HDL, the protective form of cholesterol, and also reduces the formation of clots that can block arteries in the heart, neck, and brain and ultimately cause heart attacks and the most common kind of stroke. There is good evidence that these and other effects of moderate alcohol consumption translate into protection against heart disease and ischemic strokes, and much evidence that it protects against diabetes and gallstones. Keep in mind that these benefits are almost exclusively for (and mostly harm) younger individuals.

What does *moderate* alcohol drinking actually mean? That's a tricky question and a topic that is the focus of intense research. For men, study after study has shown that men who have one or two alcoholic drinks a day are 30 to 40 percent less likely to have heart attacks than men who don't drink alcohol at all. That's about the same reduction in risk seen with the powerful cholesterol-

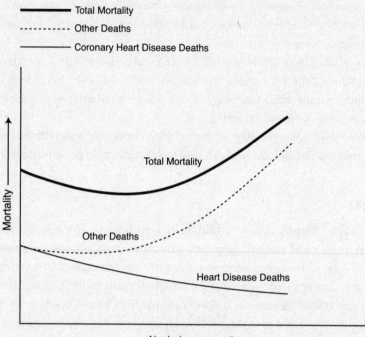

Figure 18. Alcohol and Death. Alcohol has different effects on different causes of death. As alcohol intake increases, deaths from heart disease gradually decline, while deaths from accidents, liver disease, and other causes increase, slowly at first and then sharply at high levels of consumption. The result is a J-shaped curve, with the lowest mortality associated with moderate alcohol consumption and higher mortality associated with no drinking and with excessive drinking. The optimal range for an individual depends on age, sex, folic acid intake, and other factors, but is generally considered to be one to two drinks a day for men and no more than one drink a day for women.

lowering drugs known as statins. For men with diabetes, who are at very high risk of developing heart disease, a drink or two a day has similar benefits. More than two drinks a day further increases heart and stroke protection but also increases the chances that the dark side of alcohol will emerge (see Figure 18).

For women, it is a little tougher to define moderate. Women, too, benefit from alcohol's ability to raise HDL and prevent clot formation. But the Nurses' Health Study and others have shown that two drinks a day increase the chance of developing breast cancer by 20 to 25 percent. This doesn't mean that 20 to 25 percent of women who have two drinks a day will get breast cancer. Instead it is the difference between about twelve of every hundred women developing breast cancer during their lifetimes—the current average risk in the United States—and fourteen to fifteen of every hundred women developing the disease. This is not as huge a link as that between smoking and lung cancer, but it is still enough of an increase to be worrisome.

The degree of increased risk of breast cancer is directly related to the amount of alcohol consumed. With longer follow-up in the Nurses' Health Study we detected a small increase in breast cancer even with one drink every other day.[28] It doesn't matter whether the alcohol comes from beer, wine, whiskey, or other alcoholic beverages.

Inconsistent evidence from large prospective studies of women show that the increased risk of breast cancer linked to drinking alcohol occurs mostly in women who don't consume enough of the B vitamin known as folic acid. The same applies to colon cancer, with an increased risk occurring mainly among individuals with lower intakes of folic acid. So, as I discuss in chapter eleven, taking a multivitamin that contains folic acid is especially important if you drink alcohol.

For both men and women, even moderate drinking carries some risks. Alcohol can disrupt sleep. Its ability to disrupt judgment is renowned. Alcohol, particularly in higher amounts, interacts in potentially dangerous ways with a variety of medications, including acetaminophen, antidepressants, anticonvulsants, painkillers, and sedatives. It is also addictive, especially among people with a family history of alcoholism.

So who might benefit from a daily alcoholic drink? Alcohol offers little benefit and potential risks for a pregnant woman and her unborn child, a recovering alcoholic, a person with liver disease, and individuals taking one or more medications that interact with alcohol. It doesn't benefit younger men and women, because their risk of heart disease is low and it isn't possible to bank the benefits for the future. For a sixty-year-old man with high cholesterol whose father died of a heart attack at age sixty-one, a drink a day could offer some protection against heart disease that is likely to outweigh potential harm (assuming he isn't prone to alcoholism).

The risk-benefit calculations are a bit more difficult for a sixty-year-old woman with a sister who has breast cancer. More than ten times as many women die each year from heart disease as from breast cancer—about 400,000 women a year from cardiovascular disease, compared with 40,000 a year from breast cancer. However, studies show that women are far more afraid of developing breast cancer than heart disease, something that must be factored into the equation. There's a sound basis for this fear, given that deaths from breast cancer tend to be at a younger age than those from heart disease, and that we know more about ways to help prevent heart disease than breast cancer.

The so-called French paradox—the unexpectedly low rate of heart disease in France despite a typically high-fat diet—emerged from early studies suggesting that moderate alcohol consumption could prevent heart attacks and other heart disease. Some researchers suggested that red wine was the answer, something the wine industry heavily and heartily endorsed. But red wine wasn't the only reason for lower heart disease rates in France. The overall diet and lifestyle in parts of the country, especially in the south, have much in common with other Mediterranean regions, and these almost certainly account for some of the protection against heart disease. More recent studies show that *any* alcohol-containing beverage offers the same benefits. Red or white wine, beer, cordials, or spirits such as gin or Scotch whiskey all seem to have the same effect on cardiovascular disease. Claims that the small amounts of resveratrol and other antioxidants found in red wine and grape juice prevent heart disease have yet to be proved; if they do indeed offer any extra benefit, it is likely to be small.

An individual's drinking pattern seems to be more important than the type of alcoholic beverage. My colleagues and I looked at drinking habits among almost 40,000 men whose health and lifestyles we had been following for twelve years. Those who drank alcohol at least three days a week were 30 percent less likely to have had a heart attack than men who drank less than once a week. The type of alcoholic drink and whether or not it was consumed with meals had little effect on this association.[29]

When the alcohol–heart disease connection was in its early days, the standard caution most of us used in our scientific papers and when talking to reporters or the public was that no one should start drinking alcohol just for the heart benefits. Now that these benefits are well proven and durable, I offer these more concrete guidelines:

- If you don't drink alcohol, don't feel compelled to start: you can get similar benefits by beginning to exercise (if you don't already) or boosting the intensity and duration of your activity.
- If you do drink alcohol, keep it moderate.
- A drink a day three or more times a week is far, far better for you than three or more drinks one day a week.
- If you are a man with no history of alcoholism who is at moderate to high risk for heart disease, a daily alcoholic drink may help reduce that risk.
- If you are a woman with no history of alcoholism, benefits of a drink a day may be counterbalanced by a modest increase in your chances of develop-

ing breast cancer. Getting enough folic acid (at least 400 milligrams per day) may reduce this increase in risk (see chapter eleven).

- Alcohol may be particularly beneficial if you have a low level of protective HDL cholesterol that just won't budge upward with a healthy diet and plenty of exercise.
- Talk with your health care provider to help you weigh decisions about alcohol.

PUTTING IT INTO PRACTICE

What you drink over the course of the day and your lifetime can affect your health as much as what you eat. From a purely physiological point of view, you need to drink beverages to replace the water you lose. It makes the most sense to drink water when you have a choice. Other beverages are perfectly fine as long as they don't add many calories to your diet.

- *Hydration is a day-long process.* Drink at least one glass of your beverage of choice with each meal, and one or more in between meals. Boost your fluid consumption if you are physically active or if you find yourself urinating infrequently.
- *Drink sugar-sweetened beverages such as sodas, fruit drinks, and sports drinks only occasionally, if at all.* Their liquid calories can help you unintentionally pack on extra pounds. Limit 100 percent fruit juices to one glass a day or, even better, eat the fruit whole instead of drinking its juice.
- *Adults don't need to drink milk.* Think of it as an optional part of your diet, not something you need to drink two or three times a day.
- *Coffee and tea are healthy beverages.* Just don't overload them with sugar, whipped cream, and other high-calorie additives.
- *Keep alcohol consumption moderate.* If you choose to drink alcohol, go easy—no more than one alcoholic drink a day for women, no more than two a day for men.

CHAPTER TEN

Calcium: No Emergency

F OR TWENTY YEARS THE "GOT milk?" advertising campaign urged us to drink three glasses of milk a day. Celebrities ranging from pop stars Taylor Swift and Britney Spears to Olympian Kristi Yamaguchi, model Christie Brinkley, film director Spike Lee, the Simpsons—even Superman and Batman—have sported white milk mustaches to make us aware of the dangers of not getting enough calcium while showing us the way to combat our country's "calcium emergency."

This slick, highly successful campaign was sponsored by the National Dairy

Daily Calcium Intake: Too Much?

In the United States, the current recommended daily intake of calcium intake is:

Age	Milligrams/day
1–3	700
4–8	1,000
9–18	1,300
19–50	1,000
51–70 (men)	1,000
51–70 (women)	1,200
over 70	1,200

Source: Food and Nutrition Board, Institute of Medicine. *Dietary Reference Intakes for Calcium and Vitamin D* (November 30, 2010).

Most adults don't need that much calcium, especially not from milk and other dairy foods, which also deliver unnecessary and often unhealthy extra saturated fat and calories.

Council. Too bad that its message was wrong and it ran counter to good health. For starters, there isn't a calcium emergency in the United States. In fact, Americans are near the top of the list for average daily calcium intake per person.

There's no question that calcium is an essential part of a healthy diet. But milk and dairy foods aren't necessarily the best way to get it. What's more, getting too much calcium may be harmful to long-term health for most adults.

Nutrition experts worry about calcium because they worry about the prospect of developing osteoporosis, the gradual and insidious loss of bone that often comes with old age. In the United States, osteoporosis affects 10 million women and men. Each year it causes more than 2 million fractures, including more than 250,000 broken hips. Breaking a hip in old age can be disabling, even deadly: one-quarter of older people who break a hip die in the following year, often from complications caused by their injuries.

Calcium is a key element for building and strengthening bone. But there's little evidence that boosting your calcium intake to the high level that is currently recommended will prevent broken bones. And all the high-profile attention given to calcium is distracting us from strategies that really work—like exercise, getting enough vitamin D and K, avoiding too much vitamin A, and taking certain medications.

As I describe in the next few pages, milk and dairy foods need not occupy a prominent place in your diet, nor should they be the centerpiece of the national strategy to prevent osteoporosis. Instead, the evidence shows that your dietary calcium should come from a variety of sources. And if you need more calcium, it's best to get it from an inexpensive, no-calorie, zero-saturated-fat, easy-to-take supplement. Then you can look at milk and dairy foods as an optional part of a healthy diet and take them in moderation, if at all.

WHY YOU NEED CALCIUM

Your body contains roughly two pounds of calcium, about 99 percent of it locked into bone. Think of that calcium as the mortar that cements and solidifies the components that give bone its substance and strength. The rest of your calcium is dissolved in your blood and the fluid inside and outside cells. That dissolved calcium helps conduct nerve impulses, regulates your heartbeat, and controls other cell functions.

Like an obsessive remodeler, your body constantly builds up bone and tears it down. Early in life, building up dominates. Throughout midlife, the two processes generally balance out. Later on, though, demolition may outpace construction and lead to weak or broken bones.

Calcium in Foods

Food	Amount	Milligrams	% DR*
Total cereal	1 cup	1,000	83
Milk, skim	1 cup	299	25
Orange juice, calcium fortified	6 oz.	274	23
Tofu	½ cup	253	21
Yogurt, Greek	1 container	187	16
English muffin, whole wheat	1	176	15
Collard greens, cooked	½ cup	134	11
Soybeans, boiled	½ cup	130	11
Spinach, cooked	½ cup	122	10
Almonds	1½ oz.	114	10
Whole wheat bread	2 slices	104	9
Mustard greens	½ cup	63	5
Figs, dried	4	56	5
Orange	1 medium	60	5
Swiss chard, boiled	½ cup	51	4
Kale, boiled	½ cup	47	4
Sweet potato, baked	1 medium	43	4
Butternut squash, baked	½ cup	42	4
Chickpeas, cooked	½ cup	40	3
Raisins	½ cup	41	3
Broccoli, boiled	½cup	31	3
Peanuts	1½ oz.	39	3
Black turtle beans, boiled	½ cup	23	2
Green beans, boiled	½ cup	28	2
Brussels sprouts, cooked	½ cup	28	2
White bread	2 slices	26	2
Chocolate bar	1½ oz.	10	1
Bulgur, cooked	½ cup	9	1

* Daily requirement based on 1,200 milligrams for a man or woman aged 50 years or older, but this is far higher than considered adequate by the World Health Organizaion.

Source: USDA National Nutrient Database for Standard Reference, Release 28, 2016, ndb.nal.usda.gov/ndb/foods.

Many factors influence bone remodeling. Putting a bone under repeated stress, like the stress of lifting a weight or carrying a body at a trot, triggers growth. Lack of stress, like sitting all day, leads to degeneration. Sex hormones such as estrogen and testosterone stimulate bone-building activity. The chaotic rush of these hormones during puberty sets off an adolescent's growth spurt. Their loss later in life—a gradual ebbing away in men, a more abrupt cessation in women—nudges the balance toward bone loss, a shift that can be sudden and dramatic in women. The amount of calcium available to bone-building cells, called osteoblasts, also influences bone remodeling, as do the amounts of vitamins A, D, and K. But as I will describe shortly, exactly how much calcium you need each day is a very open question.

HOW MUCH CALCIUM DO WE NEED?

We don't really know the healthiest, safest amount of dietary calcium. Different scientific approaches yield different estimates, so it's important to consider all the evidence.

Daily calcium requirements are traditionally calculated using a balance study. This is a relatively straightforward test: you assemble a group of volunteers, put them on a diet (or give them supplements) containing specific amounts of calcium for a few days or a few weeks, then measure the amount of calcium they excrete in their urine and stool. The balance point is the level at which calcium in equals calcium out. Balance studies show that about 550 milligrams of calcium a day is an optimal level for the mythical average adult.

Another route to estimating daily calcium requirements is called the maximal retention study. It, too, usually lasts only a few weeks. Volunteers take different doses of calcium and researchers try to determine the maximum amount of calcium their bodies (mainly their bones) can grab and hold on to.

Yet another piece of evidence comes from measurements of bone density using special X-ray machines before and after a year or so of calcium supplementation. These studies show an encouraging 1 to 2 percent increase in bone density. If that can be maintained for five or ten years, it would certainly help fortify the skeleton against future damage.

But there are problems with these studies. One has to do with the nature of bone itself. The small part of bone that is most able to grow and change, called the remodeling space, contains little calcium. If you greatly increased your calcium intake for a year or so—say, by drinking several glasses of milk a day or taking calcium supplements—this space would sponge up extra calcium. Your bone's calcium content would increase by a small amount, about 1 to 2 per-

Fast Fact: Osteoporosis and Men

Osteoporosis is usually portrayed as a woman's disease, but it also affects men. They make up about 2 million of the 10 million Americans with osteoporosis.

Men enter adulthood with stronger, denser bones than women, and they never face the sudden bone-draining loss of estrogen that occurs with menopause. This gives men a five- to ten-year hedge against osteoporosis, but not lifetime protection.

cent, but only temporarily. After the first year, the filled-up remodeling space wouldn't hold any more calcium, so continued calcium supplementation or a high-calcium diet would have little further effect on bone density. But it might affect other parts of the body. What's more, any gains in bone mass would be lost when the higher calcium intake stops. This phenomenon—a small, short-term increase in the calcium content of bones with no further increase after a year or so—was confirmed in a 2015 meta-analysis of fifty-nine clinical trials of calcium intake from food or from supplements. The authors concluded that the very small increases in bone density would not translate into significantly fewer spine or hip fractures.[1]

A fundamental problem is that studies lasting just a few weeks or, at most, one or two years observe only what is happening in the remodeling space—not what is really happening in the big picture of overall bone strength.

What these short-term studies fail to capture is the body's remarkable capacity to adapt. A unique study of Scandinavian prisoners, all men, shows that their bodies were still adapting after several years on a low-calcium diet (500 milligrams a day), mainly by excreting less calcium and using calcium more efficiently. In another study, conducted more than sixty years ago in Peru, prisoners who had been fed diets that gave them less than 500 milligrams of calcium a day for many years had achieved a sustainable calcium balance.

Not surprisingly, when my colleagues and I used data from a large national survey of many thousands of women and men, we saw no connection between usual calcium intake and the calcium content of bones.[2] A similar lack of association has been reported in children.

FOCUS ON BROKEN BONES

In real life, broken bones are a better measure of desirable calcium levels than the short-term flow of calcium in and out of the body or measurements of bone density.

Here's a long-recognized paradox: rates of hip fractures—the most serious type of broken bone—tend to be high in countries with high dietary calcium intake and low in countries with low calcium consumption (see Figure 19).[3]

While such country-to-country studies can't prove cause and effect, they do raise questions about the protective effects of high calcium intake. They also clearly demonstrate that a low calcium intake doesn't necessarily doom you to a broken hip.

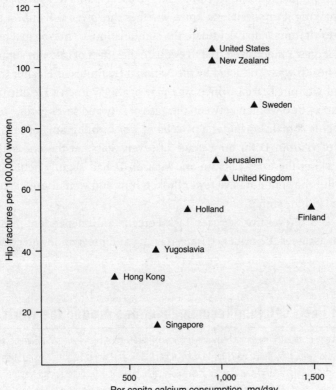

Figure 19. Calcium and Fractures. Hip fractures tend to be more common in countries with high average calcium intake, such as the United States and New Zealand, than in those with low calcium intake, such as Hong Kong and Singapore.

Some prospective cohort studies show that getting extra calcium protects against fractures, others show no benefit of getting extra calcium, and some show an *increase* in fracture risk with more calcium. The combined results from seven long-term prospective studies done in the United States, England, and Sweden that have followed large groups of people for a long time don't show any important reduction in risk of broken bones with increasing calcium intake.[4]

The findings from randomized trials are muddled, in part because some tested the effect of vitamin D in addition to calcium and others didn't. A meta-analysis of mostly small trials comparing calcium supplements without extra vitamin D to a placebo showed no real effect of extra calcium on overall risk of fractures; in fact, the risk of hip fracture was actually higher among those taking calcium supplements. In the few small trials that suggested a benefit of calcium supplements on fracture risk, the participants were also taking vitamin D, making it impossible to know whether the lower risk of broken bones was due to vitamin D, to calcium, to the combination, or maybe just to chance.

The largest randomized trial to evaluate the effect of calcium supplements on bone health was conducted by the National Institutes of Health. In the calcium and vitamin D trial, which was part of the Women's Health Initiative, more than 35,000 women between the ages of fifty and seventy-nine took daily supplements containing either a placebo or 1,000 milligrams of calcium plus 400 IU of vitamin D for an average of seven years. At the end of the trial, women taking the extra calcium and vitamin D had slightly better hip bone density. But they did not have fewer broken hips and were more likely to have developed kidney stones.[5]

The U.S. Preventive Services Task Force is an independent group of experts that assesses the evidence for screening and prevention interventions. It

Fast Fact: Calcium Recommendations Around the World

Based on essentially the same body of evidence, different countries have set different recommendations for how much calcium to take in each day. The World Health Organization says 400 to 500 milligrams of calcium a day are needed to prevent osteoporosis and fractures. The United Kingdom set the bar at 700 milligrams a day for everyone over age nineteen. Guidelines in Canada and the United States recommend that adults get between 1,000 and 1,200 milligrams a day, depending on age and gender.

recommends *against* the use of calcium supplements to prevent broken bones among postmenopausal women and says the evidence is "inconclusive" for gauging the balance of benefit and harms of calcium and vitamin D supplements among men and premenopausal women.[6]

BEYOND BONE

Although dietary calcium is mainly linked to bone strength, it plays other roles in maintaining good health.

- *Colon cancer.* Over the past two decades, studies of different types and sizes have indicated that getting more calcium from milk or supplements offers modest protection against colorectal cancer. Megadoses aren't necessary: most of the benefit comes with intakes seen in a reasonable diet, around 700 to 800 milligrams of calcium a day.
- *Blood pressure.* A calcium-rich diet or taking calcium supplements may slightly lower blood pressure, although the evidence has been inconsistent and any benefit of supplements probably applies mainly to individuals who get relatively little calcium from food.
- *Weight loss.* Drinking milk has been touted as one way to lose body fat while maintaining muscle mass. That's misleading. Scientific studies in rats and people link consuming dairy products with weight loss—*but only if calories are scaled back too.* It's the eating less, not the calcium, that's important. Not surprisingly, calcium supplements don't affect weight.[7]

THE DARK SIDE OF CALCIUM

As I described in chapter nine, drinking a lot of milk has downsides. These include consuming extra saturated fat, calories, and unneeded hormones; a likely increase in the risk of fracture later on in life when consumed during childhood and adolescence; a likely increase in the risk of prostate cancer; a possible increase in endometrial cancer; and environmental problems. Some of these findings are probably due to factors in milk other than calcium, but this is hard to determine because milk is the main source of calcium among individuals in Western countries.

How much calcium you take in matters. For example, in a 2013 meta-analysis, higher calcium intake was associated with lower risk of stroke in populations with low calcium intake, particularly in Asia, where consumption of dairy foods is low. But in populations with calcium intakes of more than 700 milligrams a day, higher intake of calcium was linked with a slightly *higher* risk of broken bones.[8] In Sweden, where consumption of milk and dairy foods is high, the risk of premature death was more than double among women with calcium intakes over 1,400 milligrams per day who also took calcium supplements.[9]

Calcium is essential for many biological functions. Humans have adapted to regulate this mineral over a wide range of intakes: If calcium intake is low, we absorb most of what we consume and excrete little in our urine. If calcium intake is high, we let much of it pass through our intestines and excrete more in urine. Aiming for 600 to 1,000 milligrams a day—a bit under the U.S recommendations—is a good target for overall health. Getting more calcium than this appears to have little or no benefit and may cause harm. I don't recommend religiously counting your milligrams of calcium each day. Later I describe how to land in this safe zone without counting.

IF NOT CALCIUM, WHAT?

Complex processes like bone health are influenced by many different factors. There's no doubt that we need some calcium to keep bones healthy. Bone health is also affected by exercise, sex hormones, and nutrients such as vitamin A, vitamin D, and vitamin K.

Exercise. A bone bends when some force is applied to it. Apply a large force and the bend turns into a break. Apply a small one and the bend is minuscule but physiologically important, especially if it is repeated again and again. That's what happens when you walk or do other exercise. Cells inside bone sense physical strain or stress and orchestrate a silent flurry of activity that remodels the bone to make it more dense and stronger. Among children and young adults, vigorous physical activity lays the foundation for a strong and healthy skeleton. The more activity and healthy stress on bones, the more bone is built. During adulthood, exercise helps maintain the balance between bone-building and bone-dissolving processes. During old age, physical activity limits bone loss.

Keep in mind that physical activity doesn't build or strengthen *all* bones, just those that are stressed. So you need a variety of exercises or activities to keep all your bones healthy.

There's no question that exercise strengthens bones and reduces risk of fractures. That has been seen consistently in study after study. What we still aren't sure of is the best combination of exercise to maintain strong bones. Some mix of weight-bearing exercises like brisk walking plus muscle-strengthening exercises like weight lifting will almost certainly turn out to be best. Not only would that combination continually stimulate bone growth, it would also strengthen muscles and improve balance and so help prevent bone-breaking falls.

Hormones. Estrogen and testosterone affect bone health. Estrogen is sometimes called the female hormone and testosterone the male hormone, even though women and men make both of them. Numerous studies have shown that these two hormones are important for building new bone early in life and for keeping it strong over the next seventy years or so. That can be a problem, because production of sex hormones plummets after menopause in women and falls off more gradually in men.

In older women, hormone therapy—usually estrogen plus a progestin—was once the first-line treatment for preventing osteoporosis and heart disease. That ended when the federally funded Women's Health Initiative showed a large increase in breast cancer, an increase in stroke, and transient elevations in heart disease with long-term use of estrogen plus progestin among postmenopausal women. Hormone therapy is still helpful in the short term for treating the symptoms of menopause, ideally without the progestin when possible. These adverse effects were not seen with estrogen alone, and estrogen alone will reduce the development of osteoporosis.

In men, the slowdown in sex hormone production isn't as abrupt or as predictable as it is in women. If there are warning signs of osteoporosis, such as an unexpected broken bone, a testosterone check is a good idea for men over age sixty-five. If the level of this hormone is low, a daily testosterone-delivering gel or patch or regular testosterone injections can bring it back up.

Don't decide to take hormones without carefully weighing the benefits and risks and sorting through the options. This is best done with a trusted health care provider.

Medications. A number of medications have been developed to shore up bone. These include bisphosphonates such as alendronate (Fosamax), etidronate (Didronel), ibandronate (Boniva), risedronate (Actonel), and zoledronic acid (Reclast); selective estrogen receptor modulators such as raloxifene (Evista); calcitonin (Fortical); a monoclonal antibody, denosumab (Prolia); and a synthetic form of parathyroid hormone, teriparatide

(Forteo). None of these work magic, restoring healthy, youthful bones, and all have their own sets of side effects. Talk with your health care provider before deciding to start taking a bone-building medication.

Limiting preformed vitamin A. You need some vitamin A for good vision, especially night vision. It's best to get it from food, not supplements.

As I describe in chapter eleven, high doses of preformed vitamin A, the kind found in many supplements, stimulate the activity of cells that break down bone. Several studies have shown that intakes of preformed vitamin A above 5,000 international units (IU)—the equivalent of 1,500 micrograms—increase the chances of losing bone density, the risk of breaking a hip or other bone, or the risk of cancer. Current guidelines recommend that men get 3,000 IU of vitamin A per day and that women get 2,333 IU.

Vitamin D. The best-known function of this fat-soluble vitamin is helping the digestive system efficiently absorb calcium and phosphorus. Vitamin D helps build and maintain healthy bones in other ways too.

Several studies have shown that vitamin D deficiencies are more common among older people with broken bones than those without them. In the Nurses' Health Study, older women who got at least 500 IU of vitamin D a day were one-third less likely to have broken a hip than women who got under 200 IU a day.[10] Results from randomized trials of vitamin D and fractures have been mixed, but trials that used 700 IU or more per day showed a benefit, while those using lower daily doses did not.[11]

The current official daily target for vitamin D intake is 600 IU (15 micrograms) between the ages of nineteen and seventy, and 800 IU (20 micrograms) after that.

Few foods naturally contain vitamin D, so you need to get most of yours from the sun or supplements. A tablespoon of cod-liver oil delivers more than 1,200 IU of vitamin D. Many multivitamins carry 1,000 IU. Some calcium supplements come with added vitamin D, which is a good idea, since there is actually better evidence for benefits from vitamin D supplements than for calcium.

Can extra vitamin D help prevent osteoporosis-related fractures? Although the evidence isn't totally consistent, extra vitamin D may be an effective way to prevent bone loss. I certainly agree with an editorial in the *New England Journal of Medicine* that succinctly concluded, "A widespread increase in vitamin D intake is likely to have a greater effect on osteoporosis and fractures than many other interventions.[12] For most people, the easiest way to do this is to take a supplement that contains vitamin D. More on this in chapter eleven.

Vitamin K. This vitamin was long thought to be needed only for the formation of proteins that regulate blood clotting. It turns out, though, that vitamin K also plays one or more roles in the regulation of calcium and the formation and stabilization of bone.[13] It is found mainly in green vegetables such as dark green lettuce, broccoli, spinach, Brussels sprouts, and kale.

Results from the Nurses' Health Study show that too little vitamin K may help set the stage for osteoporosis. Women who got slightly more than the current recommended daily intake of vitamin K each day were 30 percent less likely to break a hip than women who got less than that amount.[14]

The current recommended daily intake for vitamin K is 90 micrograms for women and 120 micrograms for men. Eating one or more servings a day of foods rich in vitamin K should give you enough of this vitamin. If you take warfarin (Coumadin) or another medication to prevent blood clots, talk with your doctor first before boosting your daily intake of vitamin K.

PUTTING IT INTO PRACTICE

The ideal prevention strategy is one that stops something bad from happening without causing other bad things to happen. Consuming plenty of calcium, mainly from milk and dairy foods, has been portrayed as a key way to prevent osteoporosis and broken bones. Not only does this fail to fit the bill as a proven prevention strategy, it doesn't even come close. The totality of evidence doesn't support the claim that getting more calcium prevents fractures over the long term, and there is plenty of evidence that drinking two or three glasses of milk a day does little to reduce the chances of breaking a bone. What's more, dairy foods pose several proven and potential problems. So if you are worried about osteoporosis, other prevention strategies make better sense than drinking more milk.

Exactly how much calcium we need for optimal health isn't completely settled. But as I described earlier, a range of 600 to 1,000 milligrams of calcium a day is a good target. Healthy people who exercise, get enough vitamin D, and have a healthy overall diet need less calcium than those on the other end of the spectrum.

Here's how to get yourself into a healthy calcium range without meticulously counting milligrams of calcium. First, almost every food you eat contains some calcium (see "Calcium in Foods" on page 194). Of course, some foods, like greens and whole grains, have more than others. A reasonable diet without milk or other dairy foods can give you about 300 milligrams of calcium a day without thinking about it. Consciously including nondairy high-calcium foods can get you into the target range. (And there are many other added benefits of eating these foods apart from their calcium content.)

Dairy is in a class by itself, with about 300 milligrams of calcium per glass of milk or the equivalent amount of cheese or yogurt. Adding one serving of milk, yogurt, or other dairy food a day will almost certainly ensure you get the calcium you need. Adding two servings a day will send you to the high end of the range, and three servings a day will put you well above the healthy range. It's one reason I don't advise drinking this much milk, along with taking in extra calories.

If you don't drink milk or eat other dairy foods, which is fine, and you worry that you aren't getting enough calcium from your diet, I suggest taking a daily calcium supplement of 500 milligrams. You don't need more than that. Keep in mind that many foods are now fortified with calcium, including breakfast cereals, orange juice, soy milk, and more. These can easily send your calcium intake above 2,000 milligrams a day. That isn't good: the National Academy of Medicine has set that as the upper limit for anyone over age fifty.

In addition, there are four things almost everyone can do to reduce the chances of developing osteoporosis and fractures:

- *Be as physically active as possible.* Engage in a variety of activities to keep your bones healthy and your muscles strong.
- *Take 800 to 1,000 IU of vitamin D a day.* Many multivitamin brands contain this much.
- *Get enough vitamin K.* You can do this by eating at least one serving of green leafy vegetables a day.
- *Don't get too much extra preformed vitamin A (retinol) unless prescribed by your doctor.* Keep your daily dose from supplements under 2,000 IU.

CHAPTER ELEVEN

Take a Multivitamin for Insurance

VITAMINS WERE ONCE THOUGHT OF as nutrients needed in small amounts to prevent diseases with exotic-sounding names like beriberi, pellagra, scurvy, and rickets. Early nutritional guidelines for vitamins focused on the amount needed to avoid these diseases. As they became rarer and rarer during the twentieth century, it seemed that the vast majority of Americans were getting enough vitamins. Getting more than the amounts needed to prevent these so-called deficiency diseases, so the thinking went, was a waste. Or, as a colleague of mine once wrote, vitamin supplements may not do much other than give Americans the "richest urine in the world."[1]

Some innovative thinking and the wonderful, logical conversation of science has been changing the way we think about vitamins, minerals, and other micronutrients. The biggest shift has been the realization that many chronic diseases, such as heart disease and some cancers, could be partly due to nutrient deficiencies, just like beriberi and scurvy. New findings suggest that some people—probably many people—don't get enough of these essential micronutrients. By increasing the amount we get, mostly from food but maybe from supplements as well, we can substantially improve our long-term health.

What blew the cover off the old vitamin-deficiency-disease connection was the discovery of a direct link between inadequate intake of the B vitamin folate (also called folic acid) and birth defects such as spina bifida and anencephaly. Both of these, collectively called neural tube defects, happen when the tissues destined to become the spinal cord, the bony tube that protects it, and the brain don't develop as they should during the first twenty-eight days of pregnancy. Spina bifida can cause paralysis and other disabilities. Children with anencephaly are born without most of the brain and spinal cord; they are either stillborn or survive for only a short time after birth. Worldwide, about 300,000 babies are born with neural tube defects each year.

Neural tube defects were most common in poor populations with poor diets. That connection prompted a search for nutritional causes. In 1976, a British team found that mothers of children with neural tube defects had relatively low levels of micronutrients.[2] Other teams discovered that drugs that interfered with folic acid also increased the risk of having a child with a neural tube defect. The not-uncommon scientific seesaw followed: some studies implicated low folic acid in these birth defects, others didn't; some small trials showed a benefit for folic acid supplements, while others didn't. In the end, two large trials gathered conclusive proof that women who didn't get enough folic acid were much more likely to have a child with spina bifida or anencephaly, and that taking folic acid supplements could prevent about 70 percent of these birth defects.[3] This was truly a remarkable achievement for a simple and cheap vitamin pill.

At first, the recommendations on folic acid were cautious. Initial guidelines from the Centers for Disease Control (CDC) in 1991 were aimed only at women who had already had a child with a neural tube defect. A year later the CDC broadened its message, recommending that *all* women who could become pregnant get 400 micrograms of folic acid a day—more than double what had been recommended before. Because many women were not heeding this advice, the U.S. Food and Drug Administration took the extraordinary step of requiring that folic acid be added to most enriched breads, flours, corn meals, pastas, rice, and other grain products along with the iron and other B vitamins that have been added for years. This has boosted the average intake of folic acid by about 100 micrograms per day.

This extra folic acid helps prevent about 1,300 neural tube defects a year.[4] There is now substantial evidence of unintended but extremely welcome side effects from folic acid fortification: less cardiovascular disease and cancer. As described later, low folic acid has been implicated in both of these.

This chapter doesn't exhaustively review all vitamins and minerals. Instead it touches on those with newly recognized or suspected roles beyond the classic deficiency diseases. Along the way, it points out how to get more vitamins and minerals in your diet and which ones you might want to, or need to, get from a supplement. The table on pages 237–239 lists the current recommended daily intake of vitamins and minerals.

WHAT ARE VITAMINS?

The classic definition of vitamin is this: a carbon-containing compound essential in small quantities for normal functioning of the body. In plainer English, vitamins are a type of nutrient your body can't make but must get from food. Vitamins are usually classified as either fat soluble or water soluble. Fat-soluble vitamins like vitamin A tend to accumulate in the body, while water-soluble vitamins like vitamin C don't.

VITAMIN A

Virtually every high school biology course covers the role that vitamin A plays in vision. It helps transform light hitting the eye's retina into electrical impulses the brain interprets as images. While that's certainly an important part of this vitamin's activity, it accounts for less than 1 percent of your body's vitamin A. Its other vital roles include helping maintain the cells that line the body's interior surfaces, boosting the production and activity of white blood cells, and directing bone remodeling. Vitamin A also helps regulate the processes by which cells split and specialize. This suggests that the body uses vitamin A to keep normal cells from turning into cancer cells and keeps cells that do become cancerous from dividing and spreading.

There are two main sources of vitamin A. Preformed vitamin A, also known as retinol, is found mainly in liver, fish oils, meat, eggs, and some vitamin supplements. The other source is fruits and vegetables rich in alpha-carotene, beta-carotene, and other so-called provitamins that your body turns into vitamin A.

Preliminary studies suggest that getting too little vitamin A may lead to a modest increase in cancer risk. They also show that once you reach a certain threshold level of vitamin A in your system, there's no benefit in getting more. That threshold appears to be in the range of the current recommended daily intakes (see "Recommended Intake" below).

As I mentioned earlier (see page 202), getting too much preformed vitamin A may harm your bones. High intakes of retinol, the active form of vitamin A, stimulates cells called osteoclasts that break down bone. Several studies have shown that intakes of preformed vitamin A (retinol) above 1,500 micrograms (5,000 IU) increase the chances of thinning bones, breaking a hip or other bone, or getting cancer.[5] Why would too much preformed vitamin A pose problems? In high amounts, vitamin A can block the effects of vitamin D, which is good for bones and muscles and has a calming effect on cancer cells.

It is easy to get too much vitamin A from supplements. I recommend avoiding vitamin A supplements unless you have a specific medical reason for them. When shopping for a multivitamin, look for one that gets all or most of its vitamin A activity from beta-carotene. Try to keep your intake of preformed vitamin A (retinol) from supplements under 2,000 IU a day.

Recommended intake: 3,000 IU for men (900 micrograms of retinol equivalents) and 2,333 IU for women (700 micrograms for retinol equivalents).

Good food sources: Food gives you either preformed, ready-to-go vitamin A or provitamin A that your body can readily convert to active vitamin A. Foods rich in preformed vitamin A—liver, fish-liver oil, eggs, and dairy products— often deliver things you don't particularly need, like extra calories and saturated fat. Provitamin A comes from several carotenoids, including alpha-carotene, beta-carotene, and beta-cryptoxanthin. Good fruit and vegetable sources of provitamin A include carrots, yellow squash, red and green peppers, spinach, kale, and other green leafy vegetables. The body absorbs carotenoids best if carotenoid-rich foods are consumed with some fat, like peppers or greens sautéed in olive oil.

Safety: Preformed vitamin A can harm bones at doses just above the recommended intake, and slightly higher amounts may increase the risks of some forms of birth defects. Considerably higher intakes have other serious effects. Provitamin A (from carotenoids in foods), on the other hand, is very safe. Taking in too much carotenoids can turn your skin orange, usually first noticeable in the palms of your hands, but this does not appear to have any serious or long-lasting implications.

THE THREE B'S: B_6, B_{12}, AND B_9 (FOLATE)

Actually there are eight B vitamins, all of them listed on the labels on cereal boxes or multivitamin supplements: thiamine, niacin, riboflavin, pantothenic acid, biotin, B_6, B_{12}, and folate (B_9). All of these help a variety of enzymes do their jobs, ranging from releasing energy from carbohydrates and fat to breaking down amino acids and transporting oxygen and energy-containing nutrients around the body. I will focus on just three of these—B_6, B_{12}, and folate—because of evidence that they may play pivotal roles in reducing heart disease and cancer.

Vitamin B_6

This vitamin is actually six related compounds. They are mostly involved with breaking down protein from food into amino acids, the building blocks used to make new proteins. Taking in too little B_6 causes a condition known as pellagra. Signs of pellagra include dermatitis (an inflammation of the skin), anemia, depression and confusion, and convulsions. Not getting enough B_6 can also increase blood levels of homocysteine, an amino acid, which may increase the risk of heart disease (see "Homocysteine and the Heart" on page 213).

Many people take extra vitamin B_6 to treat a variety of diseases and conditions, sometimes without much backing from scientific evidence. It is promoted as a remedy for premenstrual syndrome at doses far exceeding the recommended daily intake. A review of evidence suggests that 50 to 100 milligrams of vitamin B_6 a day *may* improve the physical symptoms and depression that are part of premenstrual syndrome, but the evidence for this is weak and there is no justification for higher doses.[6] Vitamin B_6 has been used off and on to treat carpal tunnel syndrome. Although there's little proof that this works, some people seem to get relief with doses of 100 to 200 milligrams.

One form of vitamin B_6 helps convert the amino acid tryptophan into serotonin, an important chemical messenger used by the brain and nervous system. Because of this connection, B_6 has been tested as a treatment for depression, attention deficit disorder, and other serotonin-related problems. Again, there's no solid evidence to show whether it works or doesn't work for these conditions.

Recommended intake: The recommended daily allowance for vitamin B_6 is between 1.3 milligrams and 1.7 milligrams/day, depending on your age and sex.

Good food sources: The average American gets much of his or her daily ration of vitamin B_6 from fortified breakfast cereals. Other good sources include meat, nuts, and beans.

Safety: Intakes of vitamin B_6 that can be achieved only by high-dose supplements—250 milligrams/day—can cause nerve damage. The Institute of Medicine (now the National Academy of Medicine) set the tolerable upper limit for vitamin B_6 at 100 milligrams/day from supplements.

VITAMIN B_{12}

Early in the twentieth century, pernicious anemia was a grim and inevitably deadly disease. It sometimes started with paleness and fatigue, which were gradually accompanied by tingling and numbness of the arms and legs, memory loss, disorientation, and even hallucinations. In some cases, memory loss, disorientation, and hallucinations were the only symptoms. In 1934, three American researchers won the Nobel Prize in medicine for their discovery that injections of liver extract effectively treated pernicious anemia. These extracts worked because liver contains large amounts of vitamin B_{12}, which is an essential ingredient for making red blood cells.

Today, full-blown pernicious anemia is uncommon. But getting too little vitamin B_{12} can still cause an array of problems, including memory loss and dementia, muscle weakness, loss of appetite, and tingling in the arms and legs. It can also lead to the accumulation of homocysteine, since vitamin B_{12} is involved in converting homocysteine into the amino acid methionine.

Because vitamin B_{12} is found only in meat and other foods from animals, deficiencies tend to crop up in vegans and strict vegetarians. In addition, as many as one in six older Americans have low blood levels of B_{12}. For many of them, the problem isn't a diet low in vitamin B_{12}. Instead, it is an inability to absorb the B_{12} in food. (The form of B_{12} in fortified food or multiple vitamins can be absorbed even when B_{12} from food is not.) By age fifty, most of us have accumulated enough B_{12} and stored it in the liver to keep us going for years, even if our capacity to extract it from food declines.

People with inflammatory bowel disease or AIDS can have problems absorbing vitamin B_{12} from food. Drinking too much alcohol can interfere with this vitamin. So do a number of drugs, including some of the acid-neutralizing drugs used to treat ulcers; colchicine, used to treat gout; and Dilantin, used to treat seizures.

Recommended intake: The current recommended daily intake for vitamin B_{12} is 2.4 micrograms/day.

Good food sources: Liver is clearly the most efficient food source of B_{12}, delivering about 23 micrograms per ounce. Other good sources include tuna, yogurt, cottage cheese, and eggs.

Safety: Although the body can handle high doses of vitamin B_{12}—the Institute of Medicine (now the National Academy of Medicine) hasn't set a tolerable upper limit—it's best not to overdo it.

Folate (Folic Acid)

Folate is the natural form of vitamin B_9. It is found in fruits, vegetables, and other foods (see "Good Sources of Folic Acid" on page 211). Folic acid is the synthetic version that's used to fortify foods like bread and cereal and is the form used to make vitamins.

As described earlier in this chapter, folate helps guide the development of the embryonic spinal cord. Pregnant women who get too little folic acid increase the chance that their babies will be born with spina bifida or anen-

Good Sources of Folic Acid

Food	Serving	Dietary Folate Equivalents*	% Daily Value**
Total cereal	¾ cup	676	169
Chicken liver, cooked	3 oz.	476	119
Centrum multivitamin	1	400	100
Cheerios	1 cup	336	84
Lentils, cooked	½ cup	179	45
Spaghetti, cooked	1 cup	148	37
Chickpeas, boiled	½ cup	141	35
Black beans, cooked	½ cup	128	32
Sunflower seeds, dry roasted	1½ oz.	101	25
Broccoli, cooked	½ cup	84	21
Lima beans, cooked	½ cup	78	20
White rice, cooked	½ cup	77	19
Beets, cooked	½ cup	68	17
Romaine lettuce	1 cup	64	16
Spinach, raw	1 cup	58	15
Orange	1 large	55	14
Wheat germ	2 tbs	53	13
Vegetable juice	1 cup	53	13
Orange juice	1 cup	47	12
Peas, frozen, cooked	½ cup	47	12
Baked beans	½ cup	46	2
Potato, russet, baked with skin	1 medium	45	11
Peanuts, dry roast	½ cup	37	9
Tofu, Firm	½ cup	37	9

* Dietary folate equivalents reflect the greater bioavailability of folic acid used to fortify foods than natural folate.

** Based on a daily value of 400 milligrams of folic acid for a 2,000-calorie-a-day diet.

Source: USDA National Nutrient Database for Standard Reference, Release 28, 2016, ndb.nal.usda.gov/ndb/foods.

cephaly. Too little folic acid also increases the likelihood of having trouble conceiving.[7]

Folate, along with vitamins B_6 and B_{12}, also helps the body break down homocysteine and so may help protect against homocysteine-related heart disease. A study from the Jean Mayer USDA Human Nutrition Research Center on Aging at Tufts University in Boston showed that, following the federal regulation that all grain products be enriched with folic acid beginning in 1998, average blood folate levels among participants in the Framingham Offspring Study (a follow-up of the famous Framingham Heart Study) more than doubled, and average homocysteine levels fell by 7 percent.[8] Folic acid deficiency, defined by blood level, has almost disappeared in the United States.

A meta-analysis of thirty randomized controlled trials that included 82,000 participants showed that getting extra folic acid from supplements decreased the risk of stroke by 10 percent and the risk of any kind of cardiovascular disease by 4 percent. The benefit was biggest among participants with low folate levels to start.[9]

Folate's key role in building DNA means that it plays a role in cell division and so may help prevent cancer as well. Getting enough folic acid seems to decrease the risk of developing colon cancer and possibly breast cancer. One of the interesting findings we have seen in the Nurses' Health Study—and that other researchers have seen in other populations—is that folic acid may temper the increase in breast cancer seen in women who average more than one alcoholic drink a day.[10] The same is true for colon cancer, another disease that is more common among alcohol drinkers than nondrinkers. People who drink alcohol and get 600 micrograms or more of folic acid each day aren't at increased risk, however.[11] This makes sense, because alcohol blocks the absorption of folic acid and also inactivates circulating folic acid.

Recommended intake: Adult women and men should get at least 400 micrograms a day of folate/folic acid, ideally from food.

Good food sources: There are many excellent sources of folate and folic acid (see the table on page 211). Most breakfast cereals are now fortified with folic acid and contain 100 micrograms per serving; some contain as much as 400 micrograms, a full day's requirement. Green leafy vegetables are an excellent source of folate, with beans, lentils, chickpeas, and black beans delivering 20 to 50 micrograms per serving. Oranges and orange juice are other good sources of folate and folic acid. Whole grains are good sources of folate, but processed grains aren't: folate is lost when grains are refined. As mentioned earlier, fortified refined flour adds about 100 micrograms per day to the average American's diet, but this varies widely depending on how much refined flour an individual consumes.

Homocysteine and the Heart

Homocysteine is a byproduct of protein digestion. High levels of it in the bloodstream have been linked to heart disease. Three B vitamins—B_6, B_{12}, and folate/folic acid—help recycle homocysteine into harmless, protein-building amino acids called methionine and cystathionine. A diet low in one or more of these vitamins leads to higher homocysteine levels and possibly an increased risk of heart disease and stroke. So getting enough folate/folic acid, vitamin B_6, and vitamin B_{12} may be one more nutritional strategy for protecting yourself against heart disease, stroke, and other forms of cardiovascular disease.

Even if homocysteine isn't a direct cause of cardiovascular disease, there's strong evidence to show that getting enough folic acid and possibly other B vitamins cuts the risk of developing this all-too-common condition.

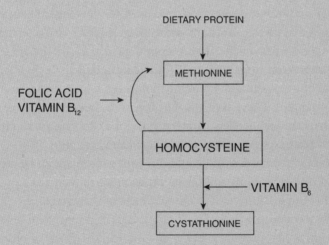

Figure 20. Homocysteine and the Three Bs. Three B vitamins—vitamin B6, vitamin B12, and folic acid—help the body turn the protein breakdown product homocysteine into less damaging substances. A buildup of homocysteine could be involved in the artery-clogging process known as atherosclerosis.

Safety: In animal studies, too little folic acid increases the development of cancer. But so does too much. These animal studies have raised a red flag that a similar effect may occur in humans. This has delayed fortification of flour with folic acid in many countries. In the United States, when folic acid fortification became mandatory in 1998, a small increase in colon cancer followed. However, this coincided with a large increase in the use of colonoscopy, which created an artificial increase in colorectal cancer due to detection of lurking tumors. Reassuringly, there was no increase in deaths from colorectal cancer. Instead, that has steadily declined, probably due in part to both colonoscopy and increased intake of folic acid. The tolerable upper limit for folic acid is 1,000 micrograms a day from supplements.

CAROTENOIDS: BETA-CAROTENE, LYCOPENE, AND MORE

Plants make hundreds of different pigments. Some trap sunlight and transform it into chemical energy; others prevent the sun's rays from damaging the plant. Some pigments advertise ripeness to the animals that will disperse the plant's seeds; others warn hungry critters that the plant contains nasty or poisonous chemicals.

One large group of plant pigments is the carotenoid family. You probably know a number of carotenoids by sight if not by name. Beta-carotene is the pigment that gives carrots and sweet potatoes their characteristic orange hues. Lycopene is responsible for the tempting red of a juicy tomato or the cool pink of watermelon flesh. Other well-studied carotenoids include lutein and zeaxanthin (the only carotenoids found in the eye's retina), alpha-carotene, and beta-cryptoxanthin. These six are just a drop in the bucket of the five hundred or so known carotenoids. Beta-carotene and alpha-carotene are vitamins, both forms of vitamin A; most others are not considered vitamins.

The human body uses carotenoids for two main functions: some of them are turned into vitamin A, and others act as powerful and adaptable antioxidants. Other important functions are waiting to be discovered.

There's a widely held notion that carotenoids in general, and several carotenoids in particular, prevent a variety of chronic ills. Dozens of observational studies show that people who choose to eat more fruits and vegetables high in carotenoids have less cardiovascular disease; cancers of the prostate, lung, stomach, colon, breast, cervix, and pancreas; memory loss; multiple sclerosis; and cataract formation and macular degeneration. Unfortunately, randomized trials in which volunteers have consumed specific antioxidants have not (so far) shown much reduction in risk of developing cancer or cardiovascular disease.

This seeming contradiction could be the result of weak studies that set up false hopes. It could mean that you need the whole complex net of antioxidants delivered by fruits and vegetables, not just one or two specific ones. It could mean that we just haven't tested the right carotenoid or carotenoid combination for long enough periods. It could also mean that many of those in the study are already consuming adequate amounts of carotenoids.

After several decades of research, some true benefits for specific carotenoids are strongly supported. There is good evidence that lutein and zeaxanthin are important for preventing macular degeneration and cataract. And a strong report from the Harvard-based Physicians' Health Study is reviving interest in beta-carotene as a supplement that can help preserve memory and thinking skills into old age (see "New Hope for Multivitamins" on page 236).

VITAMIN C

Do you reach for an orange, a glass of orange juice, or a vitamin C tablet at the first sign of a cold? If so, you aren't alone. It's an impulse nudged by *Vitamin C and the Common Cold*, written in 1970 by Linus Pauling, a double Nobel laureate and self-proclaimed champion of vitamin C. Pauling fervently believed that megadoses of vitamin C—between 1,000 and 2,000 milligrams a day (the amount in twelve to twenty-four oranges!) could prevent and abort colds . . . and could do the same for cancer.

There's no question that vitamin C plays a role in fighting infection. It helps make collagen, a substance you need for healthy bones, ligaments, teeth, gums, and blood vessels. It helps make several hormones and chemical messengers used in the brain and nerves. It is also a potent antioxidant that can neutralize the tissue-damaging free radicals that assail the body.

We've known for almost two hundred years that citrus fruits prevent scurvy, a once feared disease that killed an estimated 2 million sailors between 1500 and 1800. It wasn't until 1932, though, that vitamin C was discovered and found to be the active agent in citrus fruits responsible for fighting scurvy.

Can high doses of vitamin C fight other diseases? Not the common cold: study after study has failed to prove Pauling's proposition.[13] There's a smattering of evidence that a little extra vitamin C, about the amount found in a typical multivitamin, at the very beginning of a cold might relieve some symptoms, but there's no support for megadoses. Prevent cancer and heart disease? The evidence is thin and most studies don't support that. It's possible that some extra vitamin C might help prevent cataract formation, but here again more research is needed.

Recommended intake: The current recommended dietary allowance for vitamin C is 75 milligrams a day for women and 90 milligrams a day for men, with an extra 35 milligrams a day for smokers. As the evidence continues to unfold, I suggest getting 200 to 300 milligrams of vitamin C a day. This is easy to do with a good diet and a standard multivitamin pill.

Good food sources: Good food sources of vitamin C are citrus fruits and juices, berries, green and red peppers, tomatoes, broccoli, and spinach. Many breakfast cereals are also fortified with vitamin C.

Safety: There seems to be no harm in getting more, although the latest dietary reference intake report on vitamin C cautions against taking megadoses above 2,000 milligrams a day. But there's really no need to overdo vitamin C. Your body can't store much of it (about 1,500 to 3,000 milligrams at a time) and flushes out the excess in bright yellow urine. What's more, there's no evidence that big daily doses help. At high concentrations, vitamin C can switch roles and act like a free radical instead of an antioxidant and theoretically could cause the things you may be trying to prevent.

VITAMIN D

We are only now beginning to understand the widespread importance of vitamin D. Once known solely for its ability to help the body absorb and hold on to calcium and phosphorous, vitamin D is turning out to be far more versatile and important.

Vitamin D isn't exactly a vitamin. Instead it is a hormone made by a rather unusual gland: your skin. Sunlight striking the skin turns a cousin of cholesterol into pre–vitamin D. This is first processed by the liver and then activated by the kidneys or by cells in the heart, immune system, breast, or prostate.

Although calcium usually gets all the credit for building bones and preventing fractures, vitamin D should get equal billing. It helps on several levels. Vitamin D ensures that calcium and phosphorus (another integral part of bone) are absorbed as they pass through the digestive system. It signals the kidneys to hang on to these minerals so they aren't lost in urine. It also inhibits the breakdown of bone and boosts bone-building activity.

In chapter ten, I mentioned that many women who break a hip have an unsuspected vitamin D deficiency. A growing body of research suggests that many Americans could reduce bone loss by getting extra vitamin D. In fact, doing this more effectively reduces hip and wrist fractures in older women and men than does dramatically increasing calcium consumption.

There are other reasons to get more vitamin D besides strong bones. Here are a few of them: fewer falls, probably less cancer, as well as the possibilities of better blood pressure, a stronger heart, fewer serious infections, reduced likelihood of asthma, and protection against multiple sclerosis.

- *Stronger muscles and fewer falls.* Vitamin D signals muscle cells to make new protein. This may strengthen muscle and improve stability, especially in older people. A pooled analysis of ten randomized trials of vitamin D supplementation (200 to 1,000 IU) showed that it resulted in 14 percent fewer falls than calcium alone or a placebo.[14] However, too much vitamin D may tip the balance in the other direction. A randomized clinical trial published in 2016 showed that 60,000 IU of vitamin D given in a single dose each month increased falls compared to 24,000 IU per month.[15] Falls are the single largest cause of injuries among older people. They can lead to permanent disability, loss of independence, and even death. So determining the right dose of vitamin D is important.
- *Cancer.* In test tubes, vitamin D strongly inhibits the growth and reproduction of a variety of cancer cells, including those from the breast, ovary, colon, prostate, and brain. This means vitamin D can stifle new cancer cells much like a blanket on a small fire, snuffing out their progression to life-threatening tumors. The evidence is particularly strong for colorectal cancer. With remarkable consistency, men and women with higher blood levels of vitamin D have lower future risks of this serious cancer.[16]
- *Heart disease.* Several small studies suggest that getting more vitamin D, especially from sunlight, helps lower blood pressure. Several small and short-term trials suggest that vitamin D supplements may have some benefit for preventing heart failure—the inability of the heart to meet the body's needs for blood and oxygen—but not for preventing heart attack or stroke.[17]
- *Multiple sclerosis.* This disease, which occurs when the immune system mistakenly attacks the protective covering of nerves, is more common in countries farther from the equator, which have lower vitamin D levels. In mice, vitamin D prevents or slows the course of experimentally induced multiple sclerosis; it likely does the same thing in humans. In a study that used stored blood samples provided by 7 million men and women when they entered the U.S. armed forces, those with the highest levels of vitamin D in their blood had a 60 percent lower risk of later developing

multiple sclerosis.[18] In the Nurses' Health Study, women who took vitamin D supplements were almost half as likely to develop multiple sclerosis as those who didn't take vitamin D.[19] Also, variations in DNA that result in lower levels of vitamin D strongly predict higher risk of this disease.[20] The weight of evidence from these various lines of investigation makes a strong case that adequate vitamin D intake will reduce the risk of multiple sclerosis.

People who can bask in strong sunlight for a few minutes on most days year-round make plenty of vitamin D. That rules out everyone living north of San Francisco, Denver, Indianapolis, and Philadelphia. During the winter months, the amount of ultraviolet light hitting those northern regions (above 40 degrees latitude) isn't enough to generate vitamin D. It also rules out people who work inside all day and can't, or don't, get out for a fifteen-minute walk when the sun is high in the sky; those whose ability to get outside is limited by arthritis or other chronic diseases; and those who live in nursing homes. In other words, millions of people. Two in three Americans between the ages of fifty-one and seventy fall short of what appears to be the optimal level for vitamin D; older people fare even worse, with nine in ten not meeting this level.

The darker your skin color, the less effectively your body converts sunlight to vitamin D. In a national survey of Americans, black men and women had about half the vitamin D in their blood as their white counterparts.

The gradual loss of skin pigmentation as humans migrated northward from the so-called cradle of mankind in Africa was probably an evolutionary adaptation to capture more vitamin D from less sunlight. Yet even the near-complete loss of melanin in the skin in very fair Scandinavians isn't enough to compensate for the lack of strong sunlight, and thus many have low levels of vitamin D. Northern populations have compensated for this by eating plenty of fatty fish, including the vitamin D–rich livers, or taking cod-liver oil. The loss of such traditions may have major impacts on health.

Unless you live in the southern United States and get out in the sun most days of the week, or eat very large amounts of fish, the only way to reliably achieve the recommended intake of vitamin D is by taking a supplement. Many multiple vitamins contain only 400 IU. Don't take two a day, because the extra preformed vitamin A may work against vitamin D. Some calcium supplements contain 220 IU of vitamin D along with 500 milligrams of calcium. So one option for women is to take a standard multiple vitamin and two of these calcium pills, but this is more calcium than most women need. I don't recommend this for men because of the possible connection between high calcium intake and fatal prostate cancer. A standard multivitamin plus a specific vitamin D supplement is another option. Your best bet is to find a multivitamin that delivers 800 to 1,000 IU of vitamin D. Some of these are on the market, and I hope more will be coming soon.

Recommended intake: The current recommended dietary allowance for vitamin D for men is 600 IU a day (15 micrograms) after age nineteen. It's the same for women, except they should get 800 IU a day (20 micrograms) after age seventy. The *optimal* intake of vitamin D remains a topic of debate. I believe that the evidence shows that most people need to get at least 800 to 1,000 IU a day of vitamin D, and possibly 2,000 to 3,000 IU to get the full benefits of this vitamin. People who have darker skin or spend little time in the sun may need even more. In a 2014 study among African Americans living in Boston, increasing the daily intake to 4,000 IU offered metabolic benefits, although it did not examine actual disease risks.[21] Ongoing research will, I trust, give more precise guidance about the best daily dose of vitamin D.

You don't need regular blood tests for vitamin D, because the level varies over time and we just don't know the right target. Instead, it's best to take a vitamin D supplement to make sure you have enough on board.

Good food sources: Very few foods naturally contain vitamin D. Cold-water fish such as mackerel, salmon, sardines, and bluefish contain good doses of this fat-soluble vitamin; their livers contain very high levels. Most of what we get from food comes from dairy products (which by law must be fortified with vitamin D); vitamin-fortified breakfast cereals; and eggs from hens that are fed vitamin D.

Safety: You can't get too much vitamin D from the sun, but you can from supplements. The National Academy of Medicine says that intakes of vitamin D up to 4,000 IU a day are safe. As a fat-soluble vitamin, D can be stored and can reach very high levels in the body. Too much vitamin D can cause nonspecific symptoms such as anorexia and weight loss. It can also raise blood levels of calcium, which can, over the long term, damage the heart, blood vessels, and kidneys. In the Women's Health Initiative, use of a calcium and vitamin D supplement boosted the risk of developing kidney stones by 17 percent. This was most likely due to the calcium, as the amount of vitamin D in the supplement was low.[22]

VITAMIN E

The vitamin E story is much like the one for beta-carotene: early curiosity, intriguing laboratory results, and promising observational studies that documented a relationship between vitamin E and decreased risk of heart disease followed by disappointing clinical trials in which large groups of volunteers—mostly people already diagnosed with heart disease—were randomized to take either vitamin E or placebo pills. There are some important differences between the two stories, though. Most people get between 5 and 15 IU of vitamin E a day. Yet it takes several hundred IU a day to significantly block the oxidation of LDL cholesterol, and the biggest inhibition happens at about 800 IU a day.

Vitamin E supplements have been tested against heart disease in randomized trials such as the Cambridge Heart Antioxidant Study (CHAOS), the Gruppo Italiano per lo Studio della Sopravvivenza nell'Infarto Miocardio (known as the GISSI Prevention Trial), and the Heart Outcomes Prevention Evaluation (HOPE). Early results suggested a cardiovascular benefit of taking vitamin E supplements, but most of the later larger studies did not. For example, in the Women's Health Study, which enrolled relatively healthy middle-aged women, there was no reduction in heart attacks or cancer, among participants assigned to vitamin E, but a significantly lower risk of total cardiovascular mortality was seen.[23]

Much of the research on vitamin E has focused on its activity as an antioxidant. But it also helps reduce the tendency for clots to form in the bloodstream; such clots can trigger a heart attack or stroke. In the Women's Health Study trial, women taking vitamin E were less likely to have developed serious clots in the legs and lungs, especially those who unknowingly had a genetic predisposition to clot formation.[30]

It's hard to say why the results from randomized trials and those from observational studies don't square. There are multiple potential explanations and they will be grist for future research. With the information we have in hand right now, don't rely on high doses of vitamin E to protect you against a heart attack, stroke, or cancer.

Another possible benefit of vitamin E is protection against age-related dementia. Some early studies suggested that people who took vitamin E supplements were less likely to develop this common and troubling condition, but those findings haven't held up in further studies.[31] Another possibly promising line of research involves vitamin E and amyotrophic lateral sclerosis (also known as Lou Gehrig's disease). This rapidly progressive, invariably fatal dis-

Antioxidants: More Smoke than Fire?

On a list of the biggest nutritional buzzwords from the last couple of decades, "antioxidant" would be near the top. Before 1990 this pack of electron-donating compounds was of interest mostly to chemists and food researchers. Today antioxidants are touted in books with titles like *The Antioxidant Miracle* and *Antioxidant Smoothies*. They are promoted in herbal pharmacies and mainstream magazines as wonder substances that can prevent cancer, heart disease, memory loss, and cataracts and even reverse the aging process.

The term "antioxidant" refers to these nutrients: vitamin C, vitamin E, beta-carotene and other related carotenoids, the minerals selenium and manganese, glutathione, coenzyme Q10, lipoic acid, flavonoids, phenols, polyphenols, phytoestrogens, and more. In reality, there are probably hundreds of antioxidants in the foods we eat.

These substances guard against the constant attack of free radicals, highly reactive substances constantly generated by oxygen-using reactions such as those needed to burn fats and carbohydrates. Free radicals are present in the air you breathe, the food you eat, and the water you drink. They are plentiful in cigarette smoke, yours or someone else's. Sunlight hitting your skin or beaming into your eye also generates free radicals.

Free radicals are born missing one or more electrons, so they scavenge them from nearby DNA, important structural or functional proteins, LDL cholesterol particles, and even cell membranes. This can subtly alter the function of these substances or cell parts, or outright damage them. Over time, this damage adds up: free radicals are thought to play roles in cancer, heart disease, arthritis, cataract formation, memory loss, and aging, to name just a few health issues.

Bruce Ames, a noted molecular biologist at the University of California, Berkeley, has estimated that the genetic material in each cell of the human body gets about 10,000 "oxidative hits" a day.[24] Multiply this by the several trillion cells in your body and factor in the other cellular components that can be damaged by free radicals and oxidizing agents, and you get an idea of the magnitude of the attack.

Like marines, antioxidants stand ever ready to neutralize free radicals. Deployed strategically throughout all cells and tissues, antioxidants generously, even aggressively, give up electrons to free radicals without turning into electron-scavenging substances themselves.

No single antioxidant can do the work of the whole crowd. Taking high-dose beta-carotene or vitamin E pills is like listening to a single violin play a Mozart symphony: you get a little something but not the full, glorious effect. It's also possible that the imbalance that occurs by taking too much of any one antioxidant may be like listening to an orchestra in which one section is playing at eardrum-shattering volume.

While some initial studies were generally bullish on the benefits of antioxidants against heart disease and cancer, little or no benefit has been seen in most large, randomized controlled trials of high-dose antioxidant supplements, and harm was seen in some trials.

James Watson, who won a Nobel Prize for helping work out the structure of DNA, has even suggested that taking in loads of antioxidants from supplements may actually contribute to cancer. Free radicals help kill cancer cells. Taking an excess of antioxidants from supplements, he argues, destroys this natural anticancer activity and may prevent cancer drugs from destroying cancer cells.[25]

Two bright spots for antioxidant vitamin supplements are for eye health and brain health.

Cataracts form when damage from sunlight and free radicals clouds the clear proteins that make up the lens of the eye, much as heat clouds the clear protein in egg white. Cataracts are the leading cause of vision problems among older people. They affect more than 20 million Americans over age forty; more than half of those over age eighty have cataracts. At least 1 million cataract extraction operations are done in the United States each year, at a cost of more than $3 billion.

In the six-year Age-Related Eye Disease Study (AREDS), a combination of vitamin C, vitamin E, beta-carotene, and zinc offered some protection against the development of advanced age-related macular degeneration, but not cataracts, in people who were at high risk of the disease.[26] Lutein, a naturally occurring carotenoid found in green, leafy vegetables such as spinach and kale, and other phytonutrients may also protect vision. A new trial of the AREDS supplement regimen added lutein and the closely related carotenoid zeaxanthin.[27] Overall, lutein and zeaxanthin modestly reduced risk of advanced macular degeneration, but a large reduction in risk was seen among those who had low blood levels of lutein and zeaxanthin at the beginning of the study. Together with results from long-term cohort studies,[28] there is strong reason to get adequate lutein in our diets, but this can be achieved by including green leafy vegetables on a daily basis without supplements.

Results from the Physicians' Health Study II randomized trial showed that a beta-carotene supplement taken for more than ten years helped preserve memory and thinking skills.[29]

Bottom line: A diet naturally rich in antioxidants—meaning a diet rich in whole vegetables, fruits, grains, nuts, and other plant-based foods—will help protect you against heart disease, cancer, dementia, eye disease, and other chronic conditions. This is currently the most reliable way to get your antioxidants, along with the other beneficial components these foods contain. By relying on pills from a bottle, you run the risk of missing some important nutrients. That said, I think we should keep an open mind about other carotenoids. Supplements may be a more reliable way for many people—especially those not eating plenty of fruits and vegetables—to get healthy doses of carotenoids, Stay tuned.

ease attacks nerve cells responsible for controlling arm, leg, and other so-called voluntary muscles. In a combined analysis of large prospective studies, men and women who used vitamin E supplements for more than five years had about one-third lower risk of developing this disease compared to those who didn't take vitamin E.[32]

Recommended intake: The current recommended dietary allowance for vitamin E is 15 milligrams a day of vitamin E from food, the equivalent of 22 IU from natural-source vitamin E or 33 IU of the synthetic form. The evidence is clear that taking more than this in supplements doesn't help people with heart disease. Whether it helps otherwise healthy individuals is up in the air.

Good food sources: Some of the best sources of vitamin E are nuts, seeds, and vegetable oils such as soybean, canola, and corn oil. Green leafy vegetables and fortified cereals are also significant sources.

Safety: One meta-analysis of vitamin E trials showed that the use of high-dose vitamin E (more than 400 IU a day) might slightly *increase* death rates.[33] Headlines screamed, "Vitamin E Death Risk," but I don't believe this is so. Most of the trials in the analysis included only volunteers with heart disease. An exhaustive review of vitamin E by the Institute of Medicine concluded that vitamin E is safe up to doses of 1,000 milligrams a day (1,500 IU of natural-source vitamin E).[34] The only documented harmful effect of too much vitamin E is the worsening of a rare eye problem known as retinitis pigmentosa. One thing to be aware of: If you take a blood thinner, talk with your health care providers before starting to take a vitamin E supplement, since it can reduce the blood's ability to clot.

VITAMIN K

This fat-soluble vitamin helps make six of the thirteen proteins needed for blood clotting. Recent research showing that some of these same proteins are involved in building bone suggests another possible function: maintaining bone health. Low levels of circulating vitamin K have been linked with low bone density. A report from the Nurses' Health Study suggests that women who don't get much vitamin K are twice as likely to break a hip as women who get plenty. We estimated that eating a serving of lettuce or other green leafy vegetables a day cut the risk of hip fracture in half when compared with eating one serving a week.

According to conventional wisdom, most adults get enough vitamin K because it is found in so many foods, especially green leafy vegetables and commonly used cooking oils. That wasn't entirely backed up by a survey of vitamin K in the American diet, which showed average intakes hovering slightly under the recommended daily intake.[35] It also revealed that a fair number of Americans, particularly young ones, aren't getting the vitamin K that they need, mainly because they don't eat enough green leafy vegetables.

Recommended intake: The recommended dietary allowance for vitamin K is 90 micrograms a day for adult women and 120 micrograms a day for adult men.

Good food sources: In the United States, the most common sources of vitamin K are green leafy vegetables such as spinach, broccoli, lettuce, kale, and collard and turnip greens, as well as vegetable oils. Natto, a traditional Japanese food made by fermenting soybeans, is also rich in vitamin K.

Safety: Vitamin K from foods is very safe. The Institute of Medicine has not set a tolerable upper limit because of its low potential for toxicity. That said, people who take warfarin (Coumadin) to prevent blood clots must be careful with their vitamin K intake, because this vitamin nullifies the activity of warfarin. That doesn't mean striking green leafy vegetables from your diet. Instead, try to eat the same amount of them every day.

CALCIUM

The role of calcium, and how much of it you need, is covered in detail in chapter ten. In a nutshell, calcium is essential for health, but the high levels recommended by the Dietary Guidelines for Americans and the National Academy of Medicine aren't necessary for good bone or overall health.

Recommended intake: The current recommended daily intakes for adults are 1,000 milligrams a day for women up to age fifty and 1,200 milligrams a day after that; and 1,000 milligrams a day for men up to age seventy and 1,200 milligrams a day after that. Given the inconsistent and sometimes misleading evidence on calcium and bone health, this is probably more than enough. You certainly need some calcium each day—it's a good idea to get at least 500 milligrams—but 1,200 milligrams is probably more than you need, especially for men.

Good food sources: Contrary to the catchy milk-mustache campaign, dairy products aren't the only, or the best, way to get plenty of calcium. Other good food sources of calcium include sardines, tofu, canned salmon, turnip greens and kale, and fortified soymilk or orange juice. If you feel that you aren't getting enough calcium in your diet and want to get more, try a calcium supplement. They contain no calories and no saturated fat and are far cheaper than several daily servings of dairy products. Chewable calcium-based antacids such as Tums are a cheap and efficient way to get calcium. A calcium supplement that also includes vitamin D is even better.

Safety: A high level of calcium in the blood (hypercalcemia) can cause problems ranging from kidney stones to hardening of the arteries. Although this can happen as a result of very high calcium intake, it is usually caused by overactivity of the parathyroid glands or cancer. Consuming too much calcium can cause constipation and may interfere with the absorption of iron and zinc. As I describe in chapter ten, current evidence links higher intake of calcium from supplements with increased risk of kidney stones and prostate cancer. Calcium from foods, though, may reduce the risk of kidney stones by binding oxalate, a compound found in rhubarb, beets, spinach, nuts, tea, and a variety of chocolate and soy products, that has been linked to the formation of kidney stones.

IRON

You need iron mainly to help your red blood cells ferry oxygen from your lungs to your tissues. Iron-poor blood can leave a person pale, fatigued, and mentally sluggish. Lack of iron stunts the growth and development of children and can damage long-term thinking skills.

Iron deficiency isn't a major problem in the United States. But it is elsewhere: half of the earth's inhabitants don't get enough iron.

Most Americans get plenty of iron from eating meat and iron-fortified grain and other products. However, infants and women in their childbearing years often don't get enough iron. That's why infant formulas contain extra iron, why pregnant women are encouraged to take a multivitamin supplement with extra iron, and why women are urged to get enough iron from their diets or from supplements while they are menstruating.

There are two types of iron in food. Heme iron, which travels around the bloodstream in the oxygen-carrying protein hemoglobin, comes from red meat, poultry, and fish. Non-heme iron comes from fruits, vegetables, grains, nuts, and other plants. The body absorbs heme iron more easily than it absorbs non-heme iron, even when we already have enough iron aboard.

People who need extra iron are often advised to eat lean red meat. Meat is certainly a great source of this mineral, but it is also high in calories, saturated fat, and cholesterol. Another drawback is that your body doesn't regulate the absorption of iron from meat as carefully as it does from grains, fruits, vegetables, and supplements. If your iron storehouse is well stocked, the kind of iron in plants and supplements passes through your body. But the iron in meat slides under this mineral radar and adds to the stockpile even if your body already has plenty of iron.

That could be a problem if, as some research has shown, iron acts as a powerful generator of free radicals. A controversial "iron hypothesis" for heart disease was first floated in 1981. It suggested that the more iron you store, the higher your risk of heart disease. However, the evidence supporting this idea was weak to begin with and has gotten weaker with further studies. A similar hypothesis has been raised for cancer, and the jury is still out on that too.

Recommended intake: The current daily target for iron is 8 milligrams for men, 18 milligrams for women up until menopause, and then 8 milligrams after that. Healthy men and postmenopausal women rarely run low on iron. In fact, low iron levels in these groups are usually a tip-off of internal bleeding.

Good food sources: Good sources of heme iron include red meat, poultry, and seafood. Nuts, beans, vegetables, and fortified grain products such as breakfast cereal and bread provide non-heme iron.

Safety: If your intestinal function is normal, it's hard to get too much iron from food. However, getting big doses from supplements can irritate the stomach and cause constipation, abdominal pain, nausea, and vomiting. A large overdose can cause organ failure, coma, and even death. I recommend that men and postmenopausal women choose a supplement that doesn't contain any iron. Women in their childbearing years shouldn't take a supplement with more than the recommended amount of iron without talking with a health care provider.

MAGNESIUM

This common element is essential for hundreds of biological processes, from building substances such as DNA and proteins from scratch to releasing the energy in food, contracting muscles, and sending signals along nerves. Your heart, muscle, nerve, bone, reproductive, and other cells all depend on having enough magnesium.

In the United States, relatively few people are truly magnesium deficient. That said, Americans get less magnesium today than they did a century ago. Fewer fruits and vegetables in the diet are one reason; fewer whole grains are another. White bread and white rice, for example, contain four times less magnesium than whole wheat bread and brown rice.

Few adults meet the recommended dietary allowance for magnesium, with average intakes hovering about 100 milligrams below these targets among whites and even lower among blacks and Hispanics. Less-than-healthy magnesium levels are common among older people, who may not be getting enough in their diets or who may have trouble absorbing what they get. Magnesium deficiency can also be a problem for people taking diuretics (a type of high-blood-pressure medication) and for heavy drinkers. Diabetes speeds the loss of magnesium. So does drinking alcohol or caffeinated beverages. Caffeinated soft drinks represent a double whammy, because the phosphates found in carbonated drinks also wash magnesium from the system.

Lack of magnesium can make the body work harder to accomplish even low-intensity activities. It can also prompt abnormal heart rhythms. Some studies show that people with lower intakes or blood levels of magnesium are more likely to develop type 2 diabetes or heart disease than those who get plenty. Other studies don't show a link between low magnesium and these chronic conditions.

Recommended intake: Current nutrition guidelines recommend that men get 420 milligrams a day of magnesium and women get 320 milligrams.

Good food sources: It's fairly easy to meet your magnesium needs by food alone if you eat plenty of fruits and vegetables and whole grains. Cold breakfast cereals, which are often fortified with magnesium, are a good source. Cold cereals that are mostly whole grains are even better. Multivitamin-multimineral tablets usually contain about 100 milligrams of magnesium, which can help make up for shortfalls.

Safety: Healthy individuals have a hard time getting too much magnesium from food because the kidneys eliminate the excess in the urine. High doses of magnesium from supplements or medications can cause diarrhea, nausea, and abdominal cramping. Very large doses of magnesium, usually from laxatives and antacids, can cause dangerously low blood pressure, an irregular heartbeat, and cardiac arrest. There's no tolerable upper limit of magnesium from food. From supplements it is 350 milligrams a day for adults.

POTASSIUM

Potassium is the most abundant positively charged particle inside your cells. Your body regulates the level of potassium in your bloodstream very carefully, because too much or too little can cause problems. A drop in potassium can make you feel weak and tired, trigger extra heartbeats (especially in people who already have heart disease), and cause muscle cramps or pain. Too little potassium combined with too much sodium may also cause high blood pressure, a condition shared by more than 50 million Americans.

Most Americans would be better off getting more potassium by eating

Potassium Content of Some Foods

Food	Serving	Potassium (Milligrams)	% Daily Value*
Beet greens, cooked	½ cup	654	14
Tomato juice	1 cup	527	11
Baked beans	1 cup	509	11
Avocado	½ medium	487	0
Lima beans	½ cup	484	10
Cantaloupe	1 cup	473	10
Winter squash	½ cup	448	10
Pasta sauce, prepared	½ cup	422	9
Banana	1 medium	422	9
Spinach, cooked	½ cup	419	9
Orange juice	1 cup	378	8
Milk, 1%	1 cup	366	8
Figs, dried	large	333	7
Prunes	¼ cup	318	7
Almonds	1½ oz.	312	7
Raisins	¼ cup	309	7
Black beans, cooked	½ cup	306	7
Potatoes, russet, baked with skin	1 medium	299	6
Yogurt	7 oz.	282	6
Peanuts, dry roasted	1½ oz.	270	6
Beets, cooked	½ cup	259	6
Turkey breast, baked	3 oz.	252	5
Pumpkin seeds, roasted	¼ cup	232	5
Broccoli, cooked	½ cup	229	5
Collards, cooked	½ cup	214	5
Bran flakes	¾ cup	160	3
Wheat germ	2 tbs	150	3
Tomatoes, raw	½ medium	146	3
Coffee	1 cup	116	2

*Based on a daily value for potassium of 4,700 milligrams in a 2,000-calorie-a-day diet.

Source: USDA National Nutrient Database for Standard Reference, Release 28, 2016, ndb.nal.usda.gov/ndb/foods.

at least five servings of fruits and vegetables each day, although they may not need to hit the daily target of 4,700 milligrams recommended by the National Academy of Medicine. That target is based on very limited evidence. Low potassium is a special problem for people who take diuretics to control high blood pressure and for those who drink a lot of coffee or other caffeinated beverages, because diuretics and caffeine increase the amount of potassium lost in urine.

Getting extra potassium in your diet, from food, from potassium salt, or from supplements, can lower high blood pressure or keep blood pressure in check. In so doing, it also reduces the chances of having the kind of stroke caused by the blockage of blood flow to the brain. Although the best way to ensure an adequate potassium intake is by eating lots of fruits and vegetables. Potassium salt substitutes can be helpful to people with hypertension, those who take diuretics, and heavy coffee drinkers. Don't take potassium supplements unless you have discussed this with your physician, because they can be deadly when the kidneys aren't working properly.

Recommended intake: The recommended dietary allowance for potassium is 4,700 milligrams a day for adults.

Good food sources: Bananas are famous for the amount of potassium they contain. But many other fruits and vegetables are also good sources. These include apricots, dates, kidney beans, oranges, spinach, nuts, seeds, and whole grains (see the table on page 228).

Safety: The Food and Nutrition Board of the National Academies of Sciences, Engineering, and Medicine hasn't set an upper limit for potassium. It is almost impossible to get too much from natural foods if your kidneys are working properly. If they aren't, then you need to watch your potassium intake and have your blood level monitored. That's because too much potassium in the bloodstream can cause deadly heart rhythms.

SODIUM

Sodium has gotten more attention than almost any other micronutrient. Sodium is an essential part of our diet, but most Americans get more than they need. It's hard not to. Prepared foods are often loaded with table salt, which is one-third sodium. A cup of boxed macaroni and cheese or an order of Burger King salted french fries can deliver more than 1,000 milligrams of sodium—most of a day's healthy ration. It's also often found where you least expect it: a cup of pasta sauce can have almost half of a day's healthy salt allotment (see "Hidden Salt in Food" on page 230).

Although the "daily value" for sodium listed on food labels is 2,300 mil-

Hidden Salt in Food

Food	Serving	Sodium (Milligrams)	% Maximum Recommended Daily Limit*
Kielbasa, pan-fried	1 link	3,870	168
Arroz con grandules (restaurant)	1 order	3,807	166
Orange chicken (restaurant)	1 order	3,583	156
Applebee's crunchy onion rings	1 serving	2,916	127
Vegetable chow mein (restaurant)	1 order	2,673	116
Kung pao chicken with rice	2 cups	2,610	113
Ham sandwich with mayo and tomato	6 inches	2,130	93
Burger King Whopper with cheese	1	1,431	62
Chicken pot pie	1 small	1,187	52
Canned sauerkraut	1 cup	939	41
Baked beans, canned	1 cup	871	38
Dill pickles	1 (3 oz.)	833	36
Chicken noodle soup, canned	1 cup	831	36
Corned beef brisket	3 oz.	827	36
Tuna salad submarine sandwich	6 inches	780	34
Cheese pizza, pepperoni	1 slice	773	34
Macaroni and cheese, canned	1 cup	737	32
Lasagna, frozen	1 serving	639	28
Pasta sauce, prepared	½ cup	577	25
KFC biscuit	1	540	23
American cheese	1 slice	468	20
Green beans, canned	1 cup	461	20
Cottage cheese	½ cup	459	20
Vegetable juice cocktail	1 cup	428	19
Light tuna, canned	3 oz.	337	15
McDonald's french fries	large	290	13
Waffle, frozen	1	223	10
Raisin bran cereal	1 cup	210	9
Frozen peas	½ cup	58	3

* Based on a daily value for sodium of 2,300 milligrams in a 2,000-calorie-a-day diet.

Source: USDA National Nutrient Database for Standard Reference, Release 28, 2016, ndb.nal.usda.gov/ndb/foods.

ligrams, the average person actually needs less than 1,000 milligrams a day to keep his or her systems in good working order. That's less than half a teaspoon of salt. Yet the average American gets more than three times that amount, about 3,500 milligrams of sodium. The excess is excreted, but not always before it can do some damage. Excess sodium pulls water from cells and thus increases blood pressure, especially in people whose genes make them more sensitive to salt.

Scientists agree that consuming too much sodium promotes high blood pressure. Whether reducing sodium reduces the risk of cardiovascular disease has been controversial, but the overall evidence strongly supports a benefit of limiting sodium intake, even though the optimal target is not clear. Cutting back on sodium is often one of the first things that health care providers suggest to people who have just been diagnosed with high blood pressure, along with stopping smoking and getting more exercise. For years, the results of salt reduction studies were inconsistent and controversial. But the Dietary Approaches to Stop Hypertension (DASH) II study, which carefully controlled the amount of salt in participants' diets, showed that aggressively cutting back on salt had an important effect on blood pressure.[36] This has been supported by other carefully controlled studies. As described in chapter eight, the first DASH trial also clearly showed that eating more fruits and vegetables can substantially lower blood pressure.

Documenting the "best" sodium intake has been difficult. One reason is that it's hard to measure how much sodium individuals consume because this mineral is hidden in so many processed foods. In addition, long-term trials of sodium intake are difficult to do because keeping people on low-sodium diets is difficult in an era when high-sodium and hidden-sodium foods are everywhere.

The most effective way to keep blood pressure low combines weight loss (if needed), eating plenty of fruits and vegetables rich in potassium, and staying away from foods high in salt.

The bottom line is that a salty diet doesn't do you any good and can be harmful, so cutting out unnecessary salt makes sense.

Recommended intake: The National Academy of Medicine and the 2015–2020 *Dietary Guidelines for Americans* recommend getting no more than 2,300 milligrams of sodium a day. The American Heart Association, meanwhile, recommends getting no more than 1,500 milligrams a day. The rationale for a lower target is that further decreasing sodium intake to that level helps further reduce blood pressure, which is a strong risk factor for cardiovascular disease.

Good food sources: Sodium isn't the kind of nutrient you need to look for—it finds you. Rather than searching for foods that are *good* sources of sodium, most people need to seek low-sodium foods. Almost any unprocessed food—vegetables, fruits, grains, nuts, meats, dairy foods and the like—are low in sodium.

Safety: The Food and Nutrition Board set 2,300 milligrams of sodium a day as its upper limit. More than that isn't immediately harmful but can nudge you toward developing high blood pressure, which over a lifetime affects 90% of Americans.

SELENIUM

The mineral selenium is a potent antioxidant, but it probably doesn't contribute to good health in that way. Instead, it helps several enzymes break down peroxides, powerful oxidizing agents made throughout the body that can damage DNA and tissues.

To date, there's no convincing evidence to show that, in the United States, too little selenium increases the risk of cancer or other chronic conditions or that taking a selenium supplement prevents them. In the 1980s, selenium was added to fertilizer in Finland, where the soil level—and thus intake—were low. Although blood levels of selenium rose dramatically, cancer rates didn't budge. The Nutritional Prevention of Cancer study showed that taking extra selenium, 200 micrograms a day, may have offered some protection against skin cancer.[37] However, the Selenium and Vitamin E Cancer Prevention Trial (SELECT), established to look at prostate cancer, did not support the finding on skin cancer. It failed to answer the question about selenium and prostate cancer because only one case of fatal prostate cancer occurred during the trial.[38]

In some regions of China and other parts of the world with very low soil levels of selenium, low intakes of this mineral has led to a unique form of heart disease.

Recommended intake: The recommended dietary allowance for selenium is 55 micrograms a day for adults.

Good food sources: Many foods contain selenium. Brazil nuts, seafood, beef, eggs, and spinach are good sources, but their selenium content depends on the soil levels or feed used to produce the food.

Safety: Selenium is toxic at high doses, with a tolerable upper intake of 400 micrograms a day for adults. As with other micronutrients, it's hard to take in that much selenium from food. Getting too much from supplements can cause brittle hair and nails, upset stomach, skin rash, bad breath, and extreme exhaustion. Some types of Brazil nuts deliver a lot of selenium because of the high levels in the soil where they are produced. If you frequently consume them, try to eat a variety of nuts instead so you don't get too much selenium.

ZINC

You may have seen the "cold-fighting zinc lozenges" near the checkout counter of your local pharmacy or grocery store. These lozenges have been the topic of many trials to determine whether they truly shorten the duration of colds. More than a dozen studies have been conducted among people just developing colds, some of whom took zinc and some of whom didn't. The results have been inconsistent. However, in two recent meta-analyses, cold sufferers who popped the unpleasant-tasting zinc lozenges reduced their symptoms by about one to two days on average compared with those taking placebo lozenges.[39]

There's no question that zinc plays a key role in keeping the immune system healthy. It also acts as an antioxidant, is needed for proper vision, and is involved in blood clotting, wound healing, and the normal development of sperm cells. Does this mean you should reach for a zinc supplement? No. Despite the fact that most Americans actually get less than the recommended daily amount of zinc, there's little evidence that such low intakes cause health problems. Studies looking at colon cancer, prostate cancer, prostate inflammation (prostatitis), and macular degeneration have not shown a clear link with zinc intake.

Some people need extra zinc. Children need enough of this mineral for growth and development. Too little zinc may be one of the ways that undernourishment slows brain development and motor skills, contributes to hyperactivity, and causes problems with attention. Older people may need extra zinc for several reasons. They tend to consume less zinc than younger people. They often have trouble absorbing zinc from food. The medications they take, especially diuretics for high blood pressure, can increase zinc excretion. And the extra fiber and calcium they may take can bind zinc and make it unavailable to the digestive system. Heavy drinkers, people with digestive problems such as Crohn's disease and ulcerative colitis, and those with chronic infections also need extra zinc.

Recommended intake: The recommended dietary allowance for zinc is 8 milligrams a day for women and 11 milligrams a day for men. Women who are pregnant or breastfeeding need a bit more (12 milligrams a day instead of 8) for themselves and the children they are carrying or feeding.

Good food sources: If you like oysters, they are a go-to food for zinc. They contain more zinc per serving than any other food. Poultry, crab and lobster, beans, nuts, whole grains, fortified breakfast cereals, and dairy foods such as milk and yogurt are also good sources.

Safety: Overdosing on zinc can depress the immune system, interfere with wound healing, cause problems with taste and smell, and lead to hair loss and skin problems. High zinc intake may also promote the development or growth of prostate cancer. The advantage of getting your zinc from food, rather than from supplements or lozenges, is that it's hard to get too much from food. Getting more than 15 milligrams a day of zinc from supplements isn't a good idea unless it is for a specific medical condition.

PUTTING IT INTO PRACTICE

You pay top dollar to insure your home and your car. You may even have the kind of life insurance you'd rather not have a loved one collect. A far cheaper and more personally gratifying kind of life insurance comes from a daily multivitamin with added minerals.

Research is pointing ever more strongly to the conclusion that several ingredients in a standard multivitamin—especially vitamins B_6 and B_{12}, folic acid, vitamin D, and beta-carotene—are essential players in preventing heart disease, cancer, osteoporosis, memory loss, and other chronic diseases. A year's supply costs under $40, or about a dime a day. That's an excellent nutritional bang for your buck.

I use the term "insurance" for good reason. A multivitamin can't in any way replace healthy eating. It gives you barely a scintilla of the vast array of healthful nutrients found in food. It doesn't deliver any fiber. Or taste. Or enjoyment. The only thing it can do is offer a nutritional backup or fill in the nutrient holes that can plague even the most conscientious eaters. For example, eating more fruits and vegetables is great, but it won't give you much in the way of vitamin D. Adding more whole grains to your diet is also wonderful, but it won't net you much vitamin B_6. Older people and those with digestive problems may not be able to absorb enough vitamin B_{12} from food. Those who regularly drink alcohol may need extra folic acid to make up for alcohol's folate-reducing effects. So taking a daily multivitamin is a safe, rational plan that complements good eating but can never replace it.

Here are the eight vitamins and minerals that many people don't get enough of from their diets, so it make sense to get them via a standard multivitamin-multimineral pill:

- beta-carotene
- folic acid
- vitamin B6
- vitamin B$_{12}$
- vitamin D
- vitamin E
- iron
- zinc.

Taking a multivitamin-multimineral pill every day is a reasonable option that provides a wider nutritional safety net. For menstruating women, especially those who eat little or no red meat, a multivitamin-multimineral supplement will provide their extra iron requirements. Also, the folic acid in this pill will fulfill the recommendation by the Centers for Disease Control that all women who might possibly become pregnant should take supplemental folic acid to minimize the risk of neural tube birth defects.

You don't need a designer vitamin, a name-brand vitamin, or an "all-natural" formulation. A standard, store-brand, RDA-level multivitamin is a perfectly fine place to start. Look for labels that say the product meets the standards of the United States Pharmacopeia (USP). This organization sets manufacturing standards for medications and supplements sold in the United States. The less preformed vitamin A (retinol) in the multivitamin and the more beta-carotene, the better. Choose a supplement that contains no more than 2,000 IU of preformed vitamin A.

For most men and women, an extra vitamin E supplement is okay. Even though the ending hasn't yet been written to the vitamin E story, at least 400 milligrams a day, and possibly more, may be needed for optimal health. Standard multivitamins contain only 30 IU.

Extra vitamin D is definitely worth pursuing. Standard multivitamins offer 400 to 600 IU, half of what appears to be needed for optimal health.

Some companies make supplements that replace most of the preformed vitamin A with beta-carotene and contain adequate doses of vitamin D. I recommend looking for one of these, because it is too easy to get too much preformed vitamin A. One example is the Basic One multivitamin formulated by Dr. Kenneth Cooper, founder of the Cooper Clinic in Dallas. It contains plenty of vitamin A (2,000 IU), all in the form of beta-carotene, along with 2,000 IU of vitamin D and 200 IU of vitamin E. Menstruating women should get the version that includes iron, which men and postmenopausal women don't need.

So far there's no consensus on ideal vitamin intakes because scientific knowledge about them is still evolving. We could definitely use more evidence about the true benefits of the commonly used vitamins. At the same time, harm isn't likely when they are taken in reasonable doses, and the cost is minimal. In this situation, it seems to be a bit foolish to demand that all the evidentiary *i*'s be dotted and *t*'s be crossed before acting.

New Hope for Multivitamins

Most vitamin studies have looked at individual vitamins, like folic acid or vitamin E, or combinations of antioxidants, with or without minerals. The Physicians' Health Study II took a different path: it examined the health effects of a standard, over-the-counter, multivitamin-multimineral supplement (Centrum Silver). The results were promising.

The researchers recruited more than 14,000 older male physicians. Half took Centrum Silver for up to fourteen years, while the other half took an identical-looking placebo. At the end of the trial, there was an 8 percent reduction in the risk of developing any type of cancer in the multivitamin group compared to the placebo group.[40] Much of this was due to a reduction in risk of colorectal cancer as predicted by previous prospective cohort studies.

The multivitamin-multimineral supplement didn't appear to help prevent cardiovascular disease or protect memory or thinking skills.[41]

Two things about this trial make it noteworthy: It would never have uncovered a connection between multivitamin use and cancer, especially colorectal cancer, if the study hadn't lasted longer than ten years, which is longer than most vitamin trials. In addition, the participants were probably the best-nourished group of men ever studied, and despite that a benefit was seen for a daily multivitamin. It is likely that the benefits would have been more extensive in a group that was less well nourished.

Recommended Daily Intake of Vitamins and Minerals for Adults (Established by the Institute of Medicine)

Vitamin (Common Names)	Recommended Dietary Allowance (RDA) or Daily Adequate Intake (AI)*		Upper Limit
	Women	Men	
Vitamin A (preformed = retinol; beta-carotene can be converted to vitamin A)	700 micrograms (2,333 IU)	900 micrograms (3,000 IU)	3,000 micrograms (about 10,000 IU)
Thiamin (vitamin B₁)	1.1 milligrams	1.2 milligrams	Not known
Riboflavin (vitamin B₂)	1.1 milligrams	1.3 milligrams	Not known
Niacin (vitamin B₃, nicotinic acid)	14 milligrams	16 milligrams	35 milligrams
Pantothenic acid (vitamin B₅)	5 milligrams*	5 milligrams*	Not known
Vitamin B₆ (pyridoxal, pyridoxine, pyridoxamine)	19–50: 1.3 milligrams 51+: 1.5 milligrams	19–50: 1.3 milligrams 51+: 1.7 milligrams	100 milligrams
Vitamin B₁₂ (cobalamin)	2.4 micrograms	2.4 micrograms	Not known
Biotin	30 micrograms*	30 micrograms*	Not known
Vitamin C (ascorbic acid)	75 milligrams* *(Smokers: Add 35 milligrams)	90 milligrams*	2,000 milligrams
Choline	425 milligrams*	550 milligrams*	3,500 milligrams
Vitamin D (calciferol)	19–50: 55 micrograms (200 IU) 51–70: 10 micrograms (400 IU) 71+: 15 micrograms (600 IU)	19–50: 15 micrograms (2,000 IU) 51–70": 1- micrograms (400 IU) 71+: 15 micrograms (600 IU)	1000 micrograms (4,000 IU)

Vitamin (Common Names)	Recommended Dietary Allowance (RDA) or Daily Adequate Intake (AI)*		Upper Limit
	Women	**Men**	
Vitamin E (alpha-tocopherol)	15 milligrams (15 milligrams equals about 22 IU from natural sources of vitamin E and 33 IU from synthetic vitamin E)	15 milligrams	1,000 milligrams (nearly 1,500 IU natural vitamin E; 2,200 IU synthetic)
Folic acid (folate, folacin)	400 micrograms	400 micrograms	1,000 micrograms
Vitamin K (phylloquinone, menadione)	90 micrograms*	120 micrograms*	Not known

Mineral	Recommended Amount (Daily RDA or Daily AI)		*Upper Limit
	Women	**Men**	
Calcium	31–50: 1,000 milligrams; 51+: 1,200 milligrams	31–70: 1,000 milligrams; 51+: 1,200 milligrams	2,500 milligrams
Chloride	19–50: 2.3 grams*; 51–70: 2.0 grams*; 701+: 1.8 grams*	19–50: 2.3 grams*; 51–70: 2.0 grams*; 70+: 1.8 grams*	Not known
Chromium	31–50: 25 micrograms*; 51+: 20 micrograms*	31–50: 35 micrograms*; 51+: 30 micrograms*	Not known
Copper	900 micrograms	900 micrograms	10,000 micrograms
Fluoride	3 milligrams	4 milligrams	10 milligrams
Iodine	150 micrograms	150 micrograms	1,100 micrograms
Iron	31–50: 18 milligrams; 51+: 8 milligrams	31–50+: 8 milligrams; 51+: 8 milligrams	45 milligrams

Nutrient			
Magnesium	19-30: 310 milligrams 31-70+: 320 milligrams	19-30: 400 milligrams 31-70+: 420 milligrams	350 milligrams from supplements
Manganese	1.8 milligrams*	2.3 milligrams*	11 milligrams
Molybdenum	45 micrograms	45 micrograms	2,000 micrograms
Phosphorus	700 milligrams	700 milligrams	31-70: 4,000 milligrams 71+: 3,000 milligrams
Potassium	4,700 milligrams*	4,700 milligrams*	Not known
Selenium	55 micrograms	55 micrograms	400 micrograms
Sodium	19-50: 1,500 milligrams* 51-70: 1,300 milligrams* 70+: 1,200 milligrams*	19-50: 1,500 milligrams* 51-70: 1,300 milligrams* 70+: 1,200 milligrams*	Not determined
Zinc	8 milligrams	11 milligrams	40 milligrams

* RDA: the average daily dietary intake sufficient to meet the nutrient requirement of 97–98 percent of healthy individuals in a particular group according to stage of life and gender. AI: a recommended intake when an RDA can't be determined. Micronutrients with AIs are noted by *.

CHAPTER TWELVE

The Planet's Health Matters Too

W HAT YOU AND I EAT unquestionably affects our individual health. What we eat collectively affects the health of our planet and thus the health of our children, grandchildren, and future generations. In the first edition of this book, published sixteen years ago, climate change was becoming a global concern. I included a few paragraphs on the effects of different dietary choices on the production of greenhouse gases and other environmental impacts. What we have experienced and learned since then has made climate change a major and urgent issue. We don't need sophisticated measurements or statistical models to know this is happening; it is happening right before our eyes.

When I first worked in Tanzania as a medical student in the 1960s, the top of Mount Kilimanjaro was covered in snow year-round. Today, that snow has almost disappeared and will soon be gone. Icebergs are retreating and vanishing around the world. The Arctic Ocean is becoming open for shipping on an annual basis. Deadly storms, droughts, floods, and other extreme weather events are occurring with increasing regularity.

Why mention this in a book on healthy eating? Climate directly affects food production, and food production can affect climate and the environment.

THREE KEY ISSUES

Growing your own food in a hand-tended garden has minimal effect on the environment, especially if you use just the right amount of natural fertilizer, rely on natural strategies to control weeds and pests, and grow only as much as you need. But few of us are able to get most of the food we need this way. Understanding how food is produced, and then making small changes in the food you buy and eat, can help lighten your carbon footprint on the planet.

Farming and food production can harm the environment in many ways. Here are four of the most important:

Climate change. Fossil fuels are burned to make fertilizer and pesticides, pump irrigation water, plow fields, harvest crops, process food, and transport it—sometimes thousands of miles. Burning fossil fuels generates carbon dioxide, the main greenhouse gas responsible for trapping heat in the atmosphere. On top of this, cattle, sheep, and other ruminant animals grown for food generate and release methane as part of their natural digestive process. This gas is twenty-five times more powerful than carbon dioxide at trapping heat.

Feeding grain that has been produced by industrial farming to cattle, which convert it to meat or milk, is far less energy efficient and produces more greenhouse gases than eating that grain directly. In an American feedlot, it takes between 15 and 20 pounds of grain to produce 1 pound of beef.

Although the numbers vary depending on how emissions are calculated, the U.S. Environmental Protection Agency estimated that, in 2015, agriculture was responsible for 7.9 to 9 percent of the country's emissions of carbon dioxide and methane, the two leading greenhouse gases.[1] Between 80 and 90 percent of this is the result of food production; the rest comes from packaging, refrigeration, and transportation. The members of the 2015–2020 Dietary Guidelines Scientific Advisory Committee, after their initial report was censored by industry-influenced members of Congress, independently published an updated review on the environmental effects of dietary choices.[2]

Water contamination and depletion. American agriculture also creates water pollution. Fertilizer, herbicides, and pesticides run off farmland into rivers and lakes and eventually make their way into the oceans. Manure from animal feedlots and from fish farming does the same thing. The influx of nutrients often causes huge blooms of algae. These can produce toxins that can harm other aquatic organisms, livestock, pets, and even humans. Decomposition of dying and dead algae can use up most or all of the oxygen in the water, which kills fish and other aquatic animals. The Gulf of Mexico is just one example of this. As the Mississippi River flows from Minnesota to Louisiana, it picks up nutrient-rich runoff from much of the United States' agriculture belt and deposits it in the Gulf. In the summer of 2016, the algae bloom and subsequent die-off created a dead zone along the continental shelf along the coasts of Louisiana and east Texas that was nearly 7,000 square miles, or about the size of the state of Connecticut.

In some regions of the world, water is pulled from aquifers (underground layers of rock that hold water) to irrigate crops faster than it is replaced by rain and runoff. In parts of California and the Midwest, this is forcing farmers to drill ever-deeper wells. In India, heavy demand for this underground water is depleting the aquifers, bankrupting farmers and making it difficult for some villages to get drinking water.

Species extinction. Industrial agriculture is also contributing to the extinction crisis—the loss of species around the globe. Some of this is through the use of pesticides and herbicides. In addition, it is also turning diverse landscapes into monocultures. When visiting a meadow near our summer cabin in New Hampshire, my wife, Gail, and I could always be sure we could show our children countless monarch butterflies—until a few years ago. Despite plenty of milkweed, the favored food of these beautiful creatures, their numbers have dwindled: two years ago we found just three or four monarchs and last year saw none. Flying from the East Coast to the West on a clear day provides a picture of the problem: vast fields of crops without the natural habitat needed for monarchs to complete their yearly migration. I also see this when visiting the Willett family farm in Michigan: what were once small fields and hedgerows teeming with diverse life are now massive monocultures of corn and soy.

Monarchs are just one highly visible species in this vulnerable situation—and they still can be saved. However, scientists have documented that we are now in an age of unprecedented species extinction with somewhere between 200 and 2,000 species lost every year. This is an indication of the pressures that our agricultural system is putting on our environment. Narrowing biological diversity will reduce the resilience of ecosystems to survive.

SUSTAINABLE FOOD PRODUCTION

Climate change isn't something that will theoretically affect the way people live many generations into the future. These changes are occurring at a rate far faster than what was estimated just a few years ago and are already affecting the lives of many people today. Almost every year, with a few fluctuations, the world is setting new records for temperature. If we continue to careen down the track we are on, by 2100—well within the lifetime of the next generation—global warming will change the face of the world and the ability of many populations to survive.

One recent model predicts that current trends in temperature increases will cause sea levels to rise by six feet, possibly as soon as 2100, putting about one-third of Boston under water regularly.[3] Even half of that rise in the sea level would have enormous consequences. We can build dikes in Boston, but low-lying regions such as Florida, Malaysia, Bangladesh, Senegal, and other coastal areas can't do this for geological or financial reasons.

Climate change has already slowed the increase in food production, a worrisome trend that will only increase. The continued growth of the world's population, meaning there will be more and more people to feed, will only further stress food production and the environment. Because fertility rates haven't declined as rapidly as predicted, the United Nations now predicts that the world's population will increase to 9.7 billion people by 2050.[4]

These trends have created the triple challenge of feeding *more* people a *healthy diet* in a *sustainable* way. That's a tall order, especially when 1 billion people around the globe don't get enough food to eat and the diets of billions more in developed countries don't meet national dietary guidelines. Making more food using current agricultural practices will further degrade water and land quality and create even more greenhouse gases.

Although the challenges facing us are daunting, the Sustainable Development Goals recently released by the United Nations (https://sustainabledevel opment.un.org/sdgs) describe a way forward. I served on one of the dozen committees (focusing on health) that contributed to the creation of these goals. One of the high-priority items on the agenda is the development of sustainable food systems that can feed additional billions of people. Although details of such food systems haven't yet been proposed, a sustainable food system would be one that can maintain healthy bodies without degrading land and water resources and that reverses or eliminates greenhouse gas production.

The Paris agreement of 2015,[5] which focused on climate change, provided some specifics about sustainable food production. To avoid calamity, by 2050 food systems should have a close to zero net impact on greenhouse gas production. There's no single remedy for reining in greenhouse gas production by agriculture. One step will be limiting consumption of red meat, poultry, fish, and other food from animals, which generates far more greenhouse gases than does eating food from plants. Another step is limiting the use of fossil fuels in the production of food. Emphasizing local production of seasonal fruits and vegetables will also play a role.

That is far from the current trend of increasing production of greenhouse gases due to food production, and will be difficult to achieve as newly affluent countries like China increase their consumption of meat.

I now cochair the EAT-Lancet Commission,[6] which was assembled to investigate connections between diet, human health, and the health of the planet. We were charged with providing details on how the world can sustainably feed its growing population. Many of the solutions are based on the healthy eating principles I have been talking about in this book. What we've learned so far is that we won't be able to achieve the Sustainable Development Goals without large investments by all countries of the world in education, primary health care, clean energy, and agriculture, and with billions of small, individual investments in eating less meat and eating more sustainably produced grains, fruits, and vegetables.

CONTRIBUTE TO THE EFFORT

Although these urgent global issues can seem overwhelming, together we can make a difference. Our daily personal food choices collectively have important effects on the environment. These personal changes are the focus of this chapter. Fortunately, choices that benefit planetary health are well aligned with individual health and well-being.

Eat Less Red Meat and Dairy Foods

The single most important step you can take to limit your carbon footprint is to eat less red meat and dairy foods.

Feeding grain to cattle to make steaks and hamburgers instead of just eating that grain wastes a lot of energy. That inefficiency is less important when cattle graze on plants growing all by themselves on land that isn't usable for much else, although these cattle still produce methane every hour of every day they are alive. More and more, though, we eat beef, pork, chicken, and fish that have been grown for us. They've been fed corn and other grains sowed and reaped specifically for this purpose, which require increasingly large amounts of petroleum, fertilizers, herbicides, and pesticides to produce. The concentrated wastes from feedlots also pose substantial pollution problems. The antibiotics routinely fed to animals raised for food poses a different kind of health problem (see "Antibiotic Resistance: A New Dietary Hazard" on page 142).

While beef represents just 4 percent of the United States' retail food supply, it accounts for 36 percent of all diet-related greenhouse gas emissions.[7] Making a pound of lamb generates five times more greenhouse gases than making a pound of chicken and thirty times more than making a pound of lentils.[8]

One very persuasive number is the total environmental cost of producing protein. The Union of Concerned Scientists has calculated that one pound of beef creates seventeen times more water pollution and twenty times more habitat alteration than 1 pound of pasta.[9]

Dietary Guidelines Drop the Ball Again

The scientific panel chosen to advise the federal government for the 2015–2020 update of the *Dietary Guidelines for Americans* recommended that Americans should eat diets that require fewer resources to produce—and specifically recommended eating less red meat for both human and planetary health, exactly what I recommend in this book.[10] That statement was immediately criticized by the North American Meat Institute and other organizations, which claimed that the advisory panel had gone beyond "its scope and expertise," despite the fact that the advisory panel and its consultants included experts on the environmental impacts of diet. The powerful lobbyists for the meat industry led Congress to insert language into the final 2015 appropriations bill that made it *unlawful* to mention the environmental effects of dietary choices in the national *Dietary Guidelines*. This not only censored the Dietary Guidelines Advisory Committee, it prevented Americans from getting the best possible dietary advice.

With their hands tied by the language in the appropriations bill, the heads of the USDA and the Department of Health and Human Services, the two agencies that create the final *Dietary Guidelines*, announced that "we do not believe that the 2015 DGAs are the appropriate vehicle for this important policy conversation about sustainability."[11] Sadly, they offered no alternative "vehicle" for this essential discussion.

The final *Dietary Guidelines* for 2015–2020 made no mention of limiting red meat and actually encouraged its consumption as long as it was lean.[12]

If you are interested in the uncensored science, read the report of the Dietary Guidelines Advisory Committee—which comes very close to the recommendations in this book—instead of the final *Dietary Guidelines*. An updated review on the environmental effects of dietary choices, written by members of the Dietary Guidelines Advisory Committee after they were discharged from their official role, was eventually published.

This is one of many ways the *Dietary Guidelines* are out of step with the science and the policy of healthy eating (see chapter two).

Some argue that consuming grass-fed beef instead of feedlot beef is one way to reduce the environmental impact of eating beef. It isn't that simple (see Grass-Fed Beef or "Regular"? on page 248). If we collectively stopped feeding grain to beef cattle, the result would be far lower beef production, much less land use for grain production, less water use and contamination, and less antibiotic resistance. That's a multiple win solution. I cover the direct health effects of grass-fed versus grain-fed beef in chapter seven.

For individual and planetary health, we should be rethinking the role of beef in our diets entirely. If you like beef, think of it as an occasional splurge instead of a daily food—the way most of us think of lobster. Many people, out of interest for their health or the environment or both, are taking meat off the list of foods they eat, even if they aren't becoming vegetarians. Beef consumption has been in decline for almost 50 years, and a 2017 USDA report indicated that Americans are now eating about 12 percent less beef than we were in 2002.[13] As someone who grew up in the Midwest consuming beef twice a day, I've made this shift and my diet is much more varied—and enjoyable—than what I ate then.

Dairy foods also have a large environmental footprint, though not as much as beef. Pork has less, and poultry even less, but not quite as low as most vegetable sources of protein such as soybeans or lentils.

Fish, shrimp, and oysters can be extremely efficient converters of feed to flesh, in part because they are cold-blooded and don't need to burn calories to stay warm. Like other forms of agriculture, aquaculture can be done carefully, with minimal impact on the environment, or it can be done poorly, using industrially farmed grain, releasing highly polluting fish waste into the environ-

"Urban Local Agriculture"

Rural farms aren't the only places to grow food. More and more city dwellers and suburbanites are growing vegetables, fruits, beans, and other foods in their backyards, on balconies and rooftops, in community gardens, and in other open spaces.

Some entrepreneurs see urban farms as a business opportunity. Using hydroponics and other technologies that optimize temperature, light, moisture, and fertilizer, these "farms" produce food efficiently. A company called Gotham Greens has built and operates rooftop greenhouses in New York and Chicago. They use recirculating irrigation systems to grow leafy vegetables year-round for use in local restaurants and for sale in grocery stores. A Boston-based company, Freight Farms, recycles refrigerated shipping containers into high-tech food-growing pods that can be installed almost anywhere. The company says that an average Freight Farms box can produce nearly 50,000 mini-heads of lettuce a year, which is the equivalent of two acres of farmland. Some are parked a few feet behind the restaurants that own or rent them, ensuring a very short trip from farm to table!

This concept isn't really new. In the 1800s, Boston had a system in which horse manure, a by-product of transportation, was scooped from the streets and delivered to solar flats outside the city. There it was used to fertilize lettuce and greens during the cold months. This was the origin of Boston Bibb lettuce.

ment, and using large amounts of antibiotics. This type of food production deserves investment and monitoring to optimize production methods, because it can be an important sustainable source of protein in the future. The Monterey Bay Aquarium's Seafood Watch program (www.seafoodwatch.org) helps consumers and businesses choose seafood that's fished or farmed in ways that have less impact on the environment.

A vegetarian or vegan diet will, in general, have a lower environmental impact, although it depends on how the food is grown, transported, and processed. Eating out-of-season fruits and vegetables that are grown far across the country or overseas has a substantially greater environmental impact than eating regionally produced seasonal fruits and vegetables. Research is under way around the country to find ways to better produce local fruits and vegetables year-round.

Buy Local and Seasonal Food or Sustainably Raised Food

It makes sense to buy foods with the fewest steps from farm to plate, because processing, packaging, and transporting foods add to their carbon footprint. However, there are many exceptions. How your diet affects the environment is usually determined more by the foods you choose (for example, beef versus chicken or soy) than the effects of processing and transportation. For example, per unit of food, greenhouse gas emissions may be less for transporting carloads of fruit from Florida to Boston by train than moving a small amount by pickup truck from the western part of the state to a farmers' market. The idea of "food miles" by itself isn't a reliable indicator of environmental impact. In fact, there is no single, simple yardstick.

But combining the concept of local and seasonal may help. Flying perishable fruits across the continent so we can eat them year-round doesn't make sense. Of course there are other values that do, and should, affect our decisions, such as the quality of food and support for local communities and farmers. For example, limiting your tomato consumption to the season when they can be produced without long-distance shipping—and with more flavor—will add to your eating enjoyment and have environmental benefits.

Watch your waste

Americans throw away as much as 25 percent of the food they buy.[14] On one level, that's a huge waste of money and a lot of garbage to be buried in landfills, which emit tons of methane into the atmosphere. On another level, it's

Grass-Fed Beef or "Regular"?

Before the dawn of industrial agriculture, family farms often raised a few cows for milk and meat. These animals would graze on whatever they could, supplemented with some hay or oats if needed. Today the vast majority of our steaks, burgers, and other cuts of beef come from animals raised in large feed lots eating corn, soy, or other grains raised specifically for them.

Is so-called grass-fed beef better for you and the planet than feedlot beef? It's a hotly debated topic.

When it comes to human health, there's no evidence. No study has directly compared the effects of grass-fed beef and feedlot beef on heart disease, diabetes, cancer, and other outcomes.

Some grass-fed beef proponents say that cows grazing on their own yield more healthful meat that is leaner and health promoting, because it has higher amounts of omega-3 fats. But the amounts of omega-3 fats in beef are small—especially compared to those in fish—and they come with a large amount of saturated fat, cholesterol, and other nutrients that contribute to higher risk of heart disease. In addition, it's still unknown if the fats in beef are fully responsible for the increased risks of diabetes and heart disease linked to eating red meat. My bottom line is that grass-fed beef is probably not importantly different for your personal health than feedlot beef.

And although the concept of grass-fed beef sounds more environmentally friendly, especially with regard to greenhouse gas production, it really isn't. The environmental impact of feeding a cow or bull grain on a daily basis is definitely larger for feedlot beef than grass-fed beef. But it takes only about two years for a feedlot cow to come to market, compared to about four years for a grass-fed cow. Every day these animals are alive they are producing large amounts of methane and carbon dioxide. So the grass-fed cow produces about the same amount of greenhouse gases over its lifetime as the feedlot cow. Pound for pound, the impact on greenhouse gas production of raising grass-fed and feedlot beef is about the same.

That said, feeding grain to cattle is a hugely inefficient way of producing food, and it has major environmental impacts. Stopping this practice is one of the most important steps we can take to reduce those environmental impacts of our diets. This will also likely reduce problems of antibiotic resistance (see page 142), because huge amounts are used to deal with the unsanitary conditions and crowding in feedlots.

Eating less beef and other red meat and more poultry, fish, and plant sources of protein would lead to healthier people and a healthier planet.

a huge waste of water, fossil fuel, pesticides and herbicides, packaging, and transportation.

PUTTING IT INTO PRACTICE

Eating a diet that is largely plant based won't put an end to global warming. But it could help feed the world as we search for new and better ways to produce food and improve the health of the planet.

CHAPTER THIRTEEN

Putting It All Together

A S I HAVE LAID OUT in the preceding chapters, much of the nutrition advice we commonly hear is steering us in the wrong direction. The low-fat, high-carbohydrate approach promoted for years has been a national disaster. The high-fat, low-carb approach once known as the Atkins diet correctly identified high consumption of refined carbohydrates as a problem, but loading up with red meat and dairy fat is far from healthy. Today's gluten-free fad isn't based on evidence and has led many people to eat in unhealthy ways.

The road to good health isn't one of blandness and deprivation. Instead it's paved with hearty, tasty, and satisfying foods. The Healthy Eating Pyramid and Healthy Eating Plate, both built with the best available nutrition science as a blueprint, can guide you to better health and a satisfying diet. They recommend:

- maintaining a stable, healthy weight
- eating plenty of vegetables and fruits
- consuming more unsaturated fats, less saturated fat, and no trans fat
- eating whole grains and foods made from them in place of refined grains
- choosing healthier sources of protein by trading red meat for nuts, beans, chicken, and fish
- drinking water, tea, or coffee instead of juice or sugar-sweetened soda and, if you drink alcohol, keeping it moderate (no more than two drinks a day for men or one a day for women)
- taking a daily multivitamin for insurance.

At first glance, it might look like I am promoting a traditional Mediterranean diet. While the Mediterranean diet fits this description, and is an excellent place to start, what I suggest isn't limited to the culinary experience of just one place or time. Instead, this strategy is a science-based, multicultural approach to healthy eating.

THE HARVARD HEALTHY EATING PYRAMID

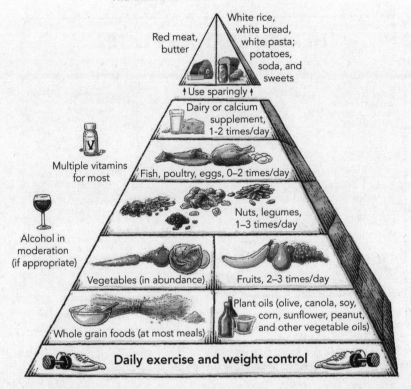

Figure 21. The Harvard Healthy Eating Pyramid, based on solid science, offers better guidance for healthy eating than advice from the USDA.

BENEFITS OF THIS EATING STRATEGY

Part of the payoff from following this healthy eating strategy comes immediately. By opening up a new world of foods, flavors, and textures, it will make eating a pleasure. It can help you break out of the often unsatisfying and not-so-healthy mealtime ruts you can fall into when following a low-fat or low-carb diet. As you gain control of your appetite and eating habits, not to mention your weight, cholesterol levels, and maybe even your blood pressure, you'll gain a sense of achievement and pride that may affect other areas of your life. You'll also have more energy and feel better right now as well as years down the road.

The other part of the payoff—protection against chronic disease—comes later. A healthful eating strategy like the one I suggest can help protect you from developing a long list of common diseases. These include heart disease, stroke, type 2 diabetes, several common cancers, cataracts, osteoporosis, de-

THE HARVARD HEALTHY EATING PLATE

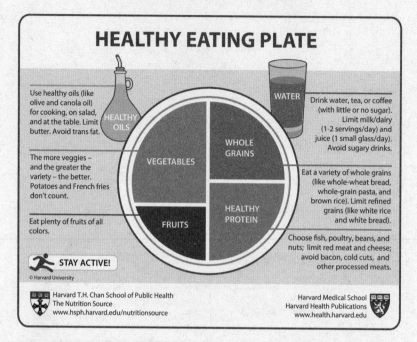

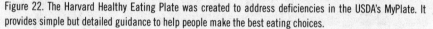

Figure 22. The Harvard Healthy Eating Plate was created to address deficiencies in the USDA's MyPlate. It provides simple but detailed guidance to help people make the best eating choices.

mentia, and other age-related diseases. It also helps prevent some types of birth defects. When combined with not smoking and regular exercise, this kind of healthy diet can reduce heart disease by 80 percent, type 2 diabetes by 90 percent, and stroke and some cancers by 70 percent, compared with average rates in the United States.[1]

To borrow a phrase from the financial world, that's a great return on investment, especially when the investment is a more flavorful and less restrictive version of what you may be eating today.

THE ROMANCE AND REALITY OF TRADITIONAL DIETS

The term "traditional diet" once meant a plain, none-too-varied regional diet that was the standard fare of farmers and laborers. Today it conjures up images of heart-healthy, cancer-free, long-lived people who understand the land, eat wonderful meals brimming with taste, and dance, drink, laugh, and love. Think Zorba the Greek meets Julia Child.

A lot of popular writing implies that the foods that go into traditional diets have been carefully chosen over the years to promote good health. That's not so. People ate what they could grow, gather, kill, or buy, and their choices were dictated by weather, geology, geography, economics, and even politics. Given these constraints, different cultures have developed various combinations of healthy (and sometimes not-so-healthy) foods. Keep in mind that these choices were made for short-term health, not for prolonging life into old age. Also keep in mind that diets that seem to be good for people whose days are full of hard physical labor aren't necessarily good for people who toil at a desk all day.

In northern Europe, for example, the short growing season makes it difficult to eat fruits and vegetables year-round. It is, however, a fine climate for raising livestock, and meat and dairy foods made a good match for the energy needs of people who had to survive long, cold winters. In the small island nation of Japan, the main components of the diet are fish, naturally, and rice, a plant that can yield large amounts of grain from small plots of land. In both these cases the traditional diet kept people healthy long enough to reproduce and raise children and also to develop complex societies. Yet their successes don't imply that either of these diets would yield the best health for contemporary people who sit most of the day.

THE MEDITERRANEAN DIET AND BEYOND

In the 1950s and 1960s, pioneering nutrition researcher Ancel Keys and his colleagues looked at eating patterns in sixteen different populations in seven countries: Greece, Finland, Italy, the Netherlands, Yugoslavia, Japan, and the United States. This landmark work, known today as the Seven Countries Study, was the first major investigation of the link between diet and heart disease. One of the more intriguing findings was that people living in Crete, other parts of Greece, and southern Italy had very high adult life expectancies (the number of years the average forty-five-year-old can expect to live) and very low rates of heart disease and some cancers, all in spite of relatively limited medical systems.[2] (See the tables on page 254.)

At the time, the traditional diet in these Mediterranean countries was mostly plant-based foods: fruits, vegetables, breads, a variety of coarsely ground grains, beans, nuts, and seeds. Olive oil was the main source of dietary fat. People regularly ate dairy foods—mostly cheese and yogurt—but not in large amounts. Fish, poultry, and red meat were eaten on special occasions, not as part of the daily fare. People, usually men, often drank wine, but typically with meals.

Keys concluded that the Mediterranean diet was an important reason for

Characteristics of Diets in the 1960s of Three Countries in the Seven Countries Study

Diet*	U.S.	Greece	Japan
Total fat (% energy)	39	37	11
Saturated fat (% energy)	18	8	3
Fruits and vegetables (grams/day)	504	654	232
Legumes (grams/day)	1	30	91
Breads, cereal grains (grams/day)	123	453	481
Meat and poultry (grams/day)	273	35	8
Fish (grams/day)	3	39	150
Eggs (grams/day)	40	15	29
Alcohol (grams/day)	6	23	22

*Since the 1960s, consumption of red meat and animal fat has greatly increased in Japan and Greece.

Comparison of Life Expectancy and Disease Rates in the 1960s of Three Countries in the Seven Countries Study*

Life Expectancy and Disease Rates	Gender	U.S.	Greece	Japan
Life expectancy at age 45 (1960s)	M	72	76	72
	F	78	79	77
Heart disease (per 100,000 people)	M	189	33	34
	F	54	14	21
Stroke (per 100,000 people)	M	30	26	102
	F	24	23	57
Colorectal cancer	M	11	3	5
	F	10	3	5
All cancers (per 100,000 people)	M	102	83	98
	F	87	61	77
Breast cancer (per 100,000 people)	F	22	8	4

*Since the 1960s the rates of stroke and stomach cancer have decreased in Japan; life expectancy at age 45 is now greatest in that country (87.7 years for females and 81.8 years for males), followed by Greece (84.6 years for females and 80.1 years for males), and the United States (83.3 years for females and 79.6 years for males).

Source: Willett, W. C., "Diet and Health: What Should We Eat?" Science 264, no. 5158 (April 22, 1994): 532–7.

the low rates of heart disease in that region. Alarmed at the epidemic of heart disease that was hitting its peak in the United States in the 1960s, Keys and his wife, Margaret, began popularizing and promoting the Mediterranean diet in a series of bestselling books.[3]

The Seven Countries study raised the possibility that the Mediterranean diet could be a cause of long life and good health. But it couldn't prove it had that effect. Other things—such as the physically active lifestyle common throughout the region, the relatively low rates of overweight and obesity, or the low rates of smoking that prevailed until the late 1960s—could have been among the causes. It was also possible that some genetic trait common among people in the Mediterranean region provided them with protection against heart disease and cancer, although this explanation was discounted by studies showing that people lose their protection when they migrate from countries where heart disease, cancer, and diabetes are rare to countries where they are common.

Evidence accumulated over the last fifty years shows that Keys and his colleagues were on the right track. My research group, for example, has documented that the main elements of the Mediterranean lifestyle are connected with lower risks of many diseases even when followed by people living away from the Mediterranean region. Results from the Nurses' Health Study document that heart disease rates in the United States could be reduced by least 80 percent by modest changes in diet and lifestyle changes.[4] The Lyon Diet Heart Study, described in chapter five, showed that a group of heart attack survivors randomly assigned to a Mediterranean-type diet were 70 percent less likely to die over a two-year period than those assigned to the low-fat diet advocated by the American Heart Association.[5] More recently, our colleagues in Spain showed in a randomized trial that a Mediterranean diet with added nuts or olive oil reduced cardiovascular disease risk by 30 percent compared to a low-fat diet.[6] Today the Mediterranean diet is often held up as a prime example of healthy eating that should be adopted by all. It was even recognized in the 2015–2020 *Dietary Guidelines for Americans* as an example of a desirable dietary pattern![7]

But the Mediterranean diet isn't necessarily perfect. It evolved out of agricultural necessities imposed by a warm and semidry climate that, by chance, favored the growth of olive trees. And it isn't the only healthy culture-based diet. A traditional Japanese diet can be quite healthy. Traditional Latin American diets, which emphasize corn, beans, and vegetables, can provide another model of healthy eating. But keep in mind that the corn we eat today is not the same as the corn eaten one hundred years ago, and that large amounts of corn may not be healthy for individuals who aren't physically active.

Along with a diverse group of colleagues, I helped Oldways Preservation and Exchange Trust create a series of food pyramids that tried to capture the traditional healthy diets of these regions (www.oldwayspt.org/traditional-diets).

As researchers continue to define more precisely the specific health-promoting elements of a Mediterranean-type diet, one thing we know for sure is that it is safe. The low rates of heart disease and cancer among people who have eaten this type of diet for thousands of years are solid proof of that. The high rate of strokes in Japan, on the other hand, suggest that some aspect of that traditional diet, possibly high carbohydrate and salt intake combined with low consumption of healthy fats, protein, fruits, and vegetables, may not be so safe.

TRADITIONAL DIETS CAN TRANSPLANT WELL

While traditional diets may have health benefits for the cultures that shaped them, a big question is whether they offer similar benefits when transplanted somewhere else, like a modern society with relatively low levels of physical activity. If traditional diets are like weeds that can grow anywhere, then an Iowa accountant should get the same benefit from a Mediterranean diet as a Greek farmer. But if traditional diets are more like painstakingly bred orchids that grow only in carefully controlled environments, then adopting a traditional diet without also taking on the other aspects of the traditional culture won't necessarily make a dent in rates of heart disease, cancer, and other chronic diseases.

Fortunately, evidence from different types of studies done in many countries shows that the components of a Mediterranean-type diet offer major benefits even for people living modern "Western" lifestyles.[8] It remains to be seen whether dining leisurely with a view of the Aegean Sea or taking a siesta after a midday meal adds an extra topping of good health.

Scientists, nutrition experts, and writers have often tried to condense the benefits of the Mediterranean or other traditional diets into one or two key elements, like olive oil or fiber or antioxidants. That's a dangerous proposition. While we know that the Mediterranean diet helps prevent chronic disease, and that olive oil is one of the reasons why, just loading up on olive oil or taking high-dose antioxidant supplements isn't a substitute for a comprehensive healthy eating strategy.

Most important, taking advantage of the Mediterranean diet isn't an all-

or-nothing proposition. We know enough about this diet to be sure that its elements can be safely and fruitfully incorporated into other healthy eating strategies.

COST OF HEALTHY EATING

Does it cost more to eat foods that promote good health than to eat those that don't? Many people believe that nutritious foods are more expensive than less healthy alternatives. They are partly right. Fats, sugar, and refined carbohydrates deliver more calories per dollar than fish or fresh vegetables.[9] Yet, when it comes to an all-around diet, cost need not stand in the way of healthy eating. And keep in mind that the traditional Mediterranean diet was originally the diet of poorer people, not the wealthy.

Following a healthy eating pattern is all about choices: picking good fats and steering clear of bad ones, adding more good sources of carbohydrate and cutting back on poor ones, opting for healthier protein packages, selecting smaller portions instead of super-sizing, and so on. Cost, along with taste and convenience, is an important factor influencing these choices.

Foods that are filling, high in calories, and satisfying are often the least expensive. In day-to-day eating and shopping, this means that a hamburger and french fries washed down with a large soda and topped off with soft-serve ice cream is a relatively inexpensive way to get calories. Foods that pack the most calories per ounce—those with the highest energy densities—tend to have the lowest cost per calorie. These include oil, margarine, sweets, and soft drinks. Healthier options, such as whole grains, fresh fruits and vegetables, and fish, cost more per calorie.

For people with limited incomes, market forces seem to conspire against healthy eating. If you're at the other end of the spectrum, you can pay top dollar for out-of-season fruits and vegetables, ready-to-eat packages of salad, top-of-the-line fish, and specialty breads. In between those extremes is the vast middle ground that most of us try to navigate as we make our way through the grocery store or market. Here are some suggestions for anyone interested in making healthy choices without breaking the bank.

Fats. There's no question that extra-virgin olive oil is more expensive than canola or soybean oil. Even so, you can find some perfectly tasty types for $8 to $10 a liter. At two tablespoons a day, that's less than 50 cents. From a health perspective, we can't say that olive oil is superior to canola or soybean oil. All are healthy fats, but we have longer-term experience with olive oil. Use olive oil where its flavor counts, such as for drizzling on vegetables or in salad dressings. Otherwise, use canola oil or other liquid plant oils for sautéing or other applications where flavor isn't as important.

Carbohydrates. White rice, pasta, and potatoes are some of the least expensive sources of carbohydrate. Whole grains, such as brown rice, bulgur, wheat berries, oat groats, and others, cost more—although they really shouldn't, because they require less processing. Yet, when you calculate the cost per serving, using whole grains adds relatively little to the food budget. Whole-grain breakfast cereals, especially oatmeal or other cooked whole grains, can be excellent choices as long as you stay away from those that deliver a lot of added sugars.

Protein. When Americans think of protein, they tend to think of meat. Beef is certainly a major protein source. Turkey and chicken offer a more healthful protein package and are typically less expensive. Roasting a whole chicken is an inexpensive main dish that also offers plenty of leftover options. Fish is an even healthier protein source. Some types, such as swordfish and sole, are budget breakers or once-in-a-while luxuries. Others are more reasonably priced and are often on sale. These include tilapia, catfish, pollock, and many types of frozen fish. Canned tuna, salmon, and mackerel—on a sandwich, in a salad, or as part of a casserole—are inexpensive ways to put fish on your plate. Canned salmon delivers the most omega-3 fats per dollar and is also very low in mercury, which is important for women who are pregnant or breastfeeding.

Eating even lower on the food chain is usually the best for your budget and your health. Making nuts, peanuts, peanut butter, beans, tofu, other vegetable sources of protein, and eggs the centerpiece of meals, instead of side dishes or garnishes, would be a boon for your budget. Don't be put off by the cost of nuts. Keep in mind that meat is two-thirds water, so nuts that cost $7.50 per pound are comparable to beef that costs $2.50 per pound. If you think about it this way, peanuts are a real bargain.

Fruits and vegetables. Even though fruits and vegetables don't deliver the cheap caloric punch of fats and sugar, they can still be a good bargain. Consider what's in season when shopping, both for price and quality. The USDA calculates that a savvy shopper can meet the recommendations for fruits and vegetables in the 2015–2020 *Dietary Guidelines for Americans* for under $3 a day.[10] My family has found that it is possible for much less. Vegetables that are quite inexpensive per serving include cabbage, winter squash, and carrots; with the right seasoning and oils, these are delicious.

Frozen fruits and vegetables are just as nutritious as fresh ones, and often cost less. Out of season, dried fruit can be a good option.

What you aren't buying. Making healthier choices usually involves cutting back or cutting out foods such as steak, potato chips, ice cream, your morning doughnut, and sweetened sodas. Savings from these can add up and may even offset the cost for fish, whole grains, and fresh fruits and vegetables. Many people spend a surprising amount on highly processed junk.

If you still think healthy eating is expensive, consider the alternative. Heart disease, stroke, diabetes, some cancers, and other diet-related chronic diseases cost far more in the long run than good nutrition. The USDA's Economic Research Service estimates that healthier eating could save Americans more than $70 billion a year in medical costs and lost productivity.[11] That's not all "invisible money" transferred from health insurance companies to doctors and hospitals. Many people pay part or all of the cost of their medications for these chronic conditions out of pocket. People who are overweight pay an average of 11 percent more in out-of-pocket medical costs than do people with healthy weights, while those who are obese have 26 percent higher out-of-pocket costs.

The bottom line: By making a few smart choices, healthy eating need not cost more than the average American diet and in the long run is a sound financial investment.

HEALTHY GLOBAL EATING

We have the good fortune to live at a time when we have seemingly unlimited choices in foods. Beside the bewildering array of junk food, grocery stores routinely carry fruits and vegetables from many countries, "new" grains are becoming easier to find, and restaurants offer an ever expanding smorgasbord of the world's cuisines. Thirty years ago in Boston, for example, Mediterranean cuisine typically meant spaghetti and meatballs. Today many local restaurants serve up a variety of vastly more interesting and healthy traditional dishes from that region as well as from other parts of the globe.

Given these choices, I don't advocate returning to a single humble diet or switching to a particular traditional diet. Instead, what I am suggesting is a flexible eating strategy based on a completely rebuilt food pyramid that incorporates elements of healthy eating patterns from around the world and leaves plenty of room for creativity and innovation. The Mediterranean diet offers a good initial blueprint for healthy eating. But there's plenty of room for fine-tuning, and other cultures also have healthy eating strategies to offer. From Japan we can incorporate the tradition of serving small portions of tasty, interesting foods instead of large helpings of the relatively bland foods that are the mainstays of U.S. and northern European diets. This approach helps keep consumption in check but doesn't make you feel deprived, as many weight-loss or weight-control diets do. From Latin America, the region that has given us corn and tomatoes, come interesting and healthy grains such as quinoa that are unfamiliar to many North Americans but deserve a place at the table. Even from Finland, the country with the most lethal diet in the Seven Countries Study, comes a great whole-grain rye bread that is much healthier and far tastier than the spongy white bread eaten by many Americans. What's more, we are learning intriguing and appetizing ways to combine and season ingredients.

A truly healthy diet for a modern age is drawn from eating strategies from around the world that have been shown to yield benefits in different populations, including Americans from all walks of life. The science has been described in the preceding sections. The global influence is unmistakable in the ingredients and recipes that follow.

PARTING WORDS

I hope the Healthy Eating Pyramid and Healthy Eating Plate, along with the eating strategies described in this book and the recipes that follow, will help you make healthy and delicious food choices that will enhance and lengthen your life. By reducing the environmental footprint of your diet, these choices can also convey a benefit to future generations.

CHAPTER FOURTEEN

Healthy Eating in Special Situations

EATING WELL CAN HELP YOU stay healthy. It's just as important, maybe even more so, when you are experiencing something out of the ordinary, such as pregnancy, heart disease, diabetes, cancer, celiac disease, and other conditions.

Each of us responds to health-related stresses in different ways. The recommendations that follow are general ones. Check with your doctor, dietitian, nutritionist, or other health care professional before making major changes to your diet.

PREGNANCY

During pregnancy, a woman needs extra nutrients for herself and her baby. That doesn't mean doubling up on food, what many call "eating for two." It *does* mean perhaps getting a few more calories, extra amounts of a few vitamins and minerals, and at least enough of the rest. A healthy diet can supply almost all of these, with the possible exceptions of folate (folic acid) and iron.

A special pregnancy diet isn't necessary. The basic eating pattern that I have described for good health will keep you and your baby healthy. That means eating *real* food: fruits, vegetables, whole grains, unsaturated fats, and healthy sources of protein. These deliver the energy, the raw materials, and the vitamins and minerals you and your baby need. Pregnancy creates a kind of "metabolic stress test." Pregnancy-related high blood pressure and diabetes represent signals of potential problems. Adopting the overall healthy diet described in this book during pregnancy—and ideally continuing it afterward—can help reduce the risk of pregnancy-related high blood pressure and diabetes.

PREGNANCY AND WEIGHT

A developing baby, the placenta that helps nourish it, the extra blood needed to provide it with oxygenated blood, and other changes add pounds to a pregnant woman's weight. She also needs to take in extra food and nutrients for her baby. Beliefs about how much weight to gain during pregnancy have changed dramatically over the last fifty years.

In 1970 the National Academy of Sciences' Food and Nutrition Board's committee on maternal nutrition concluded that "the desirable average gain is 24 pounds within a range of 20 to 25 pounds" for all pregnant women regardless of their prepregnancy weight or body mass index.[1] Today the recommended weight gain depends on a woman's starting weight. For a woman whose weight is in the healthy range and who is having one baby, the American College of Obstetricians and Gynecologists recommends a weight gain between 25 and 35 pounds during pregnancy. For a woman who is overweight, it's 15 to 25 pounds. It's even less for obese women, 11 to 20 pounds.[2]

Discuss the best weight for you with your obstetrician/gynecologist or midwife.

PUTTING IT ALL TOGETHER

The best way to get the vitamins and minerals you need during pregnancy is to follow a healthy diet and take a standard multivitamin-multimineral pill that delivers the recommended daily allowances for insurance against any dietary deficiencies in vitamins or minerals. Special prenatal supplements are available, but they can be pricey—and many don't provide anything you can't get from a standard multivitamin. Don't rely on a multivitamin-multimineral as a substitute for a good diet, because it contains only a tiny fraction of the nutrients needed for a healthy pregnancy.

It's especially important to get extra folate (also known as folic acid), a B vitamin that helps a baby's brain and spinal cord develop properly. This vitamin is so important that *all* women of childbearing age—even those who aren't planning to get pregnant—are urged to take 400 micrograms of folic acid a day, from either food or supplements, during their childbearing years.[3] That's because folic acid is needed most during the first thirty days after conception, a time when many women don't yet know they are pregnant.

Some women have trouble taking prenatal vitamins or the extra iron supplements that are sometimes needed, because these can make morning sickness worse. Instead of skipping prenatal vitamins or iron, both of which a developing baby needs, taking these supplements later in the day or after eating can help.

A developing baby needs a solid supply of omega-3 fats to make sure its brain, nervous system, eyes, and other tissues develop properly. The best way for pregnant women to get enough omega-3 fats is to eat seafood two or three times a week. Choose low-mercury types such as cod, salmon, sardines, and tilapia (see "Fish, Mercury, and Fish Oil" on page 147).

If you are looking for suggestions for healthy eating during pregnancy, check out "The Pregnancy Food Guide," developed by my colleague Kathy McManus, the nutrition team at Brigham and Women's Hospital, myself, and other experts.[4]

HIGH BLOOD PRESSURE

The term "blood pressure" has gotten a bad reputation. You need some pressure to move blood from the heart to the brain and the toes and back again. But too much pressure is harmful. It damages artery walls, which can lead to a heart attack or stroke. High blood pressure can weaken the heart muscle over time and damage other organs, like the kidneys and the eyes.

About 90 percent of Americans develop high blood pressure during their lifetimes. Most people can keep their blood pressure in the healthy range by staying lean and physically active, consuming five or more servings of fruits and vegetables daily, and keeping salt intake low. If you have been diagnosed with high blood pressure (also known as hypertension), there are several things you can do to keep your blood pressure in check without the need for medication. And even if you do need medication, these strategies can help minimize the number of drugs needed to keep blood pressure under control, which in turn will reduce both the side effects you feel and the cost of your treatment.

If you have high blood pressure and are overweight, losing just 5 to 10 percent of your starting weight can help lower your blood pressure and do much, much more for your health. Eating more fruits and vegetables delivers extra potassium, which helps control blood pressure. Aim for a minimum of five servings a day and remember: potatoes and corn don't count as vegetables.

Cutting back on sodium (a main part of table salt) will also help you control your blood pressure. Try to keep your sodium intake under 1,500 milligrams, the amount in three-quarters of a teaspoon of salt. You don't need to count milligrams of salt on a meal-by-meal basis, but it is helpful to know where most of your salt comes from, particularly because so much of it is hidden in processed and prepared foods (see "Hidden Salt in Food" on page 230). For that reason, I have included information about sodium in the recipes in chapter fifteen.

Suddenly decreasing the amount of salt (sodium) may make your diet seem bland. But if you cut back slowly, you won't notice that you are taking in less salt. Most natural foods are low in sodium, so if you limit your intake of processed foods and don't load up on salt when cooking, your sodium intake will be low without your thinking about it.

Keeping your blood pressure in check, whether by diet or drugs, is an important way to protect yourself from having a heart attack or stroke.

DIABETES

Nearly 30 million Americans have diabetes, mostly type 2 diabetes, which doesn't immediately require the use of insulin. Another 86 million have its precursor, prediabetes.

Many people have diabetes for years without knowing it. Early on, diabetes causes few if any symptoms. But years of high blood sugar eventually cause trouble. In the United States, diabetes is the leading cause of aging-related vision loss and blindness. It's the reason why more than 70,000 Americans a year have a foot or part of a leg amputated. It contributes to heart attacks and damages nerves in the feet and hands.

Maintaining a healthy weight by diet and exercise is the most important way to prevent diabetes and to treat it after it appears. Some individuals with type 2 diabetes are able to control their blood sugar by losing weight, exercising, and following a diet that focuses on vegetables, fruits, unsaturated fats, whole grains, and healthy sources of protein such as fish, poultry, and nuts, and by not eating foods made with rapidly digested carbohydrates or added sugars.

Dietary recommendations for diabetes have evolved over the last few years. They once focused on eating as few carbohydrates as possible, then moved in the direction of the ill-advised low-fat, high-carbohydrate eating pattern. Several recent studies have shown that individuals can better control type 2 diabetes when they cut back on some carbohydrate-rich foods, especially rapidly digested carbs, and eat foods that deliver unsaturated fats instead.

Eating foods that are low on the glycemic index (see "The Glycemic Index: How Carbohydrates Affect Your Body Sugar" on page 116) and high in fiber, such as intact whole grains and beans, can help control diabetes. And because people with diabetes are at high risk of having a heart attack or stroke, it's especially important for them to eat less saturated fat and more unsaturated fat. In other words, the healthy eating patterns I've laid out in this book are particularly valuable for individuals with diabetes.

Overall caloric intake—eating only as much as you burn so you don't gain weight—is even more important for people with diabetes than it is for the rest of us. As described in chapter four, the healthy eating patterns I have set out make weight control easier than focusing just on calories.

Since everyone is a bit different, it's a good idea to talk with your health care provider before choosing the diet that's right for you.

HIGH CHOLESTEROL

A high level of harmful LDL cholesterol in the bloodstream is one of several factors that can lead to heart attack, stroke, and premature death. (Total cholesterol, once the key marker, is obsolete and can be misleading, because in some people high total cholesterol is due to an abundance of protective HDL cholesterol.) High LDL cholesterol is largely driven by diet, except in the minority of people predisposed to high LDL because of their genetic makeup. A healthy diet can help prevent the emergence of high LDL cholesterol or beat it back if it does appear.

For years, the American Heart Association and others told people with high cholesterol to lower their intake of fat, especially saturated fat. But that has only a small effect on cholesterol. All too often, the diet is then declared a failure and people are simply put on drugs, usually a cholesterol-lowering statin.

In the chapters and recipes in this book, I have emphasized a broad approach of replacing saturated and trans fats with monounsaturated and polyunsaturated fats, eating whole grains instead of high-glycemic carbohydrates and sugars, weight control, and regular physical activity. This strategy can help you control your cholesterol and greatly reduce your risk of heart disease, even with medication.

Statins have gained a glowing reputation as drugs that stop heart disease. That's only partly true. There's no question that they can dramatically lower the amount of harmful LDL in the bloodstream. They reduce the risk of heart attack by about one-third. But that means most people are still at risk. So don't think of a statin as a magic bullet against heart disease; Also, high-potency statins increase the risk of diabetes, and can have other serious side effects. You can do more to prevent heart attack, stroke, and other chronic conditions by taking full advantage of the healthy eating strategies covered in this book, which work to protect your health in multiple ways besides lowering your cholesterol.

HEART ATTACK AND STROKE

Heart attacks, angina, stroke, and other cardiovascular conditions affect millions of Americans, although today they tend to appear at later ages than they did in the 1950s and 1960s. Most cases of these, as I have demonstrated in this book, can be prevented by diet and lifestyle choices.

Even after a heart attack or stroke, following the Harvard Healthy Eating Plate and the Healthy Eating Pyramid can dramatically reduce your risk of having another one. You don't need to completely reverse the damage that has been wrought to your blood vessels; you just need to stop it from getting worse.

The benefit of improving diet was dramatically demonstrated in the Lyon Heart Study, conducted among men and women who had already had a heart attack. As I describe in "Clinical Trials: Replacing Saturated Fats with Unsaturated Fats Saves Lives" on page 94, participants randomized to a Mediterranean-type diet that included getting more omega-3 fats from plant oils were 70 percent less likely to have had a repeat heart attack or to have died from one. This is truly remarkable, because statins, the powerful cholesterol-lowering agents, reduce this rate only by 30 percent or so.

This doesn't mean we shouldn't take statins—only that relying on them and not taking advantage of the full benefit of diet and lifestyle is a serious and often fatal mistake.

CANCER

A somewhat daunting discovery from the last decade of research is that cancer isn't one disease. It is *hundreds* of diseases, each with its own triggers and treatments. That means there isn't a single "treat cancer" diet.

The number one strategy to prevent cancer is not smoking or using other forms of tobacco. It's closely followed by maintaining a healthy weight. Being overweight or obese increases the risk of many cancers, including cancers of the breast, colon, endometrium, and pancreas. Because smoking is on the decline and overweight/obesity on the rise, excess weight now causes almost as many cancer deaths in the United States as smoking does.

For years a low-fat diet was promoted as the best way to *prevent* cancer. But that advice hasn't been supported by large cohort studies and randomized trials. Eating more fruits and vegetables, and less red meat will reduce the risk of some types of cancer, as will limiting alcohol consumption, if consumed at all (see chapter nine).

We are still learning about the best lifestyle strategies for keeping cancer at bay once it appears. Regular physical activity and avoiding weight gain seem to improve the odds of beating breast and colorectal cancer. When it comes to diet, though, few specific strategies have been identified.

These days, earlier diagnosis and better treatment mean that most people do not die from their cancers but instead often die from heart disease, stroke, or something else. Because of this, the healthy eating strategies described in this book have been linked to overall survival for people with cancer.

CELIAC DISEASE

If you have celiac disease, you know the problems that even a few crumbs of bread can cause: gas, bloating, abdominal cramps, diarrhea, and more. The cause is gluten, a mixture of proteins found mainly in wheat, rye, and barley. People with celiac disease can't tolerate gluten. For some reason, their immune systems see gluten as a foreign invader. Over time, the attack on gluten damages the lining of the small intestine, leading to weight loss, skin rashes, osteoporosis, infertility, nerve damage, seizures, and more.

People with celiac disease must do everything they can to avoid foods that contain gluten. Common gluten-containing foods include traditional breads and pastries made from wheat or rye, noodles and pasta, crackers and other baked goods, many breakfast foods, flour tortillas, and beer, to name just a few.

The rapid proliferation of gluten-free foods is making it easier to avoid gluten. Even so, it can lurk in unexpected foods such as soy sauce, french fries, processed meats, prepared soups and sauces, and herbal supplements.

As I described in "Gluten in Grains: A Danger for Some" on page 130, a related condition, called gluten sensitivity or non-celiac gluten sensitivity, can generate symptoms similar to celiac disease but without the intestinal damage.

If you need to go gluten free, or decide to do it, try to find new ways to get folic acid, other B vitamins, and dietary fiber, which the bowels need to work properly. You can do this by eating fruits, vegetables, beans, and non-gluten grains such as brown rice or quinoa.

DEPRESSION

Many people are afflicted with depression at some point in their lifetimes. Globally, it is among the most important causes of disability. Depression can be mild and brief or prolonged and severe. Seeking professional help is important in any case.

Maintaining overall wellness through diet and regular physical activity can help promote good mental health. One specific aspect of diet linked to mental health is consumption of caffeinated coffee, which is strongly related to lower risk of depression and suicide.[5] In both the Nurses' Health Study and Health Professionals Follow-Up Study, women and men who consumed three or more cups of coffee per day had about half the risk of suicide compared with those who didn't drink coffee. This isn't surprising, because coffee has long been known to have mild mood-elevating effects. We also found that consumption of flavonoid-containing fruits and vegetables, especially citrus fruits and juices, was associated with lower risk of depression.[6]

In spite of intense interest in the possibility that higher intake of omega-3 fats might prevent depression, the evidence for this is weak. Some researchers have hypothesized that higher dietary intakes of omega-6 fatty acids, found in many plant oils like soybean and corn oil, could increase the risk of depression by boosting inflammation throughout the body. But higher intake of omega-6 fats may actually *reduce* inflammation.[7] In our investigation of suicide risk, we saw no evidence of a reduction in suicide with a higher intake of omega-3 fats or lower intake of omega-6 fats.[8]

MEMORY LOSS

Because the average American is living longer—thanks mainly to reductions in smoking, improvements in diet, and earlier diagnosis and better treatments of medical conditions—age-related memory loss (dementia) is an increasing burden on individuals and family members. However, there is good news in the trend seen over the last few decades. When comparing people of similar ages, the incidence of dementia has decreased by more than 40 percent since the late 1970s.[9] But because our population is aging, the actual number of people with dementia is increasing, and there is currently no satisfactory medical treatment for it.

There is exciting evidence that a Mediterranean-type dietary pattern can reduce the risk of memory loss and slow the course of this process. This isn't completely surprising, because the factors that lead to memory loss and dementia include damage to the brain's blood supply and the occurrence of multiple small strokes. A poor diet may also promote processes in the brain related to Alzheimer's disease, a common form of dementia. Both cardiovascular disease and Alzheimer's disease develop slowly over many decades, providing major opportunities for prevention by diet. A Mediterranean-type diet pattern is proven to reduce these and other forms of cardiovascular disease. But even once memory loss has begun, slowing its progression through diet can be valuable.

Many types of studies, including long-term epidemiologic studies, have examined the connection between diet, memory loss, and dementia. These were recently reviewed by my colleague, Martha Clare Morris, and her team. They identified a variety of foods that were related to better thinking skills. These include vegetables, especially green leafy vegetables, berries, nuts, olive oil, whole grains, fish, poultry, and wine taken moderately. Foods linked to *poorer* thinking skills included red meat, fast fried food, pastries, and sweets. Sound familiar?

Morris created a score based on these foods, which she called the MIND diet score, and tested it in a group of almost 1,000 older men and women taking part in the Memory and Aging Project at Rush University Medical Center in Chicago. Over a five-year period, higher MIND scores—meaning healthier eating—were associated with better scores on thinking and memory tests.[10] As is the case for cardiovascular disease, the strong benefit of the MIND dietary pattern likely comes from multiple foods, not a single nutrient. However, we do know that beta-carotene is one of the contributors to a healthier brain because of its beneficial effect on cognitive function when given as a supplement in the Physicians' Health Study (see "New Hope for Multivitamins" on page 236). Further support for the connection between healthy eating and preserved memory and thinking skills comes from the PREDIMED randomized trial, in which participants who followed a Mediterranean-type dietary pattern experienced better cognitive function compared to those on a control diet.[11]

It only makes sense that a diet that is good for many other organs is also good for the brain. While ongoing research aims to understand the effects of specific dietary factors on the brain, adopting a Mediterranean-type diet that includes a variety of foods high in carotenoids will put you on a path to better long-term cognitive function. Starting on this path as early in life as possible is best, but from what we have seen in other health outcomes, you can still reap the benefits of a healthy diet even if you start once symptoms have developed.

CHAPTER FIFTEEN

Shopping Tips, Recipes, and Menus

E ATING HEALTHFULLY, AS YOU'VE LEARNED earlier in this book, is not a complicated concept. Simply put, it involves building an eating style that is based on whole grains, fresh produce, good fats, and healthy protein "packages." To get you started in the right direction, my wife, Gail, and I have developed a group of seventy-seven recipes, everything from Curried Winter Squash Soup to Fruit 'n' Spicy Nut Trail Mix, that will tempt your taste buds and renew your faith that eating for good health can be a delicious endeavor. Some of the recipes are quick fixes that can go from preparation to table in under thirty minutes. Others take a bit more time, but include classic favorites like multigrain hotcakes, chili, and fried rice.

In general, these recipes represent just good, healthy food and so don't require any major manipulations. Although the recipes aren't specifically geared toward weight loss and require no special culinary skills, just the fact that they emphasize whole grains, fruits, vegetables, nuts, seeds, and legumes should make it easy to work these recipes into a weight-loss plan, because the *quality* of your diet is as important to long-term weight control as the *quantity* of your diet.

If you are battling with excess weight, you already know there is no quick fix. As discussed in chapter four, you'll need to become more active, find a diet that's right for you, and practice defensive eating (see pages 64 to 66). This section of the book will give you an easy, delicious way to find foods that are right for you.

If you are looking to lose weight, at the bottom of each day's menu is some advice on how to adapt the menu to a reduced-calorie plan. Losing weight isn't about deprivation. It's about moderation and choosing high-quality food. So don't put favorite foods on a taboo list; just learn to eat them in smaller portions and less frequently. At the same time, take delight in truly good, fresh food. A just-picked juicy sweet peach. Steamed fresh green beans with a squeeze of lemon juice and a sprinkle of pepper. A hot-off-the-grill salmon steak. Your tastes may eventually start shifting away from salty, sugary, overprocessed foods and wake up to a whole wonderful world of fresh, clean flavors. Who knows, your list of favorites might just change completely.

This section also includes a week's worth of menus to help you get started planning healthful meals.

CHOOSE NUTRITION-PACKED FOODS

While there are no superfoods that contain every single nutrient needed for good health, some foods pack more nutrients per calorie than others. By choosing nutrient-dense foods, the overall quality of your diet will improve practically overnight. For the most part, that means eating whole grains, fruits, and vegetables at every meal. Here are some tips to get you started.

Add dark leafy greens to salads. Dark leafy greens contain more nutrients than iceberg lettuce. Spinach, kale, and romaine lettuce, for example, contain everything from iron to folate to fiber. Iceberg lettuce, on the other hand, is mostly water. A good rule of thumb: The darker the green, the more nutrients a leafy vegetable contains.

Sprinkle wheat germ on cereals, casseroles, or yogurt. Adding 2 tablespoons of wheat germ boosts the fiber nearly 2 grams but adds only 51 calories. Use the toasted variety for a nuttier flavor.

Serve a whole grain as a side dish instead of potatoes. White potatoes and grains like bulgur and wheat berries are considered starchy side dishes. But the potatoes have nowhere near as much fiber and are not as nutrient dense as whole grains. In addition, the body quickly turns the starch in white potatoes into sugar, causing a quick spike in blood sugar and insulin. Whole grains are digested more slowly, causing a lower and more even rise in blood sugar.

Snack on whole-grain crackers rather than those made with processed flour. Whole-grain crackers such as Triscuit or Ak-mak contain more fiber than those made with refined flour. That fiber can add up if you're a regular snacker. Even better, think of nuts as an alternative. They are probably the healthiest hunger-blunting snack you could have.

Try the "three pleasures" for dessert instead of ice cream or cake. Instead of a traditional calorie-laden dessert, create one from three of the healthiest foods you can eat: fruit, nuts, and dark chocolate. This offers a sweet, delicious way to end a meal that's also good for your health and your waistline. When Gail

Making Better Food Choices

Eat This	Not That
whole grain bread	white bread
brown rice or other intact grains	white rice or potatoes
olive or other liquid oils	butter
peanut butter	cheese or bologna for a sandwich
nuts on a salad	cheese on a salad
nuts as a snack	sweets as a snack
Three Pleasures for dessert	cheesecake, ice cream, or other usual desserts
beans, soy, fish, or poultry	red meat
plain yogurt with added fruit and nuts	ice cream

and I have dessert at home, this is usually what we make. When we dine out, I have been challenging chefs around the country to redesign dessert to focus on these foods, which I call the Three Pleasures. We have experienced many wonderful creations. You can find more details and "business cards" to give to your waiter at Google hsph.me/3fordessert.

HEALTHFUL SUBSTITUTIONS

No single food will make or break good health. But the overall quality of your diet—the kinds of foods you choose to eat day in and day out—does have a major impact. Good diets, ones that promote well-being, are built mainly on nutrient-dense choices: foods that contain healthful fats, fiber, and a whole host of other nutrients and phytochemicals. I urge you to enjoy food. But when push comes to shove, make choices that are high in flavor *and* good for health.

One important step is to replace unhealthy saturated and trans fats with healthful unsaturated fats (see "Replacing Unhealthy Fats with Healthier Ones" on page 106). And make it a point to start adding more whole grains, fruits, and vegetables to meals. Here are some suggestions for achieving those goals.

Directory of Whole or Intact Grains

Grains have nourished humans since early times. But somewhere along the way most of us have lost touch with their goodness. Here's a brief overview

Intact Grain Versus Whole Grain

Grains are the seeds of plants that are mostly in the grass family. Each intact grain has three parts: the bran, the germ, and the endosperm.

The bran surrounds the grain. It provides protection so the seed can endure harsh conditions and still germinate many months or years later. Even though the brain is mostly indigestible fiber, many minerals and vitamins are closely attached to it.

The germ is the embryonic plant that will sprout and grow when the temperature and moisture conditions are right. The delicate living tissues in the germ are bathed in unsaturated oil, which also contains a large amount of fat-soluble antioxidants, such as vitamin E, to protect the oil from becoming oxidized.

The endosperm provides energy for the germinating seed until it can begin to make its own food through photosynthesis. It is mainly starch. Over the years, grains have been bred to grow larger and larger endosperms, meaning more and more starch. Although the endosperm contains other nutrients, too, the amounts are low compared to the calories from starch.

Intact grains are grains that have been minimally processed to remove them from the seed head and to remove grit and other impurities. They have not been smashed, pulverized, steamed, or undergone other processing. Examples of intact grains include wheat berries, brown rice, millet, oat groats, and quinoa.

Whole grains, and foods made from them, are intact grains that have been processed in one way or another, often by milling, which grinds up the grain. They still contain the bran, germ, and endosperm.

In contrast, refined grains such as wheat flour (not "whole wheat" flour), have had the bran and germ removed. Vitamins and minerals are often added to this depleted flour, which is then sold as "enriched" flour. While that may sound healthy, what's added is only a small fraction of the many nutrients and phytochemicals that the original grain contained.

Whole grains are significantly better for you than refined grains because they deliver all the nutrients that were in the intact grain. But they aren't as good as intact grains. One reason is that milling chops up the grains, disrupting the bran layer. It no longer covers the endosperm, opening it up to faster attack by starch-digesting enzymes. This speeds the conversion of starch to blood sugar. Grinding the endosperm into fine particles also makes it easier for starch-digesting enzymes to do their job. The result is that intact grains have a lower glycemic index (see page 117), which results in slower and lower rises in blood glucose, less demand for insulin, and lower risk of type 2 diabetes. The lower glycemic index of intact grains helps you feel full longer after a meal or snack and delays the onset of hunger.

of whole and intact grains, an A-to-Z list with what you need to know about cooking techniques, storage guidelines, and taste. Remember, whole grains are unrefined but can be available as flour; intact grains are just that.

Amaranth

Cultivated by the Aztecs, this yellow-gold seed has a crunchy texture that softens only slightly when cooked. In fact, its creamy-crunchy texture is so much like the consistency of hot cereals that this is the way the grain is most often eaten. For the adventurous, amaranth (pronounced AM-uh-ranth) can be tucked into baked goods (see Banana-Apricot Nut Bread, page 306) or mixed with other grains to make a pilaf or casserole. Try toasting the seeds in a dry skillet; they expand and "pop" just like corn. Sprinkle the crunchy popped kernels on salads, vegetables, and pizza.

Cooking rating: Easy but time-consuming. Amaranth must be simmered in a large amount of water (1 part grain to 3 parts water) for twenty-five to thirty minutes to eat as cereal. To use in baked goods, presoak in boiling water.

Nutritional benefits: Cholesterol-free with a small amount of fat, most of it unsaturated. Rich in iron, with 60 percent of the required amount in ¼ cup of the dry seed. Good source of fiber—3 grams per ¼ cup dry—but not as high in fiber as some other whole grains. Also a good source of calcium, with small amounts of B vitamins.

Shopping tip: It's unlikely you will find this grain at the supermarket. It can be found in most specialty stores or ordered online. (See website information in the section that follows this dictionary.)

Barley

This nutty-flavored whole grain is sold in many different forms: hulled, pearled, flakes, and grits. The pearled variety is the most common and most versatile. It retains a chewy texture even after long periods of cooking. That makes it a good candidate for soups, casseroles, and even a whole-grain risotto (see Wild Mushroom–Barley Risotto, page 367).

Cooking rating: Easy but time-consuming.

Whole hulled barley: Must be soaked overnight and then simmered for an hour or more.

Pearled barley: Made from grains that are split but still contain the center, or "pearl." Thanks to the refining, you can skip the soaking step and shave thirty minutes off the cooking time. If that's not fast enough, look for quick-cooking pearl barley, which cooks in ten minutes.

Flakes/grits: Barley flakes, which resemble rolled oats, can be made into hot cereal or soup. Barley "grits" are a fine grind of the grain used for hot cereal.

Nutritional benefits: Cholesterol-free, with a tiny amount of healthy fat. Good source of protein, with decent amounts of iron, potassium, and magnesium. Excellent source of fiber: about 8 grams per ¼ cup dry.

Shopping tip: Pearl and instant barley are found in most supermarkets. Whole hulled barley, barley flakes, and barley grits can be found in specialty stores or ordered online.

Brown Rice

Brown rice gets its characteristic brown color and nutty flavor from the fact that the grain's outer layer, the bran, is left on when the rice is harvested. It can be found in short, medium, or long grains, each of which has different uses. Brown basmati rice, a special type of long-grain brown rice, has a particularly nutty flavor and gives off a wonderful aroma as it cooks. Since it still contains the bran layer, which has small amounts of oil, brown rice is best used within a few weeks of purchase. Or keep it refrigerated in an airtight container.

Cooking rating: Easy but time-consuming. Needs to simmer for forty to forty-five minutes.

Nutritional benefits: Cholesterol-free with only a small amount of healthy mostly unsaturated fat. Twice as high in fiber as white rice; rich in vitamin E and other nutrients.

Shopping tip: The quality and flavor of brown rice can vary by brand. Most supermarkets carry a variety of brown rices, including store brands and specialty blends. Several companies now market instant brown rice; it typically isn't as flavorful as "regular" brown rice and tends to have a higher glycemic index.

Buckwheat

Buckwheat is one of several grain-like foods that isn't technically a grain. It is actually a distant cousin of rhubarb. Buckwheat is typically roasted and then used either whole or ground. Whole or cracked buckwheat seeds (buckwheat groats), once they have been toasted, are sometimes called kasha. In eastern Europe, kasha is routinely used in cooking in much the same way that Americans use potatoes.

Cooking rating: Very easy.

Nutritional benefits: Buckwheat is not as stellar a source of fiber and nutrients as most whole grains, but it can be combined with other grains to make a healthy pilaf.

Bulgur (Bulghur)

This whole grain is actually a form of wheat. A staple in the eastern Mediterranean, bulgur (pronounced BUHL-guhr) is made by steaming or boiling kernels of wheat, called wheat berries, and then crushing them. Bulgur comes in fine, medium, or coarse grind, although the most common form is the medium grind. It can be made from either red wheat (dark brown grain) or white wheat (golden-brown grain). Bulgur can be used in everything from salads and soups to veggie burgers.

Cooking rating: Very easy. Just add boiling water to the fine or medium grain and allow it to soak for twenty to thirty minutes or until tender. (Coarse-textured bulgur must be simmered instead of soaked.)

Nutritional benefits: Cholesterol-free, high fiber (5 grams per ¼ cup dry), and relatively high protein (4 grams per ¼ cup dry).

Shopping tip: Easy to find at most supermarkets.

Corn

This native American grain comes in many different packages. The most obvious is fresh corn on the cob. But the grain can be ground and dried and made into grits, cornmeal, flour, and pasta. The less it's processed, the more flavor and nutrients it will contain.

Cooking rating: Very easy.

Cornmeal: Regular (degerminated) cornmeal is made by stripping dried corn kernels of their outer husk and the germ, which causes loss of nutrients. However, it is usually enriched with some of these lost nutrients. The grain is then ground into a fine, medium, or coarse texture. Polenta is made from a coarse-grain cornmeal. Finely ground cornmeal is called corn flour; masa harina is a type of corn flour used to make corn tortillas. Look for the stone-ground variety if possible, as it contains more nutrients than other varieties of cornmeal. Note that degerminated cornmeal is not whole grain.

Hominy: Corn kernels that are soaked in a weak solution of lye. Since it's degermed and hulled after soaking, hominy isn't as nutritious as fresh corn, but it still contains fiber.

Grits: This southern specialty is made from coarsely ground dried hominy.

Nutritional benefits: Cholesterol-free and rich in fiber. A fair source of vitamin A (yellow corn only), with traces of iron and vitamin C.

Shopping tip: Found in virtually every supermarket.

Whole Wheat Couscous

Couscous (pronounced KOOS-koos) is not technically a whole grain, but when this tiny, golden-colored pasta is made from whole-grain flour, it has quite a few nutritional benefits—not to mention a superfast cooking time.

Cooking rating: Quick and easy. Since couscous is precooked, you'll just need to combine it with water, bring the mixture to a boil, remove from the heat, and let stand, covered, for five minutes. If seasonings (salt, olive oil, herbs) are mixed into the water or the cooking liquid is flavored (chicken broth, tomato juice), the couscous will take on these flavors.

Nutritional benefits: One cup of prepared whole wheat couscous has 2 grams of fiber; regular couscous has none. High in protein, with 8 grams per 1 cup cooked. Small amounts of iron.

Shopping tip: Couscous can be found in many supermarkets.

Flaxseed

This tiny reddish-brown seed has a wonderfully nutty flavor that works well in baked goods. In fact, in many European countries, bakers routinely use this grain in everything from cookies and cakes to bread.

Cooking rating: Very easy. Flaxseed has a tough outer coating that must be partly crushed or ground (in either a clean coffee grinder or blender) in order to unlock the nutritional benefits. The crushed seeds or ground meal can then be added to breads and muffins or used as a topping for yogurt or cereal. Left whole, the seeds pass through the body undigested.

Nutritional benefits: Cholesterol-free. High in fiber and rich in omega-3 fatty acids, fats that help protect against heart disease and other chronic ills.

Shopping tip: Although flaxseeds and ground flaxseed meal are starting to show up in many large supermarkets, the grain is still easier to find in specialty stores or online. Store whole seeds in an airtight container at room temperature for up to a year. Keep the ground seeds in the refrigerator for up to thirty days.

Millet

Yes, this is the same tiny yellow-gold grain that's sold in the United States as bird food. But in other parts of the world, particularly in Africa and Asia, this crunchy, nutty-flavored grain is eaten by humans and highly prized for both its flavor and its strong nutritional profile. Most often cooked as a hot cereal, millet (pronounced MIHL-leht) can also be an ingredient in puddings (used like rice in rice pudding) or mixed into pilafs, pancakes (see the recipe for Multigrain Hotcakes with Warm Apple Syrup on page 309), soups, or stews.

Cooking rating: Easy but time-consuming. To shorten the time, use a two-step process. First toast the grain in a heavy skillet for two to three minutes. Then place it in a saucepan (1 part grain to 2 parts water) and simmer for twenty-five to thirty minutes.

Nutritional benefits: Cholesterol-free, with a tiny amount of healthy fat from the whole grain. Incredibly rich in thiamin and iron, providing 20 to 25 percent of the recommended requirement for these two nutrients. Millett also delivers significant amounts of protein, fiber, and potassium.

Shopping tip: You probably won't be able to find millet in a regular supermarket (except in the pet food aisle). But it's easily purchased at specialty stores and online.

Oats

One of the world's most popular grains—half of the farmland in Ireland and one-third in Scotland is devoted to growing it—oats are valued for their flavor, versatility, and medical prowess. The latter is due to the fact that oats are one of the top sources of soluble fiber, a type of fiber that can help lower blood cholesterol levels. Oats can be purchased as the whole grain—oat groats—or as processed oat flour, oat bran, and oatmeal.

Cooking rating: Easy to very easy, depending on variety.

Oatmeal: Made from whole-grain oats that have been husked or stripped of their outer coat. Some varieties of oatmeal are steamed and rolled flat (old-fashioned or quick-cooking rolled oats) before being thinly sliced. Others, like Scotch oats and Irish oatmeal, are simply sliced thin with steel blades.

Rolled oats: Unless they're the instant variety, rolled oats need to be simmered for about ten minutes. Instant varieties are precooked and dried to make cooking times shorter. Quick-cooking oats are more thinly sliced than old-fashioned rolled oats and cook in only three to five minutes.

Steel-cut oats: Firmer and nuttier tasting than the steam-processed varieties, steel-cut oats make a creamier oatmeal but require a longer cooking time, up to forty minutes. If you like oatmeal for breakfast, a good idea is to make six or seven servings of steel-cut oats on a Saturday or Sunday morning. When cooled, spoon the oatmeal into single-serve containers and microwave as needed.

Oat bran: The outer coating of the oat seed is high in fiber and many nutrients, including iron, potassium, and thiamin. Like wheat bran, this fiber can be added to baked goods or cereal.

Oat groats: An excellent intact grain, these whole-oat kernels must be simmered for thirty-to forty-five minutes. The nutty-flavored groats can also be toasted and added to baked goods (see Whole Wheat Pizza Crust on page 337).

Oat flour: Sold in many supermarkets, the flour made from husked oats can sometimes be highly refined, but most varieties are richer in fiber than white flour. While it works well in thickening sauces, oat flour lacks gluten, the protein that helps yeast breads rise. Small amounts of oat flour can be used in baked goods, but bread, pizza dough, or cake made with all oat flour will turn out poorly.

Nutritional benefits: Cholesterol-free, with small amounts of healthy fat from the whole grain. Rich in soluble fiber. Steel-cut oats have a lower glycemic index than standard rolled oats.

Shopping tip: Oatmeal, even the Irish steel-cut variety, is readily found in supermarkets. Oat bran and oat flour can be found in many larger supermarkets. But the more specialized products, like oat groats, are found mainly in specialty stores and online.

Quinoa

This South American "grain," grown for generations in the Andes Mountains of Peru, has come stateside big time. And that's good news. Quinoa (pronounced KEEN-wah), with its distinctively nutty flavor and pearly appearance, is quite the nutrition powerhouse. Fully cooked quinoa has an almost translucent quality except for the germ of the grain, which is visible as a white crescent.

Cooking rating: Easy. Simmers for ten to fifteen minutes.

Nutritional benefits: Has the distinction of being a complete protein. In other words, it is a "high-quality" protein comparable to the protein found in meat and eggs.

Shopping tip: Available in many supermarkets.

Rye

Once referred to as "the grain of poverty," rye is a hearty cereal grain that can grow just about anywhere. Poor soil, high altitudes, harsh climates—none of these seem to stop this grain from taking hold. In fact, rye first appeared as a weed that overran fields of wheat nearly 2,000 years ago. This grain is sold in several forms. The berries, which look like wheat berries and can be used like them, are available mainly in specialty stores and online. Rye flour, because it's low in gluten (the protein that helps bread to rise), makes dense loaves of bread. It's usually used in combination with a higher-protein flour like wheat or with gluten powder.

Cooking rating: Easy but time-consuming. Simmers for thirty to forty minutes.

Nutritional benefits: Lower in protein than wheat.

Shopping tip: Look for the whole kernels or berries at specialty stores. A medium grind of rye flour is sold in many supermarkets. Dark rye flour or the more coarsely ground pumpernickel flour is usually available mainly at specialty stores or online.

Spelt

An ancient cousin to wheat, these large brown kernels look nearly identical to wheat berries (whole kernels of wheat) and, in fact, are pretty much interchangeable with wheat berries in recipes. Spelt, however, is slightly higher in protein than wheat and may be tolerated by people with wheat allergies. Either the berries or the flaked form of spelt can be used for hot cereal or in granola mixtures (see Apple Crunch Oatmeal on page 303). They're also good cooked into soups, salads, and casseroles. Spelt flour can be used in place of wheat flour. See the cooking instructions for wheat berries.

Triticale

This slightly sweet hybrid of two other grains—wheat and rye—is found mainly in specialty stores. You can cook the whole berries, which look like wheat berries and can be used much the same way, or buy triticale (pronounced triht-ih-KAY-lee) flakes to use as cereal or for baking. Triticale flour, like the whole grain, is low in gluten, the protein that gives yeast breads their lift, so triticale flour is used in combination with wheat flour to make acceptably textured baked goods.

Cooking rating: Easy but time-consuming. The whole berries must be simmered thirty to forty minutes.

Nutritional benefits: Cholesterol-free, with a small amount of healthy fat from the whole grain. Higher in protein than wheat, but lower in gluten. (Rye is low in gluten, so this hybrid has some of its characteristics.)

Shopping tip: Look for this grain in health or natural food stores.

Wheat Berries

These whole kernels of wheat contain all the goodness of the wheat grain. Wheat berries come in soft and hard varieties, but the soft and hard moniker has nothing to do with tenderness. The difference between the two varieties is gluten (protein) content. Soft wheat is low in gluten and is ground into pastry flour. Hard wheat is high in gluten and is ground into regular or hearty flours.

Very nutty in flavor, cooked wheat berries make a wonderful breakfast cereal or a crunchy addition to breads and baked goods. They even make a chewy-crunchy substitute for pasta in cold salads.

Cooking rating: Easy but time-consuming. Wheat berries must be simmered for thirty minutes or so. They can be toasted in the oven or in a dry skillet beforehand to shorten the cooking time.

Nutritional benefits: Cholesterol-free and high in fiber; 16 percent of calories from protein. Small amounts of minerals, including iron and zinc.

Shopping tip: Wheat berries can be found in specialty or whole-food grocery stores.

Wild Rice

Technically not a type of rice but the seed of an aquatic grass, this grain rates attention for its stellar fiber content, not to mention an intensely nutty flavor. Because it is so intense—and quite expensive—wild rice is often paired with milder-flavored grains (see Wild Rice–Quinoa Pilaf on page 365). Like its grain counterparts, wild rice is cholesterol-free and has a small amount of healthy fat. Quality can vary, with the more expensive brands typically having a larger percentage of well-shaped, uncrushed grains. Use more expensive varieties in dishes where appearance is important and less expensive ones in soups or stuffings. Steer clear of instant varieties: they may save you time but don't look quite so appetizing.

Cooking rating: Easy but time-consuming. Wild rice must be simmered for 40 to 45 minutes.

Nutritional benefits: Wild rice contains more protein than brown rice. It's a good source of vitamins A, C, and E, as well as phosphorus, zinc, and folate.

Shopping tip: Wild rice can be found in specialty or whole-food grocery stores but is also showing up in mainstream grocery stores.

Whole-Grain Cooking and Storage Tips

Here are some general points to keep in mind when storing and cooking whole grains.

- *Soaking intact whole grains, either for just a few hours or overnight, helps reduce cooking time.*
- *Toasting whole grains intensifies their nutty flavor.* Toasting can also reduce the cooking time for some grains, including barley, spelt, wheat berries, and oat groats.

- *Cooking times aren't carved in stone.* Grains, like legumes, may cook faster or slower depending on how long they have been in storage. Just-harvested grains cook quicker than grains that have been stored for a long time. Tenderness is the best measure of doneness.
- *Store whole grains in airtight containers, preferably in the refrigerator.* All whole grains carry small amounts of natural oils, which can spoil quickly, particularly during hot weather.
- *Cooked whole grains will keep in the refrigerator for two to three days.* They also freeze well. So you might want to consider simmering large batches of grains and packaging them for the freezer. That way you can pull them out and drop them in a soup, a casserole, or a salad without investing a lot of time in the kitchen.

FILLING THE HEALTHY SHOPPING BAG

Now that you're committed to eating more whole grains, fresh produce, unsaturated fats, and healthy protein packages, chances are your shopping list has a few new additions. And you may have questions about where and how to find these foods. Will you need to make routine pilgrimages to specialty stores? How do organic foods fit into the overall picture? Which whole-food products taste best? These questions aren't difficult to answer, but they do involve some individual preference.

The organic issue, for example, has more to do with personal choice than nutrition. There is no evidence that organic produce, grains, or meat are nutritionally superior to produce and grains grown by traditional farming methods.[1] The key difference is what other things they contain—or don't contain—like pesticides and antibiotics. Organic foods come out on top in that category because they are grown without pesticides and antibiotics.

If you decide to make a commitment to organic foods, keep in mind that these products are not always widely available. One of the best strategies is to consider locally grown produce. When you shop at a local farmers' market, farm stand, or small supermarket that carries local produce, you'll be rewarded by some of the best-tasting fruits and vegetables around, organic or not. Produce that is shipped from long distances may have lost some of its flavor or nutritional value because it can take many days to reach the supermarket. Locally grown fruits and vegetables, picked at the height of ripeness, have incredible flavors and nutrition profiles. So, rather than look for asparagus to make the Asparagus, Tofu, Shiitake, and Cashew Stir-Fry (page 336) in July when it's out of season, find a vegetable that's being harvested. Green beans are a summertime crop; they can make a nice stand-in for asparagus in the stir-fry recipe. Learn to cook with the seasons. You'll be rewarded with fruits and vegetables that are at their flavor and nutritional peak.

Also, keep in mind that organic doesn't equate with healthy. The shelves and freezers at Whole Foods and related stores are loaded with organic foods high in sugar, refined starch, and unhealthy fats, and eating organic bacon will still increase your risks of heart disease and diabetes.

As for whole-grain products, locating them is now a lot easier than it used to be. Many whole-grain foods are now firmly entrenched in regular supermarkets. Look for them either in a special aisle with organic and health foods or in the regular flour, cereal, and rice/pasta aisles. Owing to a burgeoning interest in whole foods, the natural-food sections of many supermarkets are growing larger, and whole-food markets are becoming a familiar option in many cities. Then there's the Internet. Many of the larger companies that market whole-grain products have comprehensive websites and efficient mail-order systems. Many company websites have a store locator or "Where to Find" button that lets you locate nearby stores that sell their products.

Just in case you're having trouble locating some of the whole grains used in the following recipes, I've included names and Web addresses of a sampling of the companies that market these foods. This is by no means either a comprehensive list or an endorsement. There are many small companies that produce or import whole-grain foods, but since their availability is limited and varies from region to region, I've focused on some of the national brands. If nothing else, this list should help get you started. Then you can branch out on

Splurge on Quality Ingredients

Eating healthy doesn't mean that food has to be less satisfying. Learn what chefs have known all along: a little bit of a high-quality ingredient goes a long way toward boosting flavor. A good-quality flavored vinegar (balsamic, sherry) can make a potent vinaigrette. A small sprinkling of fresh grated Parmesan cheese, rather than the powdered stuff in the can, can top off a pizza or a salad with a burst of salty, nutty flavor. An extra-virgin olive oil, a roasted peanut oil, a sesame-flavored oil—just small amounts of these high-flavored ingredients can put the finishing touches on a recipe and elevate it from average to sublime.

your own, checking out local stores and ethnic markets for all kinds of wonderful whole-grain foods. Since taste is a personal thing, chances are you'll need a bit of trial and error to find the foods that suit your palate.

Arrowhead Mills, Inc.
Hereford, Texas
www.arrowheadmills.com

Product line: Arrowhead Mills sells organic whole grains, whole-grain cereals and flours, and more mostly through supermarkets and specialty stores.

Bob's Red Mill
Milwaukie, Oregon
www.bobsredmill.com

Product line: Selections include whole grains, whole-grain cereals, whole-grain flours, and whole-grain pastry flours.

Eden Foods, Inc.
Clinton, Michigan
www.edenfoods.com

Product line: Selections range from whole-grain pastas to canned organic tomatoes, legumes, and soy milks. Most, but not all, of the selections are organic.

Hodgson Mill, Inc.
Effingham, Illinois
www.hodgsonmill.com

Product line: Whole-grain pastas, baking mixes, cereals, flours, and cornmeal, with many organic choices. Available in some supermarkets and specialty stores and online.

King Arthur Flour
Norwich, Vermont
www.kingarthurflour.com

Product line: Specialty flours, including whole-grain flours.

Lundberg Family Farms
Richvale, California
www.lundberg.com

Product line: Wide assortment of whole-grain rice products, including brown rice pasta and brown rice blends with names like black Japonica (a blend of short-grain black rice and medium-grain mahogany rice), Christmas blend, and Wehani. Often sold in bulk in specialty stores, available prepackaged in many supermarkets, and also online.

Westbrae Natural Foods
Garden City, New York
www.westbrae.com

Product line: Foods "to support a nutritionally well-rounded vegetarian diet" including organic canned beans and vegetables, organic whole-grain pastas, condiments, and more.

DECIPHERING FOOD LABELS

Federal regulations require food makers to include on a label information about the food's nutrition profile, as well as the ingredients contained in said food. Both of these parts of the label offer valuable information, if you know how to use them. Here's a rundown of key points to consider.

Nutrition Facts Label

The nutrition facts label gives a detailed accounting of how a serving of the food rates nutritionally, first by providing information about calorie content and key nutrients and then by comparing that information to reference values or standard requirements. In 2016, the FDA updated the food label to "make it easier for consumers to make better informed food choices."

- *Serving size.* Don't lose sight of this amount. All the other information on the panel is meaningless if you can't put portion size into perspective. Unfortunately, the portion size listed is often far smaller than what most people might eat. For example, an oversize cookie may list the calories and fat for one-fifth of the cookie as a serving rather than list calories, fat, and nutrients for the whole cookie. Or what looks like a single-serving entrée of frozen lasagna, upon closer inspection, turns out to be 2.5 servings.

SIDE-BY-SIDE COMPARISON

Original Label

Nutrition Facts
Serving Size 2/3 cup (55g)
Servings Per Container About 8

Amount Per Serving

Calories 230 Calories from Fat 72

% Daily Value*

Total Fat 8g	12%
Saturated Fat 1g	5%
Trans Fat 0g	
Cholesterol 0mg	0%
Sodium 160mg	7%
Total Carbohydrate 37g	12%
Dietary Fiber 4g	16%
Sugars 1g	
Protein 3g	

Vitamin A	10%
Vitamin C	8%
Calcium	20%
Iron	45%

* Percent Daily Values are based on a 2,000 calorie diet. Your daily value may be higher or lower depending on your calorie needs.

		Calories:	2,000	2,500
Total Fat	Less than		65g	80g
Sat Fat	Less than		20g	25g
Cholesterol	Less than		300mg	300mg
Sodium	Less than		2,400mg	2,400mg
Total Carbohydrate			300g	375g
Dietary Fiber			25g	30g

New Label

Nutrition Facts
8 servings per container
Serving size 2/3 cup (55g)

Amount per serving
Calories 230

% Daily Value*

Total Fat 8g	10%
Saturated Fat 1g	5%
Trans Fat 0g	
Cholesterol 0mg	0%
Sodium 160mg	7%
Total Carbohydrate 37g	13%
Dietary Fiber 4g	14%
Total Sugars 12g	
Includes 10g Added Sugars	20%
Protein 3g	

Vitamin D 2mcg	10%
Calcium 260mg	20%
Iron 8mg	45%
Potassium 235mg	6%

* The % Daily Value (DV) tells you how much a nutrient in a serving of food contributes to a daily diet. 2,000 calories a day is used for general nutrition advice.

Note: The images above are meant for illustrative purposes to show how the new Nutrition Facts label might look compared to the old label. Both labels represent fictional products. When the original hypothetical label was developed in 2014 (the image on the left-hand side), added sugars was not yet proposed so the "original" label shows 1g of sugar as an example. The image created for the "new" label (shown on the right-hand side) lists 12g total sugar and 10g added sugar to give an example of how added sugars would be broken out with a % Daily Value.

- *Calories.* Calories count. Yet the numbers may not be as important as the quality of those calories. If the calories come mainly from healthy fats and whole grains, then higher numbers aren't a problem, particularly if you're not trying to lose weight. If the calories come mainly from added sugars and saturated fats, then the food is one that's better to pass by.
- *Total fat.* This listing provides the total grams of fat per serving. Again, the number is not as important as the type of fat. Read farther down the panel to find out how much of that fat is saturated and how much is monounsaturated or polyunsaturated. This section of the label also includes infor-

mation on trans fats, the unhealthy fats formed when liquid oils are made into solid shortenings.

- *Cholesterol.* This is one number you shouldn't have trouble with, not if you're searching out whole grains, fruits, and vegetables—all foods that are cholesterol-free. Keep in mind that the American Heart Association recommends eating less than 300 milligrams of cholesterol per day.
- *Sodium.* Look to this section of the food label if you need to restrict salt or sodium in your diet. General guidelines encourage 1,200–1,300 milligrams of sodium per day, with an upper limit of 2,300 milligrams (about the amount found in 1 teaspoon of salt).
- *Total carbohydrates.* Rather than live by numbers, it's best to emphasize whole grains. A listing of the grams of sugar and grams of fiber helps put into context the type of carbohydrate the food contains. The 2016 update of the label requires food companies to list the amount of sugar that has been added to the food, in addition to the amount of naturally occurring sugar it contains. Added sugars deliver calories but few, if any, nutrients.
- *Protein.* Most Americans, even those on vegetarian diets, eat more protein than the body requires. Don't spend much time with this number.
- *Daily values.* The old label listed vitamins A and C, calcium, and iron. The new one lists vitamin D, calcium, iron, and potassium. Keep in mind that it's based on a person who requires two thousand calories per day. That means your needs may be different if you're eating fewer calories or your energy requirements are higher.

Ingredient List

This item-by-item list offers the most detailed accounting of what a product contains. While it doesn't give exact amounts of each ingredient, it does list them in descending order by weight. At the top of the list is the main or most predominant ingredient.

Say you're looking at a juice drink label. The first two ingredients might be water and high-fructose corn syrup. Farther down the list, about three or four ingredients later, a fruit juice like grape or apple might be mentioned. This lets you know that the drink is mostly water and sugar with a tiny amount of fruit juice. An ingredient label on orange juice, on the other hand, will list the first ingredient as orange juice or orange juice from concentrate.

The ingredient list is also where you'll find information about the use of hydrogenated and partially hydrogenated oils, a tipoff about trans fat content.

STOCKING A HEALTHY KITCHEN

Here are some tips for items you'll want to have on hand for your healthy kitchen:

Produce

Whenever possible, choose locally grown fruits and vegetables. Aim for a variety of colors, from red and orange peppers through green kale and spinach to purple plums. The more choices the better: no single food provides all of the nutrients you need to be healthy.

Grains

Once you've used up the white rice in your pantry, replace it with whole grains such as barley, bulgur, millet, quinoa, and more. If your grocery store sells grain in bulk bins, buy small amounts of unfamiliar ones to discover delicious new choices that are often simple to prepare. Keep in mind that whole grains, particularly if milled, can lose their freshness and become rancid if stored at room temperature too long. Keeping them in the refrigerator or freezer will greatly lengthen their shelf life.

Fats and Oils

Stock your pantry with olive oil plus one or more of the following: canola, sunflower, corn, soybean, and peanut oil. Use these oils to sauté vegetables, to stir-fry fish or chicken, and as the base of salad dressings. At the table, try dipping bread into olive oil or drizzling oil onto the bread instead of using butter or margarine.

Protein

The best choices for protein are beans, nuts, tofu and other soy foods, fish, chicken, or turkey. Balance them with plenty of vegetables and fruits, whole grains, and healthy fats.

Other Essentials

Have on hand high-quality basics like extra-virgin olive oil, balsamic vinegar, fresh and dried herbs, plus different types of nuts. Along with the essentials above, you'll have what you need to build virtually any healthy recipe.

ONE WEEK OF MENUS

To give you some idea of how meals might shape up when you're dining according to the Healthy Eating Pyramid and Healthy Eating Plate, I've developed a sample week of menus. These Monday-through-Sunday food plans are meant simply as a guideline, one that illustrates how to put into practice the principles talked about in the preceding chapters. Each day's menu is based on 2,000 calories, the reference figure that health professionals and the food industry use as a benchmark for the energy needs of the average American. Granted, not every individual needs exactly 2,000 calories each day. Most of us have varying energy needs based on age, size, activity level, and how effectively we burn energy. But this figure is a good starting point.

No doubt you'll want to make adjustments to these meal plans based on your own needs. In fact, an addendum at the end of each day explains how to easily convert the menus into a 1,600-calorie plan, a realistic amount of calories if you're looking to lose weight or are just a petite, less active person. We haven't built alcohol into these daily menus; if you are drinking a glass of wine or beer with your evening meal, you will need to figure in an additional 100 to 200 calories a day.

Rather than agonize over daily calorie numbers, however, think about your current situation. Are you maintaining a healthy weight? If you are, then you're no doubt eating the right amount of food for you. Look to these menu plans to guide you in the direction of healthy food choices, letting your natural instincts guide portion size. If you need to lose weight, follow the 1,600-calorie plan or just begin cutting back on what you currently eat. Weight will come off naturally as you begin to cut back and become more active.

The menus run the gamut of choices. One day's lunch looks at how a fast-food restaurant meal (grilled chicken sandwich) can fit into the average day. A weekend supper suggests what you might pull together and eat at your own Cinco de Mayo party, a meal based entirely on selections from our recipe section. There's also a day with six small meals, a style of eating that is just as healthy as three squares a day and, in fact, may be better at helping some people keep their appetite under control and blood sugar on an even keel.

All in all, with the help of these menus and the eighty recipes that follow this section, you'll find that eating healthfully is a simple concept, one that you can put into practice from Monday through Sunday with very little effort.

Recipes for italicized items can be found in the following pages. Those marked with an asterisk (*) are Fast Fix Foods.

SUNDAY

Breakfast

Fresh-Squeezed Orange Juice, 4 ounces
Multigrain Hotcakes with Warm Apple Syrup, 2 servings
Hot Brewed Coffee

Lunch

Herb-Crusted Grilled Chicken Breast
Fresh Cantaloupe (¼)
Sliced Strawberries (½ cup)

Supper

Double Mushroom Meat Loaf
Roasted Winter Vegetable Medley, 2 servings
Mixed Salad Greens, 2 cups with 1½ tablespoons Extra-Virgin Olive Oil
Spiced Poached Pear

Adjustments and variations

For 1,600 calories: Reduce to 1 serving of hotcakes (2 hotcakes with 3 tablespoons of syrup) at breakfast; subtract 259 calories. Omit one tablespoon of olive oil at supper; subtract 126 calories.

MONDAY

Breakfast

Bran Flakes, 2 cups Skim or Soy Milk, 1 cup Banana, sliced
Whole Wheat Toast
Apricot Fruit Spread, 1 tablespoon

Lunch

Oldways Sweet Potato Peanut Stew ("Mafe")
Hearty Wheat Berry–Oat Groat Bread
Fresh Orange Sections

Supper

Grilled Salmon Steaks with Papaya-Mint Salsa
Green Snap Beans
Steamed Whole Wheat Couscous
Fresh-Baked Pumpernickel Roll
Snack
Easy Peach, Pineapple, and Apricot Crisp

Adjustments and variations

For 1,600 calories: Omit whole wheat toast and fruit spread; subtract 166 calories. Omit pumpernickel roll at supper; subtract 65 calories. Omit fruit crisp at snack time; subtract 212 calories. Munch on a ripe fresh peach instead; add 60 calories.

TUESDAY

Breakfast

("grab-and-go" items)
Mango Energy Blitz*
Banana-Apricot Nut Bread, 2 slices
(Fast-food restaurant)
Grilled Chicken Sandwich (with Whole Wheat Bun if possible)
Mixed Green Salad
Vinaigrette Salad Dressing
Large Apple

Supper

Chicken and Vegetable Stir Fry
Wild Rice–Quinoa Pilaf
Steamed Fresh Asparagus
Cinnamon Applesauce
Snack
Whole-Grain Crackers (3)
Natural-Style Peanut Butter, 1½ tablespoons

Adjustments and variations

For 1,600 calories: Omit sandwich bun at lunch; subtract 135 calories. Omit snack; subtract 249 calories. If you are hungry in the evening, munch on raw vegetables (carrots, celery, cherry tomatoes) instead.

WEDNESDAY

Breakfast

Fried Egg Sandwich on Grilled Whole Wheat English Muffin
Ruby Red Grapefruit
*Blackberry-Banana Smoothie**

Lunch

Onion–Crusted Tofu–Steak Sandwich
*Seven-Vegetable Slaw,** 1 cup
Sliced Kiwi with Fresh Blueberries

Supper

*Curried Winter Squash Soup**
Cracked Wheat Peasant Bread, large chunk
Spinach and Mushroom Salad, with Vinaigrette
Snack
*Fruit 'n' Spicy Nut Trail Mix,** ½ cup
Orange Juice Spritzer

Adjustments and variations

For 1,600 calories: Cut down to 1 teaspoon of oil at breakfast to cook egg (toast English muffin or grill it dry); subtract 84 calories. Cut smoothie portion in half (6 ounces); subtract 92 calories. Cut down to a small wedge of bread; subtract 65 calories. Omit night snack; subtract 182 calories.

THURSDAY

Breakfast

Whole Wheat Toast, 2 slices
Natural-Style Peanut Butter
Strawberry Fruit Spread
Apple-Cranberry Juice

Lunch

Chipotle Chicken Chili
Baked Tortilla Chips
Fruit Cocktail in Juice
Oatmeal-Raisin Cookie

Supper

(Restaurant dinner) Crostini with Olive Oil
Oven-Roasted Sea Bass
Wild Rice Pilaf
Steamed Broccoli
Fruit Sorbet with Almond Biscotti
Espresso

Adjustments and variations

For 1,600 calories: Omit apple-cranberry juice at breakfast; subtract 128 calories. Omit cookie at lunch; subtract 74 calories. Omit biscotti at supper; subtract 180 calories.

FRIDAY

Six Small Meals

Early Morning (1)

Apple Crunch Oatmeal
Chilled Pineapple Juice, 6 ounces
Fresh Brewed Coffee or Tea

Midmorning (2)

Carrot–Wheat Germ Muffin
Hard-boiled Egg with Coarse Salt and Pepper
Sweet Black Grapes, 12

Noon (3)

*California Chicken Salad**
Large Banana

Midafternoon (4)

Spicy Shrimp and Peanut Noodle Salad
Celery Sticks
Sparkling Water with Lime

Evening (5)

Lemon-Oregano Grouper with Vegetables
Chopped Romaine Lettuce Salad with Light Balsamic Vinaigrette
Orange Juice Sorbet

Mid-evening (6)

Blackberry-Banana Smoothie*
Roasted Salted Cashews, 6 small

Adjustments and variations

For 1,600 calories: Replace pineapple juice with 4 ounces of orange juice at breakfast; subtract 49 calories. Omit carrot–wheat germ muffin midmorning and save for evening snack; no calorie change. Cut down to a small banana at lunch; subtract 59 calories. Omit sorbet at supper; subtract 68 calories. Omit smoothie and cashews at midevening snack and eat carrot–wheat germ muffin instead; subtract 254 calories.

SATURDAY

Breakfast

Fresh-Squeezed White Grapefruit Juice, 1 cup
Scrambled Eggs, 2 (cooked with 2 teaspoons oil)
Whole-Grain Toast, 2 slices
Pineapple Fruit Spread
Fresh Brewed Coffee or Tea

Lunch

California Chicken Salad*
Hearty Wheat Berry–Oat Groat Bread
Iced Tea with Lemon

Supper

(Cinco de Mayo party)
*Avocado-Shrimp Salsa**
*Sun-Dried Tomato Dip with Oven-Roasted Corn Chips,** 2 servings
Chipotle Chicken Chili
Mexican Beer, 12 ounces
Midnight movie snack
Popcorn Popped in Oil, 2 cups
*Fruit 'n' Spicy Nut Trail Mix**

Adjustments and variations

For 1,600 calories: Use 1 teaspoon of oil to cook eggs (instead of 2); subtract 40 calories. Cut down to half a slice of bread at lunch; subtract 75 calories. Omit beer at supper; subtract 140 calories. Choose one appetizer at supper: either the salsa or the dip and chips; subtract 90 calories. Switch to air-popped popcorn instead of oil-popped (you can still include the trail mix); subtract 50 calories.

Busy Day Menu

It isn't always easy to combine healthy eating with an intense work schedule and busy family life. Here's how I try to do it on busy days, a plan that can be varied in an almost infinite number of ways.

Wake up, boil water, and dump in steel-cut oats or a packet of Kashi pilaf, a mix of intact oats, brown rice, wheat, and other grains. While this is cooking, I exercise. When the grains are almost done, I add dried fruit or fresh fruit in season and some nuts plus a bit of yogurt on top. Orange juice diluted with carbonated water provides fresh-tasting but low-calorie hydration at breakfast. With this breakfast I'm never hungry before noon, so a snack never enters my mind. (For days with early meetings, Kashi can be cooked the night before.)

Leftover Kashi provides the beginning of a lunch that can be prepared in five minutes. To a base of Kashi in a glass or plastic container, add whatever sounds good. It might be a salad or a mix of fruits or leftover bits of chicken or fish. Most of the time I also add one or more types of nuts. A few generous dashes of a flavorful olive oil with vinegar or a seasoning make almost any of these endless combinations taste good. My favorite is when our peaches, blueberries, and grapes are all ripe at the same time: with roasted almonds and olive oil, this is hard to beat. Snap on a cover and slip it in a bag with an apple, fork, and napkin; this is quicker than waiting in a cafeteria line. I put all this in my backpack, dash out the door with my bike, and I'm in my office in the Harvard Medical area in fifteen minutes, faster than I can get there by driving and parking.

In the evening, if I'm lucky, my wife, Gail, may have made one of the entrées from this book, or one of countless other healthy creations, for dinner. If not, a stop at the fish market provides a quick beginning for a meal. Broil with some lemon, add a salad and maybe some whole-grain bread with a little olive oil for dipping, and in fifteen minutes we can have a fresh, satisfying, and healthy meal.

Recipes

Roasted Portobello Mushrooms with Hazelnut Buckwheat Stuffing

Maria Speck, award-winning author of Simply Ancient Grains *(Ten Speed Press, 2015) and* Ancient Grains for Modern Meals (Ten Speed Press, 2011)

Nonstick cooking spray (optional)
4 large portobello mushrooms with 5-inch-diameter caps (about 1 pound), wiped clean
3 tablespoons olive oil
¾ teaspoon fine sea salt
½ teaspoon freshly ground black pepper, plus more as needed
¾ cup kasha (whole toasted buckwheat, not raw groats)
Heaping ⅓ cup coarsely chopped hazelnuts
2 garlic cloves, pressed or minced
1 tablespoon fresh thyme leaves, or 1 teaspoon dried, plus 4 small sprigs for garnish
½ teaspoon Aleppo pepper, or ¼ teaspoon crushed red pepper flakes (optional)
2 ounces Parmesan cheese, finely grated (about ½ cup)
Balsamic vinegar, for drizzling

1. Place a rack about 6 inches away from the heat and preheat the broiler on high for about 5 minutes. Grease a large rimmed baking sheet with olive oil or cooking spray.
2. Remove the stems of the mushrooms, slicing close to the base (reserve for another use such as in a broth or vegetable stir-fry). Rub the mushrooms, inside and out, with 2 tablespoons of the olive oil. Season with ½ teaspoon of the salt and the black pepper.

3. Place the mushrooms, gill-side up, on the prepared baking sheet and broil for 5 minutes (7 minutes for thick mushrooms).

4. Meanwhile, in a medium bowl, combine the kasha, hazelnuts, garlic, thyme, Aleppo pepper, and remaining ¼ teaspoon salt. Drizzle with the remaining 1 tablespoon olive oil and stir with a fork to combine well.

5. Remove the baking sheet with the mushrooms from the oven and carefully heap about ¼ cup of the buckwheat filling into the center of each mushroom. Spread the filling with the back of a spoon, gently pressing it down. Sprinkle the Parmesan across the top.

6. Rotate the baking sheet and return it to the oven. Broil until the mushrooms are tender and the cheese becomes crisp and starts to brown, 3 to 5 minutes more, watching closely so as not to burn the Parmesan (this can happen within 30 seconds—I've been there!).

7. To finish, remove the baking sheet from the oven. Garnish each mushroom with a sprig of thyme, drizzle with balsamic vinegar, and grind a bit of black pepper on top. Serve right away.

Note: Large portobello mushrooms are key here so you have enough room for the filling.

Yield: 4 servings as a light meal, or 8 as an appetizer

Calories: 349; Protein: 13 g; Carbohydrate: 15 g; Fiber: 2 g; Sodium: 808 mg; Fat: 27 g (Sat: 7 g, Mono: 17 g, Poly: 3 g, Trans: 0 g); Cholesterol: 22 mg

Avocado-Shrimp Salsa (FAST FIX)

The buttery rich texture of avocado pairs nicely with shrimp in this guacamole-style salsa. To save time, buy cooked, peeled shrimp. If all you can find are large shrimp, cut them in half or into thirds. Try this salsa with the Oven-Roasted Corn Chips (page 299) or use as a filling for a wrap-style sandwich made with shredded romaine lettuce.

½ pound medium shrimp (about 20)

2 small avocados, pitted, peeled, and coarsely chopped

2 plum tomatoes, seeded and chopped (about 1 cup)

2 tablespoons minced red onion

1 tablespoon fresh lime juice

Coarse salt
32 baked tortilla chips, for serving

Place the shrimp, avocados, tomatoes, onion, and lime juice in a medium bowl. Season with salt. Toss gently to mix; let stand 5 to 10 minutes. Serve at room temperature with the tortilla chips.

Yield: 3 cups (12 servings); Serving: ¼ cup salsa, 4 tortilla chips

Calories: 86; Protein: 6.5 g; Carbohydrate: 9.7 g; Fiber: 1.6 g; Sodium: 100 mg; Fat 3.0 g (Sat: 0.38 g, Mono: 1.47 g, Poly: 0.33 g, Trans: 0 g); Cholesterol: 46 mg

Sun-Dried Tomato Dip with Oven-Roasted Corn Chips (FAST FIX)

Sun-dried tomatoes can be found either in the produce section of the super-market or next to the canned tomato sauces. If you can only find sun-dried tomatoes packed in oil, go ahead and use them and omit some of the oil used in the dip.

CHIPS

Nonstick cooking spray (optional)
1 tablespoon canola oil, plus more if needed for the baking sheet
6 (6-inch) corn tortillas
¼ teaspoon coarse salt

DIP

1 (15-ounce) can cannellini (white kidney beans) or other white beans
1 tablespoon canola oil
1 to 2 garlic cloves, minced
2 tablespoons fresh lime juice
3 tablespoons coarsely chopped sun-dried tomatoes
Coarse salt

1. Preheat the oven to 400°F. Lightly coat a nonstick baking sheet with cooking spray or oil.
2. To make the chips, brush each tortilla with ½ teaspoon of the canola oil and stack the rounds on top of one another. Cut the stack in half and then

into quarters; you will have 24 large triangles. Place the triangles oiled side up on the baking sheet. Sprinkle with the salt and bake for 8 to 12 minutes, or until crisp.

3. To make the dip, drain the beans through a sieve set over a bowl, reserving ¼ cup of the liquid. Place the beans, 1 tablespoon oil, garlic, lime juice, and sun-dried tomatoes in a food processor and process until the mixture resembles coarse meal. Add the reserved bean liquid and process into a smooth paste. (If the mixture is too thick, add water until the desired consistency is reached.) Taste for seasoning and add salt, if desired.

4. Transfer to a serving bowl and serve with the chips.

Note: Make this dip the night before a party, if possible. Flavors will improve if left to chill overnight.

Yield: 1½ cups dip, 24 large chips; Serving: 1 tablespoon dip and 1 chip

Calories: 45; Protein: 1.3 g; Carbohydrate: 6.5 g; Fiber: 1.2 g; Sodium: 75 mg; Fat: 1.7 g (Sat: 0.13 g, Mono: 0.88 g, Poly: 0.58 g, Trans: 0 g); Cholesterol: 0 mg

Fruit 'n' Spicy Nut Trail Mix (FAST FIX)

Buying roasted soy nuts and sunflower seeds helps save some time. The dried corn adds a nice bit of sweetness and crunch to this mix. Look for it at health food stores, which have a large selection of fruits and vegetables that are dried without sugar.

SPICY NUTS

½ cup raw cashews
½ cup raw whole almonds with skin
1½ teaspoons canola or olive oil
1 teaspoon chili powder
½ teaspoon coarse salt
½ teaspoon dried oregano
½ teaspoon paprika
¼ teaspoon onion powder
¼ teaspoon freshly ground black pepper

TRAIL MIX

1 cup salted roasted soy nuts
¼ cup salted roasted sunflower seeds

1 cup coarsely chopped unsweetened dried apricots

1 cup unsweetened dried apple slices, chopped

½ cup dried corn (such as Just Corn)

1. Preheat the oven to 375°F.
2. To make the spicy nuts, combine all the ingredients for the nuts in a small bowl and toss until blended. Place the coated nuts on a small nonstick baking sheet and bake for 7 to 10 minutes, or until roasted, turning the nuts once about halfway through.
3. To make the trail mix, transfer the spicy nuts when cool to a medium bowl and add the remaining ingredients. Stir to combine. Store the trail mix in an airtight container at room temperature.

Yield: 4½ cups; Serving: ¼ cup

Calories: 117; Protein: 4.0 g; Carbohydrate: 15 g; Fiber: 1.7 g; Sodium: 122 mg; Fat: 5.4 g (Sat: 0.7 g, Mono: 1.33 g, Poly: 0.52 g, Trans: 0 g); Cholesterol: 0 mg

Blackberry-Banana Smoothie (FAST FIX)

The flavors for a fruit smoothie are nearly limitless. But naturally sweet blackberries and bananas—a great thickener for smoothies—are a delicious match. Try raspberries, blueberries, or strawberries in place of the blackberries.

2 cups frozen unsweetened blackberries (about 8 ounces)

1 large banana, peeled and cut into 4 sections

1 cup vanilla soy milk (such as Eden Soy)

½ cup apple juice

½ cup soft silken reduced-fat tofu (such as Mori-Nu Lite)

Place all the ingredients in a blender or food processor and process until smooth. Pour into chilled glasses and serve.

Note: Leftovers will keep in the refrigerator for up to 24 hours. Be sure to use silken-style tofu. Water-packed tofu is too firm in texture to make a smooth blend.

Yield: 2½ cups (3 servings); Serving: ¾ cup

Calories: 185; Protein: 5.9 g; Carbohydrate: 38 g; Fiber: 6.4 g; Sodium: 2 mg; Fat: 1.8 g (Sat: 0.07 g, Mono: 0.09 g, Poly: 0.43 g, Trans: 0 g); Cholesterol: 0 mg

General: This liquid refreshment has more fiber than most breakfast cereals and small amounts of many other nutrients, everything from vitamin E to calcium to phosphorus.

Strawberry-Almond Shake (FAST FIX)

I f the thick texture of a smoothie isn't to your liking, this blended drink has a smooth, frothy texture similar to that of a milk shake. Vary the fruit and add ingredients like wheat germ and bran to give the shake more fiber.

1 cup frozen unsweetened strawberries
1 cup plain soy milk
2 tablespoons sliced almonds
1 tablespoon ground flaxseed
¼ teaspoon finely grated orange zest
3 ice cubes
Dash of almond extract
2 fresh strawberries (optional)

1. Place the frozen strawberries, soy milk, almonds, flaxseed, orange zest, ice cubes, and almond extract in a blender. Blend until smooth.
2. Pour into two glasses. Garnish each with a fresh strawberry, if desired.

Yield: 2 servings; Serving: about ¾ cup

Calories: 131; Protein: 5.9 g; Carbohydrate: 13.3 g; Fiber: 3.3 g; Sodium: 41 mg: Fat: 6.8 g (Sat: 0.3, Mono: 2.4, Poly: 1.3 g, Trans: 0 g); Cholesterol 0 mg

Mango Energy Blitz (FAST FIX)

W ith a small amount of caffeine from the brewed tea, and the natural energy from carrot juice and three kinds of fruits, this sweet drink can give a nutritious jump-start to your day. Make the tea the night before so it will be chilled and ready to go in the morning. And try freezing the banana and mango in plastic freezer bags so that you can be ready to make this delicious beverage whenever you feel your energy waning. Pure carrot juice can be found in health food stores.

1 tea bag kiwi-pear green tea (such as Republic of Tea) or Earl Grey tea
½ cup boiling water

1 mango, peeled and chopped (about 1 cup)

1 large banana, peeled and cut into sections

1 cup apricot nectar (such as R. W. Knudsen), chilled

½ cup carrot juice, chilled

⅛ teaspoon freshly grated nutmeg

1. Steep the tea bag in the boiling water for 3 minutes or according to the package directions. Remove the tea bag and refrigerate the tea until chilled.

2. Combine the mango, banana, and chilled tea in a blender or food processor and process until smooth. Add the apricot nectar, carrot juice, and nutmeg and pulse to mix. Pour into chilled glasses and serve.

Note: Leftovers will keep in the refrigerator for up to 24 hours. For a variation, consider adding ¼ cup toasted wheat germ for an extra dose of fiber.

Yield: 4 cups; Serving: 1 cup

Calories: 98; Protein: 0.7 g; Carbohydrate: 25.2 g; Fiber: 2 g; Sodium: 27 mg; Fat: 0.2 g (Sat: 0.06 g, Mono: 0.06 g, Poly: 0.05 g, Trans: 0 g); Cholesterol: 0 mg

BREADS AND GRAINS

Apple Crunch Oatmeal

Be sure to choose a sweet red apple rather than a tart variety like Granny Smith for this cereal. To save time in the morning, you can cook the spelt or wheat berries (kernels of wheat) the night before. Spelt and wheat berries are interchangeable in recipes, as both are just different strains of wheat. Either can be found in health food stores or on the internet.

½ cup spelt berries or soft wheat berries

3½ cups water

½ teaspoon coarse salt, plus more as needed

1½ cups rolled oats

2 large red apples (such as McIntosh or Rome), halved and cored

1 teaspoon ground cinnamon

½ teaspoon pure vanilla extract

2 tablespoons thawed frozen unsweetened apple juice concentrate

4 tablespoons chopped walnuts, toasted
Brown sugar (optional)

1. Put the spelt, water, and salt in a medium saucepan. Bring to a boil, reduce the heat, and simmer for 12 to 15 minutes, or until the berries are tender-crunchy. Return the mixture to a boil. Add the oats. Reduce the heat to medium and cook, stirring continuously to prevent lumps from forming, until the oatmeal is thick and creamy, 6 to 8 minutes.
2. Grate the apples, including the skin, directly into the pan. (Alternatively, leave the apples whole and grate over a plate using a box grater.) Stir in the cinnamon, vanilla, and apple juice concentrate. Taste for seasoning and add more salt if needed. Divide the oatmeal among four serving bowls and top each with 1 tablespoon of the toasted nuts and a sprinkling of brown sugar, if desired. Serve immediately.

Note: Steel cut oats—Irish and Scottish oatmeals are made with these—can be substituted for the rolled oats; they take much longer to cook (about 40 minutes) but make a nuttier, creamier cereal. A small sprinkling of brown sugar makes a nice finish for this dish.

Yield: 4½ cups (6 servings); Serving: ¾ cup

Calories: 260; Protein: 8.63 g; Carbohydrate: 45 g; Fiber: 6.3 g; Sodium: 160 mg; Fat: 6.1 g (Sat: 0.76 g, Mono: 1.56 g, Poly: 2.95 g, Trans: 0 g); Cholesterol: 0 mg

Carrot–Wheat Germ Muffins

This light, moist, slightly sweet muffin is made even tastier by the addition of freshly grated carrots, golden raisins, and chopped walnuts. Leftovers freeze well in zip-top bags; take them out one by one and reheat them in the oven or microwave for fresh-baked flavor.

Nonstick cooking spray or canola oil
2 cups whole wheat flour
1 cup toasted wheat germ
1 tablespoon baking powder
½ teaspoon coarse salt
2 large eggs, lightly beaten

2 tablespoons vegetable oil

1 cup unsweetened apple juice

½ cup thawed frozen unsweetened apple juice concentrate

⅓ cup unsweetened applesauce

1 cup grated carrots (about 2 medium)

½ cup tightly packed golden raisins

⅓ cup chopped walnuts

1. Preheat the oven to 375°F. Lightly coat a 12-cup muffin pan with cooking spray or oil.

2. Combine the flour, wheat germ, baking powder, and salt in a small bowl; whisk well.

3. Combine the eggs, vegetable oil, apple juice, apple juice concentrate, and applesauce in a large bowl; using a hand mixer, beat well on medium speed. Add the dry ingredients and stir by hand until just moist. Fold in the carrots, raisins, and walnuts.

4. Spoon the batter into the muffin pan, filling the cups about two-thirds full. Bake for 25 to 30 minutes, or until a wooden pick inserted into the center of a muffin comes out clean. Place the muffin pan on a wire rack and let cool for 10 minutes; remove from the pan and let cool completely on the rack.

Yield: 12 muffins; Serving: 1 muffin

Calories: 216; Protein: 7.4 g; Carbohydrate: 34 g; Fiber: 4.5 g; Sodium: 156 mg; Fat: 6.7 g (Sat: 0.88 g, Mono: 2.34 g, Poly: 2.91 g, Trans: 0.01 g); Cholesterol: 35 mg

Carrot-Apple-Ginger-Nut Muffins

Didi Emmons, caterer, personal chef, and author of Wild Flavors *(Chelsea Green Publishing, 2011)*

A real mouthful! This nutrient-packed muffin has so much flavor you don't need lots of sugar.

Nonstick cooking spray

⅓ cup sugar

½ cup safflower or expeller-pressed canola oil

1½ tablespoons grated fresh ginger

2 large eggs

¼ cup water

1½ cups white whole wheat or whole wheat flour

2 teaspoons baking powder

1 teaspoon ground allspice

2½ cups loosely packed grated carrots (about 5 to 6 medium)

1 cup grated unpeeled apple (about 1 medium)

½ cup raisins

½ cup dried unsweetened shredded coconut

½ cup chopped walnuts or pecans, toasted

1. Preheat the oven to 350°F. Lightly coat a 12-cup muffin pan with cooking spray.
2. In a small bowl, whisk together the sugar, oil, ginger, eggs, and water.
3. In a large bowl, mix together the flour, baking powder, allspice, carrots, and apple. Make a well in the center and pour in the egg mixture. Stir the egg mixture, gradually incorporating it with the flour mixture. Stir in the raisins, coconut, and walnuts. The batter will be chunky.
4. Spoon the batter into the muffin pan, filling the cups to the rim to make a large cap (the batter does not overflow). Bake for 25 to 30 minutes, or until a knife inserted into the center of a muffin comes out clean.
5. Take the muffin pans out of the oven. Run a paring knife carefully around each muffin and invert the pan, knocking it against the edge of your work surface to release the muffins.
6. Eat right away or once cool, cover with plastic wrap.

Yield: 12 muffins; Serving: 1 muffin

Calories: 433; Protein: 4 g; Carbohydrate: 79 g; Fiber: 4 g; Sodium: 45 mg; Fat: 15 g (Sat: 1 g, Mono: 1 g, Poly: 3 g, Trans: 0 g); Cholesterol: 31 mg

Banana-Apricot Nut Bread

Amaranth, a tiny golden-yellow grain with lots of protein and calcium, adds a crunchy texture and wonderful speckled appearance to this quick bread. Be sure to leave the walnuts in fairly big pieces, as that makes for a spectacular-looking topping. And if you have a real sweet tooth, try spreading apple butter (the kind sweetened with just apples and apple juice) or an all-fruit spread onto slices.

1 cup unsweetened apple juice

½ cup all-fruit apricot spread or jam

⅔ cup dried apricots, chopped

½ cup amaranth

Nonstick cooking spray (optional)

⅓ cup canola oil, plus more if needed for the pan

2 large eggs, lightly beaten

1 large ripe banana, mashed (about ½ cup)

2 tablespoons honey

2 cups whole wheat flour

1 teaspoon baking powder

1 teaspoon ground cinnamon

¼ teaspoon coarse salt

¼ cup coarsely chopped walnuts or other nut

1. Bring the apple juice to a boil in a small saucepan. Remove from the heat and add the apricot spread, apricots, and amaranth; let stand for 20 minutes.
2. Preheat the oven to 350°F. Lightly coat a 9 x 5-inch loaf pan with cooking spray or oil.
3. Combine the oil, eggs, banana, and honey in a large bowl; using a hand mixer, beat well on medium speed. Add the apple juice mixture to the egg mixture and beat well. In a separate bowl, combine the flour, baking powder, cinnamon, and salt; whisk well. Add the dry ingredients to the egg mixture and stir until just moist. (Do not overmix.)
4. Spoon the batter into the pan and sprinkle top with nuts. Bake for 55 to 65 minutes, or until a wooden pick inserted into the center of the loaf comes out clean. Let cool in the pan on a wire rack for 5 minutes; remove from the pan and let cool completely on the wire rack.

Yield: 1 loaf, 12 servings; Serving: 1 slice

Calories: 227; Protein: 5.87 g; Carbohydrate: 39 g; Fiber: 4.8 g; Sodium: 74 mg; Fat: 9.4 g (Sat: 1.05 g, Mono: 4.42 g, Poly: 3.30 g, Trans: 0.01 g); Cholesterol: 35 mg

Hearty Wheat Berry–Oat Groat Bread

This bread is 100% whole grain, made with whole wheat flour and both wheat berries (kernels of wheat) and oats (oat groats.) Sunflower seeds are thrown in to enhance the nuttiness of the whole grains. Keep in mind that whole grain breads don't rise as high as breads made with all white flour. But the rich, wheaty flavor is superior. Look for wheat berries and oat groats in health food stores.

2 tablespoons raw sunflower seeds

2 tablespoons wheat berries

2 tablespoons oat groats

2 teaspoons active dry yeast

½ cup warm water (105° to 115°F)

2 tablespoons molasses

1½ teaspoons coarse salt

2 tablespoons canola or other oil, plus more for the pan

2½ to 3 cups whole wheat flour, plus more for dusting

Nonstick cooking spray (optional)

1. Place the sunflower seeds, wheat berries, and oat groats in a dry nonstick skillet over medium heat. Toast, stirring frequently to prevent scorching, for 3 to 6 minutes, or until lightly browned.

2. Combine the yeast and the warm water in a large bowl; let stand for 5 minutes. Stir in the molasses, salt, and oil. Add 2½ cups of the flour and stir to form a soft dough. Turn the dough out onto a lightly floured surface and knead until smooth and elastic, 6 to 8 minutes, adding enough of the remaining flour, 1 tablespoon at a time, to prevent the dough from sticking to your hands. Knead the sunflower seeds, wheat berries, and oat groats into the dough until well dispersed, 1 to 2 minutes.

3. Place the dough in a large bowl lightly coated with oil or cooking spray, turning to coat the top. Cover and let rise in a warm place (85°F), free from drafts, for 1 to 2 hours, or until doubled in bulk. Punch down the dough and turn it out onto a lightly floured surface. Roll the dough into a 12 x 7-inch rectangle. Roll up the rectangle tightly, starting with the short edge; press firmly to eliminate air pockets; pinch the seam and ends to seal. Place the roll, seam side down, in an 8 x 5-inch nonstick loaf pan lightly

coated with oil or cooking spray. Cover and let rise until the dough reaches the top of the pan, 50 to 60 minutes.

4. Preheat the oven to 350°F.
5. Bake for 45 minutes, or until the loaf sounds hollow when tapped. Remove from the pan immediately; let cool on a wire rack.

Note: To make this in a bread machine, use bread machine yeast and a large-capacity bread machine. Follow the manufacturer's instructions for whole wheat or specialty loaves.

Yield: 1 loaf (12 servings); Serving: 1 slice

Calories: 149; Protein: 5.1 g; Carbohydrate: 26 g; Fiber: 3.9 g; Sodium: 239 mg; Fat: 3.6 g (Sat: 0.32 g, Mono: 1.42 g, Poly: 0.95 g, Trans: 0.01 g); Cholesterol: o mg

Multigrain Hotcakes with Warm Apple Syrup

These multigrain pancakes have a nutty flavor and crunchy texture due to toasted sunflower seeds and several whole grains—millet, barley, wheat. The addition of reduced-fat buttermilk makes for a light, tender texture, but you can substitute apple juice if necessary. Also, these pancakes cook perfectly well in a nonstick skillet without a drop of oil. But if you like a crispy edge on your hotcakes, add some oil to the griddle before cooking.

SYRUP

1½ cups thawed frozen unsweetened apple juice concentrate

1 stick cinnamon, or ¼ teaspoon ground cinnamon

2 whole cloves (optional)

⅓ cup unsweetened applesauce

HOTCAKES

2 tablespoons raw sunflower seeds

2 tablespoons millet

⅓ cup quick-cooking barley (such as Mother's)

1⅓ cups fat-free or reduced-fat buttermilk

2 large eggs, lightly beaten

2 tablespoons canola oil

2 tablespoons thawed frozen unsweetened apple juice concentrate

1 cup bran flakes cereal

½ cup whole wheat flour

½ cup all-purpose flour

1½ teaspoons baking soda

1 teaspoon baking powder

½ teaspoon coarse salt

½ teaspoon ground cinnamon

¼ teaspoon freshly grated nutmeg

1. To make the syrup, place the juice concentrate, cinnamon stick, and cloves, if using, in a small saucepan over medium-high heat. Bring to a boil, reduce the heat to medium, and simmer for 5 to 10 minutes, or until the mixture is reduced by about a third. Remove the cinnamon stick and cloves with a slotted spoon. Stir in the applesauce. Reduce the heat to low and keep warm.

2. To make the pancakes, place a large nonstick skillet over medium to medium-high heat. Add the sunflower seeds and millet. Toast the sunflower seeds for 3 to 6 minutes or until lightly browned, stirring occasionally to prevent scorching. Remove from the heat and set aside. (You will use this same skillet to cook the hotcakes.)

3. Place the barley (do not use pearl barley) and buttermilk in a mixing bowl and let stand for 30 minutes. Add the eggs, oil, apple juice concentrate, and bran flakes, mixing until just blended.

4. Combine the wheat and white flours, baking soda, baking powder, salt, cinnamon, nutmeg, and the sunflower seed and millet mixture in a medium mixing bowl. Whisk until well blended. Add the buttermilk mixture to the flour mixture and stir until just moist.

5. Heat a large nonstick skillet or griddle over medium to medium-high heat. Pour ¼ cup batter into the skillet for each pancake (do not crowd) and cook for 2 to 3 minutes until tops bubble and edges look dry. Turn the pancakes and cook for 1 to 2 minutes more until the undersides are golden brown. Repeat with the remaining batter. Serve with Warm Apple Syrup.

Note: To keep the pancakes warm, preheat the oven to 200°F. Place the pancakes on a nonstick baking sheet and cover loosely with aluminum foil. Keep in the oven until ready to serve. Also, these pancakes freeze well. Pop them in the microwave or toaster to reheat.

Yield: 12 hotcakes, 1⅛ cups syrup; Serving: 2 hotcakes and 3 tablespoons syrup

Calories: 282; Protein: 9 g; Carbohydrate: 43.7 g; Fiber: 4.4 g; Sodium: 502 mg; Fat: 8.9 g (Sat: 0.76 g, Mono: 1.56 g, Poly: 2.95 g, Trans: 0 g); Cholesterol: 0 mg

Griddle-Baked Semolina Pancakes with Sweet Date-Orange Filling

Nancy Harmon Jenkins, author of Virgin Territory: Exploring the World of Olive Oil
(Houghton Mifflin Harcourt, 2015)

In the summer, Tunisian cooks solve the hot kitchen dilemma by griddle baking, toasting these delicious cakes on a stovetop griddle instead of lighting the oven. These griddle cakes derive their sweetness solely from the dates in the filling, and with the pleasant crunch of semolina, they are a lovely surprise for Sunday breakfast. Any leftovers are also delicious with afternoon tea or midmorning coffee. Made with a combination of high-protein durum wheat semolina and whole wheat flour, they are a healthy antidote to more conventional pancakes and need no infusion of syrup to make them tasty.

If you don't have a griddle on your stovetop, you can easily make the cakes in a cast-iron skillet, preheated until it's very hot.

12 ounces dates, pitted
1¼ cups extra-virgin olive oil, plus more for the griddle
2 tablespoons crumbled dried orange peel
2 tablespoons freshly grated orange zest
Juice of ½ orange
Sea salt
¾ cup warm water
2 cups whole wheat flour, plus more for dusting
2 cups semolina

1. Process the dates in the bowl of a food processor until they are quite smooth, then, with the motor running, slowly pour in ¼ cup of the oil. Add the dried orange peel, fresh orange zest, and orange juice and process until you have a smooth paste. Set aside. (This can be done well ahead; the date paste need not be refrigerated except on very hot days.)
2. Add about 1 teaspoon salt to the warm water and set aside to dissolve.
3. Place the flour and semolina in a large bowl. Add the remaining 1 cup oil, working the semolina thoroughly with a wooden spoon until the oil has been absorbed. Slowly add the salty water to the dough, continuing to work it in the bowl until you have a kneadable consistency. Knead in the bowl briefly, then transfer to a board, lightly dusted with additional flour, and knead with your hands until the dough is quite smooth.

4. When the dough is well kneaded, it should feel soft but not at all sticky. Set aside, covered with plastic wrap or a kitchen towel, to rest for about 30 minutes.

5. When ready to proceed, heat a griddle or skillet over medium-low heat. Divide the dough into quarters. Shape a quarter into a ball, then, using your hands, pat it out into a circle on the lightly floured board. (For best results, pat the dough out on a sheet of parchment paper.) Use a rolling pin to roll an even circle 8 to 9 inches in diameter and ⅛ to ¼ inch thick. Spread half the date mixture over the circle, dotting it liberally all over the top. Set the circle aside on its parchment paper and roll out another quarter of the dough, making a circle on parchment to match the first. Flip the second circle over the top of the first one and press gently so that the top and bottom circles adhere lightly all the way around, sealing in the date mixture.

6. When the griddle or skillet is hot, brush it lightly with a very little bit of oil—not more than ½ teaspoon or so. Turn the griddle cake onto the hot surface and adjust the heat so that it toasts golden on both sides, turning it once, about 4 minutes per side, until the surfaces are golden and crisp and the inside is cooked through. Be careful not to burn the cake.

7. When done, remove the griddle cake and use the remaining dough and date mixture to make a second griddle cake. Serve the cakes immediately, cut into pie-shaped wedges. The griddle cakes are also very good set aside and served later at room temperature.

Note: The round cakes may also be cut up before cooking, if you prefer. Just slice through all the layers to make lozenges, squares, or rectangles, sort of like elegant Fig Newtons.

Yield: 6 servings; Servings: ⅓ of a griddle cake

Calories: 549; Protein: 5 g; Carbohydrate: 118 g; Fiber: 11 g; Sodium: 39 mg; Fat: 5 g (Sat: 1 g, Mono: 3 g, Poly: 1 g, Trans: 0 g); Cholesterol: 0 mg

Menemen (Turkish–Style Scrambled Eggs) with Pita Bread

Ana Sortun, executive chef and owner Oleana and Sofra Bakery and Cafe; author of Spice: Flavors of the Eastern Mediterranean *(HarperCollins, 2006)*

> 2 large greenhouse or beefsteak tomatoes, halved, most of the seeds removed
> 2 tablespoons olive oil
> 1 green bell pepper, cut into ½-inch dice
> 1 Hungarian hot wax pepper, seeded and cut into ½-inch dice
> ¼ cup finely chopped scallions
> 2 teaspoons tomato paste
> 1 teaspoon red pepper paste or harissa
> Coarse salt
> 8 large eggs
> 2 tablespoons chopped fresh parsley
> ½ teaspoon Aleppo or Maras pepper
> 4 small (7-inch) pita breads
> 2 mini cucumbers, or ½ English cucumber, thinly sliced

1. Holding the tomato halves cut side out, grate the tomato over a shallow dish on the large holes of a box grater until there is nothing but skin left in your hand. Set aside.
2. Heat the oil in a medium skillet over medium heat. Add the bell pepper, wax pepper, and scallions and cook, stirring occasionally, until the peppers are tender, about 4 minutes. Add the grated tomato, tomato paste, and red pepper paste. Season with salt. Cook until the sauce thickens slightly, 2 to 3 minutes.
3. In a medium bowl, beat the eggs with ½ teaspoon salt. Stir the eggs into the sauce gently and as they start to scramble, stir in the parsley and Aleppo pepper. Cook and gently stir until the eggs are scrambled to your liking.
4. Spread the egg mixture on the pitas. Keep warm in a toaster oven until ready to serve and then serve each pita with 5 or 6 slices of cucumber.

Yield: 6 servings

Calories: 323; Protein: 15 g; Carbohydrate: 34 g; Fiber: 3 g; Sodium: 626 mg; Fat: 14 g (Sat: 3 g, Mono: 5 g, Poly: 4 g, Trans: 0 g); Cholesterol: 248 mg

ENTRÉES

Mediterranean Stuffed Breast of Chicken (FAST FIX)

The filling for these chicken breasts is simple to put together: canned artichoke hearts, jarred roasted peppers, and already-crumbled feta cheese combined with some fresh basil and toasted pine nuts. Toast the pine nuts in a dry skillet on the stove; it will take just 2 to 3 minutes.

¼ cup water-packed artichoke hearts, drained and finely chopped
1 (7-ounce) jar roasted red peppers, drained and chopped
½ cup crumbled feta cheese (about 2 ounces)
2 tablespoons chopped fresh basil
2 tablespoons pine nuts, toasted
2 teaspoons red wine vinegar
1½ tablespoons garlic olive oil
4 (5-ounce) boneless, skinless chicken breasts
Coarse salt and freshly ground black pepper

1. Combine the artichoke hearts, roasted peppers, feta, basil, pine nuts, and vinegar in a small bowl. Stir in 1 tablespoon of the oil and set aside.
2. Using a thin, sharp knife (such as a boning knife), cut a 2-inch horizontal slit in the thickest part of each chicken breast, cutting to but not through, the opposite side of the breast. Hold the knife blade parallel to the cutting board and guide the blade around inside the breast to create a pocket. Stuff ¼ cup of the artichoke mixture into each pocket. Sprinkle the chicken with salt and black pepper.
3. In a skillet, heat the remaining ½ tablespoon oil over medium-high heat. Add the chicken and cook for 5 to 6 minutes on each side, or until cooked through.

Note: Don't be put off by the idea of cutting pockets into a chicken breast. If you start with a plump breast and use a sharp knife, the task is quite easy. If you accidentally cut through a side or bottom of the breast, a toothpick can help seal the pocket during cooking. Remove it before serving and no one will be the wiser.

Yield: 4 servings; Serving: 1 stuffed chicken breast

Calories: 261; Protein: 31 g; Carbohydrate: 4.5 g; Fiber: 0.8 g; Sodium: 283 mg; Fat: 12.6 g (Sat: 4.18 g, Mono: 5.75 g, Poly: 1.76 g, Trans: .050 g); Cholesterol: 82 mg

Chicken Enchilada Casserole

This casserole uses already-prepared enchilada sauce (the Hatch brand is made with wheat flour instead of white), store-bought rotisserie chicken, and canned beans and chilies. If you can, buy the organic canned beans; they're worth the extra cost: better flavor, less salt, and a firm texture.

CASSEROLE

2 tablespoons canola or olive oil
2 cups chopped white or yellow onions (about 1 large)
2 garlic cloves, minced
1 cup thinly sliced scallions
1 teaspoon dried oregano
¼ cup fresh cilantro, finely chopped
2 cups skinless roasted chicken breast (about 8 ounces)
1 cup jarred roasted red peppers, chopped
1 (4.5-ounce) can chopped green chilies, drained
2 tablespoons fresh lime juice
Coarse salt and freshly ground black pepper (optional)
1 (15-ounce) can enchilada sauce (such as Hatch)
1 (15-ounce) can diced tomatoes
½ cup defatted chicken stock or broth, preferably low-sodium
Nonstick cooking spray or canola oil
6 (6-inch) corn tortillas, torn or cut into thirds
1 (15-ounce) can black beans, rinsed and drained

TOPPING

¼ cup shredded sharp cheddar cheese (about 1 ounce)
4 tablespoons finely chopped black olives
Cilantro sprigs (optional)

1. Preheat the oven to 350°F.
2. To make the casserole, in a large skillet, heat the oil over medium to

medium-high heat. Add the onion; cook, stirring, for 5 to 8 minutes, or until the onion is tender-crisp. Stir in the garlic, scallions, oregano, and cilantro; cook for 1 minute. Remove from the heat and add the chicken, red peppers, chilies, and lime juice. Taste and season with salt and black pepper, if desired.

3. Lightly coat an 11 x 7-inch baking dish with cooking spray or oil. Combine the enchilada sauce, tomatoes, and stock in a medium bowl. Place ½ cup of the sauce into the bottom of the baking dish. Arrange 6 tortilla pieces over the sauce. Top with one-third of the onion-chicken mixture, one-third of the black beans, and ¾ cup sauce. Repeat the layers, ending with the sauce. Bake for 45 to 50 minutes, or until bubbling. Remove from the oven and sprinkle with the cheese, 1 tablespoon at a time, making four diagonal rows across the casserole. Sprinkle 1 tablespoon of olives next to each row of cheese, following the same diagonal pattern. Let stand for 10 minutes before serving.

Yield: 6 servings; Serving: 1 (3.5-inch) square

Calories: 381; Protein: 23.8 g; Carbohydrate: 40.5 g; Fiber: 9.2 g; Sodium: 876 mg; Fat: 13.7 g (Sat: 2.45 g, Mono: 5.67 g, Poly: 2.85 g, Trans: 0.05 g); Cholesterol: 44 mg

California Chicken Salad (FAST FIX)

This cool summer salad is very versatile; substitute whole wheat couscous for the bulgur if you'd like a milder flavor, and vary the greens (arugula instead of spinach). Leave out the chicken for a vegetarian meal.

LEMON-BASIL VINAIGRETTE

1 tablespoon chopped fresh basil, or 1 teaspoon dried
¼ cup extra-virgin olive oil
⅓ cup fresh lemon juice
¼ teaspoon garlic powder
Coarse salt and freshly ground black pepper

SALAD

1 cup bulgur
1 cup boiling water
2 cups chopped fresh spinach
1 cup shredded roasted chicken (about 4 ounces)

1 medium avocado, pitted, peeled, and chopped (about 1 cup)

¼ cup thinly sliced scallions

¼ cup fresh parsley, chopped

12 Kalamata olives, pitted and quartered

1. To make the vinaigrette, whisk together all the vinaigrette ingredients in a small bowl.
2. To make the salad, place the bulgur in a large bowl and pour over the boiling water. Let stand for 30 minutes, or until the liquid has been completely absorbed. Stir in the spinach, chicken, avocado, scallions, parsley, and olives. Add the vinaigrette and toss gently. Serve at room temperature.

Yield: 8 cups (5 servings); Serving: about 1½ cups

Calories: 355; Protein: 19.7 g; Carbohydrate: 34 g; Fiber: 10.6 g; Sodium: 51 mg; Fat: 17.2 g (Sat: 3.19 g, Mono: 7.42 g, Poly: 1.66 g, Trans: 0.08 g); Cholesterol: 38 mg

Moroccan Chicken Tagine

Charles Burke, MD, president of the New Hampshire Farm to Restaurant Connection

This recipe is a take on traditional Moroccan tagines, the name for both the cooking vessel, a glazed clay low-rimmed bottom with a conical lid, and for the recipe cooked in it. This preparation requires a little effort, but the layers of flavor and colorful presentation result in a somewhat exotic meal suitable for guests or a special family dinner. Traditionally, it is served with bread or couscous, replaced here with chickpeas.

½ cup pine nuts or almonds

2 teaspoons coriander seed, or 1 teaspoon ground coriander

2 teaspoons cumin seed, or 1 teaspoon ground cumin

2 teaspoons whole black or white peppercorns, or 1 teaspoon freshly ground

½ cinnamon stick, or 1 teaspoon ground cinnamon

1½ tablespoons olive or canola oil

3 garlic cloves, thinly sliced

1 medium sweet yellow onion, sliced

1 red bell pepper, seeded and thinly sliced lengthwise

1 yellow bell pepper, seeded and thinly sliced lengthwise

8 (6-ounce) bone-in, skinless chicken thighs

2 lemons, zest removed and reserved, fruit very thinly sliced and seeded

1 tablespoon finely chopped fresh ginger, or 2 teaspoons ground ginger

¾ cup small whole cherry tomatoes

1½ cups no-salt-added canned chickpeas, rinsed and drained

⅓ cup pitted green olives, sliced crosswise

⅓ cup currants or other unsweetened dried fruit

2 teaspoons ground turmeric

½ teaspoon saffron (optional)

2 teaspoons crushed red pepper flakes

1½ cups chicken stock

1. Preheat the oven to 350°F.
2. In a heavy-bottomed skillet, toast the pine nuts over medium heat, stirring frequently, until slightly browned. Transfer to a plate and set aside.
3. If using whole spices, place the coriander seed, cumin seed, peppercorns, and cinnamon stick in the same skillet and toast over medium heat until fragrant, 2 to 3 minutes. Transfer to a plate and let cool. When cooled, grind the spices in a spice grinder or using a mortar and pestle.
4. In a tagine or medium Dutch oven, heat the oil over medium-low heat. Add the garlic, onion, and bell peppers and cook, stirring, until soft.
5. Remove from the heat and place the chicken thighs over the bell peppers and onion. Arrange the lemon slices over the chicken. Spoon some of the sautéed vegetables over the chicken, along with the ginger, tomatoes, chickpeas, olives, currants, and pine nuts.
6. Add the toasted spices, turmeric, saffron, red pepper flakes, and lemon zest to the stock and mix well. Pour the stock mixture over the chicken.
7. Return the tagine to the stovetop over medium heat and bring the liquid to a boil.
8. Cover and place the tagine in the lower third of the oven and cook for 35 to 45 minutes, until the internal temperature of the chicken reaches 160°F or the juices run clear.
9. Remove from the oven and let sit for 10 minutes before serving.

Note: Bone-in chicken thighs are used in this recipe because they remain moist and have a longer cooking time, permitting flavors to develop fully. Boneless thighs are an option, but the cooking time will be shorter. If chicken breasts are substituted, they should be pounded to a uniform thickness because their irregular shape prevents uniform cooking. The skin is removed from all because the moist heat in this recipe results in poor texture and flavor. Average chicken thighs weigh about 6 ounces, yielding 2½ to 3 ounces of meat after removing the bone and skin.

Yield: 4 servings

Calories: 591; Protein: 39 g; Carbohydrate: 42 g; Fiber: 8 g; Sodium: 369 mg; Fat: 31 g (Sat: 5 g, Mono: 12 g, Poly: 10 g, Trans: 0 g); Cholesterol: 103 mg

Chicken and Vegetable Stir-Fry

Ming Tsai, chef/owner Blue Dragon (Boston, Massachusetts); author of Simply Ming in Your Kitchen *(Kyle Books, 2012)*

2 pounds boneless, skinless chicken thighs, cut into ½-inch dice

2 tablespoons cornstarch

1 teaspoon untoasted sesame oil (optional)

Salt and freshly ground black pepper

2 tablespoons grapeseed oil

1 cup sliced white or yellow onions (about 1 medium)

2 cups sliced carrots, cut ¼-inch thick (about 2 large)

5 celery stalks, cut into ½-inch dice

2 tablespoons minced fresh ginger

3 tablespoons minced garlic

2 tablespoons reduced-sodium soy sauce

Juice of 1 lime

Zest and juice of 1 lemon

½ cup defatted chicken stock, preferably low-sodium

1 cup shelled edamame

4 cups cooked brown rice (see Note), for serving

1. In a large bowl, combine the chicken, cornstarch, and sesame oil (if using). Season with salt and pepper and set aside.
2. Heat a large nonstick wok or nonstick skillet over high heat. Add 1 tablespoon of the grapeseed oil and swirl to coat the wok. When the oil is hot, add the chicken and stir-fry, separating the pieces, until the chicken is cooked through, 4 to 5 minutes. Transfer the chicken to a plate.
3. Add the remaining 1 tablespoon grapeseed oil and swirl to coat the wok. When the oil is hot, add the onions, carrots, celery, ginger, and garlic. Stir-

fry for 2 minutes, until the flavors have combined and the vegetables begin to soften.

4. Add the soy sauce, lime juice, lemon zest, lemon juice, and stock. Reduce the heat to a simmer and return the chicken to the wok. Cook to thicken slightly, about 2 minutes. Finish with the edamame at the last minute.

5. Make a bed of the rice on a platter, top with the stir-fry, and serve.

Note: For the best brown rice, soak the rice in water to cover for 1 hour before cooking.

Yield: 4 servings

Calories: 682; Protein: 57 g; Carbohydrate: 70 g; Fiber: 7 g; Sodium: 562 mg; Fat: 25 g (Sat: 1 g, Mono: 2 g, Poly: 6 g, Trans: 0 g); Cholesterol: 185 mg

Thai Basil Chicken with Long Beans

Mai Pham, chef/owner, Lemon Grass Kitchen; author of Pleasures of the Vietnamese Table *(HarperCollins, 2001)*

If you love chilies and Thai basil, you'll love this quick, simple, and utterly delicious dish, especially if you cook it the Thai way: start with a hot pan, go heavy on the chilies and basil, and don't overcook.

2 tablespoons canola oil

2 tablespoons minced garlic

2 to 4 Thai bird chilies, or 1 red serrano chile, sliced on an angle, or to taste

⅔ cup fresh Thai basil leaves

1 teaspoon fish sauce

⅔ pound coarsely ground chicken thighs

2 teaspoons oyster sauce

½ cup diced red bell peppers, cut into ½-inch pieces (about 1 medium)

1 cup sliced long beans, cut into 1-inch pieces, blanched (about 4 ounces)

2 to 3 tablespoons chicken stock or water (optional)

Cilantro sprigs for garnish

1. In a wok or skillet, heat the oil over medium-high heat. Add the garlic, chilies, and basil and cook until the garlic is golden and the wok is very fragrant, about 1 minute. Drizzle the fish sauce into the wok.

2. Add the ground chicken and, using a wooden spoon or chopsticks, stir to loosen and separate. Cook, undisturbed, for 1 minute to brown on the bottom.

3. Add the oyster sauce, bell peppers, and long beans. Cook until the vegetables are thoroughly hot and the chicken is cooked through.

4. If the wok is dry, add the stock. Taste and adjust the seasonings to your palate. Transfer to a serving dish, garnish with cilantro, and serve.

Yield: 3 servings

Calories: 323; Protein: 29 g; Carbohydrate: 15 g; Fiber: 1 g; Sodium: 707 mg; Fat: 16 g (Sat: 1 g, Mono: 7 g, Poly: 3 g, Trans: 0 g); Cholesterol: 90 mg

Tandoori Tuna (FAST FIX)

This spicy fish takes its flavor cues from India, where savory and sweet spices are blended and used on every thing from meat to vegetables to seafood. The tuna is marinated briefly in the tandoori spice mixture and then cooked in a skillet. Fix some citrus-flavored couscous as a side dish.

4 (5-ounce) tuna steaks, about ½-inch thick
¾ cup pineapple juice
1 tablespoon fresh lemon juice
1 tablespoon minced fresh ginger
1 tablespoon minced fresh garlic
1 tablespoon ground coriander
1 tablespoon paprika
1½ teaspoons ground cumin
1 teaspoon coarse salt
1 teaspoon cumin seed
1 teaspoon chili garlic sauce
¼ teaspoon ground cinnamon
⅛ teaspoon ground cloves
1 tablespoon canola or other oil

1. Combine all the ingredients except the oil in a large zip-top bag. Press the air out of the bag and seal; refrigerate for 15 minutes, turning once or twice.

2. In a large cast-iron or nonstick skillet, heat the oil over medium heat.

Remove the tuna from the marinade; discard the marinade. Place the tuna in the hot skillet; cook for 4 to 5 minutes on each side or until cooked to your liking.

Note: Tuna can be grilled or broiled. Prepare a grill or preheat the broiler. Brush the tuna with the oil and cook as directed above. Look for chili garlic sauce in the Asian section of most supermarkets.

Yield: 4 servings; Serving: 1 tuna steak

Calories: 195; Protein: 33 g; Carbohydrate: 2.5 g; Fiber: 0.3 g; Sodium: 67 mg; Fat: 4.9 g (Sat: 0.59 g, Mono: 2.30 g, Poly: 1.46 g, Trans: 0.01 g); Cholesterol: 64 mg

Lemon–Oregano Grouper with Vegetables

When you use the French technique of oven-steaming single servings of fish, seasonings, and vegetables in individual packages, the reward is twofold: very little to clean up and lots of flavor. Any white fish, such as mahi-mahi, pollock, wahoo, or cod will work in this recipe. Whole wheat couscous makes a quick side dish for this fish; prepare it while the fish is cooking.

2 tablespoons olive oil
2 small zucchini, julienned (about 2 cups)
1 cup fresh or frozen corn kernels
¼ cup diced red bell peppers (about 1 small)
½ teaspoon coarse salt, plus more as needed
4 (5-ounce) grouper fillets, about 1-inch thick
Freshly ground black pepper
2 teaspoons fresh lemon juice
2 tablespoons fresh oregano, coarsely chopped
4 paper-thin slices lemon, halved

1. Preheat the oven to 375°F.
2. Combine 1 tablespoon of the olive oil, the zucchini, corn, bell peppers, and salt in a medium bowl; toss to coat. Divide this vegetable mixture among four large pieces of aluminum foil, placing the vegetables in the center of each piece. Sprinkle each fillet with salt and black pepper and place the fish on top of the vegetables.
3. Combine the remaining 1 tablespoon oil, the lemon juice, and the oregano

in a small bowl. Drizzle one-quarter of this mixture over each fillet and top with 2 lemon-slice halves. Seal the package by rolling up the top and sides. Put the packets on a baking sheet and bake for 16 to 20 minutes, or until the fish flakes easily with a fork. Place each foil package on a serving plate, carefully open the package (the steam will be hot), and serve.

Yield: 4 servings; Serving: 1 grouper fillet with vegetables

Calories: 239; Protein: 30.4 g; Carbohydrate: 10 g; Fiber: 1.8 g; Sodium: 318 mg; Fat: 9 g (Sat: 1.36 g, Mono: 5.41 g, Poly: 1.34 g, Trans: 0.07 g); Cholesterol: 52 mg

Pad Thai–Style Fried Rice

One of the most popular menu choices at a Thai restaurant is a noodle dish with Thai spices, shrimp, eggs, and Thai rice noodles. Here's a version of that popular dish made with brown rice, which is easier to find and higher in fiber than the rice noodles. The secret to making a great fried rice is to cook the rice the night before and to use a little bit less liquid than is called for on the package directions. Rice that's cooked a bit on the "dry" side won't become mushy when stir-fried.

PEANUT SAUCE

2 tablespoons fish sauce or tamari soy sauce

2 tablespoons defatted chicken stock or broth, preferably low-sodium

1 tablespoon ketchup sweetened with fruit juice, or plain ketchup

1 tablespoon natural-style peanut butter

1 tablespoon fresh lime juice

FRIED RICE

3 tablespoons roasted peanut oil or canola oil

2 large eggs, lightly beaten

½ cup shredded carrots (about 1 medium)

2 large garlic cloves, minced

1 teaspoon minced fresh ginger

1 cup thinly sliced scallions

½ cup diced red bell peppers (about 1 medium)

¼ teaspoon crushed red pepper flakes

4 cups cooked brown rice, chilled

½ pound cooked and peeled medium shrimp (about 20)

10 fresh Thai or regular basil leaves, chopped
¼ cup fresh cilantro, minced
Salt
½ cup fresh bean sprouts (optional)
Chopped peanuts (optional)

1. To make the peanut sauce, combine all the sauce ingredients in a small bowl. Set aside.
2. To make the fried rice, in a large nonstick skillet, heat 1 teaspoon of the oil over medium-high heat. Add the eggs, stirring to scramble them loosely; cook until done, 1 to 2 minutes. Transfer the eggs to a plate. Add 2 teaspoons of the oil to the skillet, then add the carrots; cook for 2 to 3 minutes, or until the carrots begin to soften. Remove from the skillet. Add the remaining 2 tablespoons oil to the skillet, then add the garlic, ginger, scallions, bell peppers, and red pepper flakes. Cook for 1 to 2 minutes, or until the vegetables begin to soften. Reduce the heat to low and add the cooked rice. Cook for 1 to 2 minutes; stir in the eggs, shrimp, basil, cilantro, and peanut sauce; cook until heated through. Taste and season with salt if needed. Garnish with the bean sprouts and chopped peanuts, if using. Serve immediately.

Note: Look for fish sauce and tamari soy sauce in the Asian section of most supermarkets.

Yield: 6 servings; Serving: about 1 cup

Calories: 303; Protein: 14.9 g; Carbohydrate: 35 g; Fiber: 3.9 g; Sodium: 634 mg; Fat: 11.5 g (Sat: 2.11 g, Mono: 4.89 g, Poly: 3.26 g, Trans: 0 g); Cholesterol: 145 mg

Grilled Salmon Steaks with Papaya-Mint Salsa

S almon is perfectly great just plain off the grill. But this tart-sweet fruit salsa complements the richness of the fatty fish. Make the salsa earlier in the day to allow the flavors to blend. Be sure to cut down on the amount of jalapeño or leave it out altogether if you don't like hot peppers.

SALSA

¾ cup chopped peeled papaya
¼ cup chopped yellow bell peppers (about 1 small)

¼ cup thinly sliced scallions

1 tablespoon chopped pimiento

1 tablespoon chopped fresh mint

1 tablespoon rice vinegar

1 tablespoon fresh lime juice

1 teaspoon grated fresh ginger

1 teaspoon minced seeded jalapeño

SALMON

Nonstick cooking spray or oil

4 (5-ounce) salmon steaks or fillets, about 1 to 1¼ inches thick

Coarse salt and freshly ground black pepper

1. To make the salsa, combine all the salsa ingredients in a small bowl. Cover and refrigerate for at least 30 minutes to allow the flavors to blend.
2. To make the salmon, prepare a grill or preheat the broiler. Lightly coat the grill or broiler pan with cooking spray to prevent the fish from sticking. Sprinkle both sides of the fish with salt and pepper. Grill the fish for 5 minutes on each side or until cooked through. Top the salmon with the salsa and serve.

Yield: 4 servings; Serving: 1 salmon fillet and ¼ cup salsa

Calories: 281; Protein: 28.8 g; Carbohydrate: 4.9 g; Fiber: 0.9 g; Sodium: 86 mg; Fat: 15.6 g (Sat: 3.1 g, Mono: 5.5 g, Poly: 5.6 g, Trans: 0 g); Cholesterol: 84 mg

Spicy Shrimp and Peanut Noodle Salad

Typically, this Asian noodle salad is made with soba (buckwheat) noodles. Here we've substituted whole wheat spaghetti for a little extra fiber. The change is hardly noticeable, since the flavors in the spicy peanut sauce are the most predominant. Don't be put off by the ingredients list; most of the items are seasonings that can be quickly measured and mixed together for the sauce. To save time, buy precooked shrimp and precut veggies so the only cooking you'll be doing is boiling a few noodles.

PEANUT SAUCE

2 garlic cloves, minced

2 teaspoons minced fresh ginger

3 tablespoons natural chunky-style peanut butter

2 tablespoons tamari soy sauce

2 tablespoons rice vinegar

2 tablespoons water

2 tablespoons untoasted sesame oil

1 to 2 teaspoons chili garlic sauce

SALAD

1 pound cooked and peeled medium shrimp (about 40)

1 large red bell pepper, julienned (about 1 cup)

1 cup shredded carrots (about 2 medium)

¼ pound snow peas, trimmed and halved

1 cup sliced scallions

¼ cup fresh cilantro, chopped

4 cups cooked whole wheat spaghetti or soba (buckwheat) noodles

Chopped peanuts (optional)

1. To make the peanut sauce, whisk together all the sauce ingredients in a small bowl and set aside.
2. To make the salad, combine the shrimp, bell pepper, carrots, snow peas, scallions, and cilantro in a large serving bowl. Add the spaghetti and peanut sauce and toss gently to mix. Sprinkle with peanuts, if desired. Serve at room temperature.

Note: The salad is versatile: switch to chicken or pork instead of shrimp or just leave the meat out altogether for a vegetarian noodle dish. Look for the chili garlic sauce in the Asian section of most supermarkets. Brand names vary, but the basic ingredients are similar from sauce to sauce.

Yield: 6 servings; Serving: 1½ cups

Calories: 337; Protein: 27.7 g; Carbohydrate: 33.7 g; Fiber: 6.8 g; Sodium: 545 mg

Double Mushroom Meat Loaf

Dried and fresh mushrooms give this beef-and-turkey meat loaf a wonderful rich flavor. Be sure to use lean ground turkey and not ground turkey breast in this loaf; the ground breast (all white meat) has very little fat and makes a dry loaf. Substitute lean ground turkey for the beef if you'd like.

½ ounce dried mixed mushroom blend (shiitake, oyster, porcini) or dried shiitakes

1 cup boiling water

1 pound 93% lean ground beef or lean ground round

½ pound lean ground turkey

1 cup chopped white or yellow onions (abou 1 medium)

¼ cup chopped fresh parsley

½ cup diced button mushrooms (about 2 ounces)

¼ cup rolled oats

1 large egg, lightly beaten

2½ tablespoons tomato paste

¾ teaspoon coarse salt

2 teaspoons dried basil

1 teaspoon dried oregano

1. Combine the dried mushrooms and boiling water in a small bowl and let stand for 30 minutes, or until the mushrooms are soft. Drain and finely chop the mushrooms, reserving the soaking liquid. Strain the soaking liquid through cheesecloth or a fine sieve to remove any grit.

2. Preheat the oven to 325°F.

3. Combine the ground beef, turkey, rehydrated mushrooms, 2 tablespoons of the reserved mushroom soaking liquid, the onions, parsley, button mushrooms, oats, egg, tomato paste, salt, basil, and oregano and mix until well blended. Place the meat mixture in a nonstick 9 x 5-inch loaf pan and bake for 45 to 50 minutes or until cooked through.

Yield: 10 servings; Serving: 1 slice (about 3 ounces)

Calories: 161; Protein: 15.9 g; Carbohydrate: 7.0 g; Fiber: 1.6 g; Sodium: 254 mg; Fat: 7.6 g (Sat: 2.48 g, Mono: 2.79 g, Poly: 0.88 g, Trans: 0.04 g); Cholesterol: 56 mg

VEGETARIAN ENTRÉES

Radicchio Leaves and Walnut, Red Pepper, and Feta Salad

Ana Sortun, executive chef and owner Oleana and Sofra Bakery and Cafe; author of Spice: Flavors of the Eastern Mediterranean *(HarperCollins, 2006)*

I love all the popping flavors in this salad and the texture from the crisp bread and walnuts. Pomegranate molasses is easy to find these days in specialty grocery stores like Whole Foods or in any Middle Eastern market. It's got a lovely depth, sourness, and acidity. You can substitute an aged balsamic vinegar if you have trouble finding pomegranate molasses near you.

> 1 cup lightly toasted walnuts, coarsely chopped
> 1 cup jarred piquillo peppers (preferably not from a can), cut into ¼-inch dice
> ½ cup whole wheat croutons, preferably homemade
> 3 ounces barrel-aged feta (look for a harder cheese that crumbles well and is not creamy), cut into ½-inch cubes
> 1 tablespoon finely minced scallions
> 1 tablespoon finely chopped fresh parsley
> 2 tablespoons fresh lemon juice
> 1 tablespoon pomegranate molasses
> 1½ teaspoons ground cumin
> 2 garlic cloves, grated with a Microplane
> 2 tablespoons extra-virgin olive oil
> 1 teaspoon Aleppo or Maras pepper
> Salt
> 1 medium or 2 small heads radicchio, or 3 endives, cored and broken into leaves for scooping (about 24 leaves total)

1. In a small bowl, combine the walnuts and piquillo peppers.
2. Crush the croutons using your hands until they are roughly the same size as the walnuts and add them to the bowl. Add the feta (don't stir anything yet), scallions, and parsley.
3. In a separate small bowl, whisk together the lemon juice, pomegranate molasses, cumin, and garlic. While whisking, slowly add the oil. Season with the Aleppo pepper and salt to taste.
4. Arrange the leaves on six plates. Season very lightly with salt.
5. Spoon half the dressing into the red pepper mixture and stir to coat everything and until everything is well combined.
6. Spoon over the leaves on the plates and drizzle with the remaining dressing. Serve immediately.

Yield: 6 servings

Calories: 311; Protein: 11 g; Carbohydrate: 12 g; Fiber: 3 g; Sodium: 345 mg; Fat: 27 g (Sat: 4 g, Mono: 3 g, Poly: 1 g, Trans: 0 g); Cholesterol: 8 mg

Spicy Tofu Salad

Anna Thomas, author of Vegan Vegetarian Omnivore *(W. W. Norton, 2016)*

This intensely flavored salad is tasty when first made and gets even better as the tofu absorbs the flavors of the sesame oil, soy sauce, and chile sambal. Serve the spicy tofu over cold soba noodles in orange-ginger glaze for a beautiful lunch, or serve it with plain steamed rice or a mixed salad.

   1 pound extra-firm tofu, cut into thick slices
   1½ teaspoons dark sesame oil
   1 tablespoon sambal oelek or other hot red chili paste
   1 tablespoon tamari or soy sauce
   ½ cup chopped fresh cilantro, plus extra sprigs for garnish
   ⅓ cup thinly sliced scallions or spring onions
   Cold Soba Noodles with Orange-Ginger Glaze (page 330), for serving

1. Drain the tofu and press out the excess moisture: Arrange the tofu slices on a plate lined with a triple layer of paper towels. Cover the tofu with additional paper towels, place a small cutting board on top of them, and weight it down with a pot, or anything for a few pounds of weight. After a few minutes, change the paper towels and repeat until the towels are damp, not soaking wet. You can also simply press tofu slices by hand, squeezing them between your palms over the sink, but do this carefully, so as not to crumble the tofu. Cut the pressed tofu into ¾-inch cubes.
2. In a small bowl, whisk together the sesame oil, sambal oelek, and tamari. Add the tofu cubes and mix gently. Add the cilantro and scallions and toss again, but don't break the tofu cubes into bits.
3. Serve immediately, or cover and refrigerate for a few hours before serving. For an elegant look, use tongs to twist glazed soba noodles into little nests on the plates, then pile some spicy tofu into each nest and garnish with a sprig or two of cilantro.

Note: Sambal oelek, a paste of red chilies in vinegar and salt, is the heat that ignites this pretty salad. It's used in Vietnamese and Thai food, and you can find it in the Asian section of your supermarket—or substitute any simple red chili paste.

Yield: 4 to 6 as a lunch in combination with noodles, or 6 to 8 as an appetizer

Calories: 110; Protein: 10 g; Carbohydrate: 5 g; Fiber: 1 g; Sodium: 219 mg; Fat: 6 g (Sat: 1 g, Mono: 2 g, Poly: 3 g, Trans: 0 g); Cholesterol: 0 mg

Cold Soba Noodles with Orange-Ginger Glaze

Anna Thomas, author of Vegan Vegetarian Omnivore *(W. W. Norton, 2016)*

12 ounces soba noodles
½ cup fresh orange juice
1 tablespoon rice vinegar
1½ tablespoons finely grated fresh ginger
1 scant teaspoon finely grated orange zest
¼ teaspoon sea salt, plus more to taste
⅓ cup peanut oil
2 tablespoons black sesame seed

1. Cook the noodles in boiling salted water according to package directions, 3 or 4 minutes. Drain them and immediately plunge them into a bowl of ice water to cool them, then drain again.
2. Whisk together the orange juice, vinegar, ginger, orange zest, sea salt, and peanut oil. Spoon 5 to 6 tablespoons of the mixture over the noodles and lift them gently with tongs or with your hands until they are evenly glazed. Taste, and adjust the seasoning by adding as much of the glaze as you like, or another pinch of sea salt. (Reserve extra orange-ginger glaze to add to a stir-fry.) Sprinkle on the sesame seed, give the noodles a few more turns, and serve.

Note: These noodles can be kept in the refrigerator, tightly covered, for several hours.

Yield: 5 servings

Calories: 404; Protein: 8 g; Carbohydrate: 56 g; Fiber: 4 g; Sodium: 143 mg; Fat: 17 g (Sat: 3 g, Mono: 7 g, Poly: 6 g, Trans: 0 g); Cholesterol: 0 mg

Watercress Salad with Currants and Walnuts

Mollie Katzen, author and illustrator of numerous cookbooks for adults and children. Adapted from her Still Life With Menu Cookbook *(Ten Speed Press, 1988)*

This is a subtle and elegant salad with small touches of scallions, walnuts, and currants. Balsamic vinegar is the first choice to use here, but champagne vinegar or raspberry vinegar will be just as effective. If you clean and dry the greens ahead of time, the salad will take just minutes to prepare. Wrap the cleaned greens in paper towels, then refrigerate in a plastic bag until ready to use.

1 medium head butter lettuce or a similar soft-leaf variety
1 small bunch fresh watercress
1 to 2 small scallions, or about 6 chives, finely minced
Handful of currants
2 handfuls chopped walnuts, lightly toasted
2 to 3 tablespoons extra-virgin olive or walnut oil
Scant 1 teaspoon balsamic vinegar
Salt and freshly ground black pepper

1. Clean, thoroughly dry, and chill the lettuce and watercress. Tear into bite-size pieces and place them in a large bowl.
2. Add the scallions, currants, and walnuts.
3. Drizzle in the oil and toss well. Sprinkle with the vinegar and a little salt and pepper. Toss again and serve immediately.

Yield: 4 servings

Calories: 284; Protein: 5 g; Carbohydrate: 18 g; Fiber: 3 g; Sodium: 78 mg; Fat: 24 g (Sat: 3 g, Mono: 9 g, Poly: 10 g, Trans: 0 g); Cholesterol: 0 mg

Tempeh Salad with Pita and Pine Nuts

The addition of tempeh, nuts, and pita makes this Greek-style salad a main course rather than a side dish. If the weather is good, consider grilling the pita bread and tempeh to add a wonderful smoky flavor to the dish.

2 tablespoons oil

2 (2-ounce) whole wheat pita breads

1 (8-ounce) package five-grain tempeh

4 plum tomatoes, seeded and diced (about 2 cups)

2 small cucumbers, peeled, seeded, and diced (about 2 cups)

⅓ cup thinly sliced red onions (about 1 small)

¼ cup diced green bell peppers (about 1 small)

½ cup pine nuts, toasted

2 tablespoons chopped fresh basil

2 tablespoons fresh oregano leaves

1 tablespoon fresh lemon juice

¼ teaspoon Dijon mustard

½ teaspoon coarse salt

¼ teaspoon freshly ground black pepper

1. Preheat the broiler or prepare a grill.
2. Brush ½ teaspoon of the oil onto the pita breads and broil or grill for 2 minutes per side, or until they begin to brown. Let cool and cut each pita into 8 wedges or triangles.
3. In a large nonstick skillet, heat 1½ teaspoons of the oil over medium-high heat. Add the tempeh and cook, stirring, for 3 to 4 minutes, or until nicely browned.
4. Combine the tomatoes, cucumbers, tempeh, pita, onions, bell peppers, pine nuts, basil, and oregano in a large bowl; toss gently to mix.
5. Combine the lemon juice and mustard in a small bowl. Whisk to blend. Gradually stir in remaining oil and the salt and black pepper. Pour the vinaigrette over the cucumber mixture. Toss gently to blend and serve.

Yield: 4 servings; Serving: 1½ cups

Calories: 372; Protein: 14.8 g; Carbohydrate: 39.6 g; Fiber: 10.7 g; Sodium: 428 mg; Fat: 19 g (Sat: 2.3 g, Mono: 6.8 g, Poly: 4.1 g, Trans: 0 g); Cholesterol 0 mg

Onion-Crusted Tofu-Steak Sandwich

Panfried tofu steaks make a delicious and quick sandwich filling. Splurge with a nice whole grain bakery bun and top with a buttery lettuce such as Boston, a thick slice of fresh tomato, and a quick flavored mayonnaise spread that's created from store-bought mayonnaise. The Seven-Vegetable Slaw (page 355) makes a nice accompaniment for this sandwich. In fact, you can omit the aioli and top the tofu with slaw for another version of this sandwich.

LEMON-CILANTRO AIOLI

⅓ cup canola or soybean oil mayonnaise
2 tablespoons minced fresh cilantro
1 small garlic clove, minced
1 teaspoon untoasted sesame oil
¼ teaspoon grated lemon zest

SANDWICH

1 (16-ounce) package extra-firm tofu, cut crosswise into 12 slices
¼ cup oat flour or all-purpose flour
¼ cup minced dried onion
2 tablespoons sesame seed
½ teaspoon paprika
Coarse salt and freshly ground black pepper
1 large egg, lightly beaten
2 tablespoons water
2 tablespoons roasted peanut oil or canola oil
6 whole grain sandwich buns
1½ cups shredded butterhead (Boston or Bibb) lettuce
6 (½-inch-thick) slices ripe yellow or red tomato

1. To make the aioli, combine all the aioli ingredients in a small bowl and set aside to let the flavors blend.
2. To make the sandwiches, place the tofu slices on a double thickness of paper towels and let sit for 5 minutes.
3. Combine the flour, dried onion, sesame seed, paprika, and salt and pepper to taste in a shallow bowl. Place the egg in another shallow bowl and whisk in the water. Dip the tofu slices into the egg mixture and then dredge one at a time in the flour mixture.

4. In a large nonstick skillet, heat 1 tablespoon of the peanut oil over medium heat. Add 6 tofu slices and cook for 2 to 3 minutes on each side, or until lightly browned. Remove from the skillet. Repeat with the remaining 1 tablespoon peanut oil and tofu. Place 2 tofu slices on the bottom half of a bun. Top with ¼ cup of the lettuce and a tomato slice. Spread 1 tablespoon of the aioli on each top bun half and place the bun over the tomato. Serve immediately.

Note: Tofu packed in water makes the best tofu "steak." The texture is firmer, which makes it much easier to work with when breading and dipping. You can certainly use silken or reduced-fat tofu in this recipe; you'll just need to be more careful since its delicate nature causes it to break apart more easily.

Yield: 6 sandwiches; Serving: 1 sandwich

Calories: 420; Protein: 20.3 g; Carbohydrate: 33.7 g; Fiber: 6 g; Sodium: 344 mg; Fat: 18.1 g (Sat: 3.1 g, Mono: 9.9 g, Poly: 8.1 g, Trans: 0 g); Cholesterol: 40 mg

Farro and Mushroom Burgers

Suvir Saran, chef, author, public speaker, hobby farmer, and author of Masala Farm: Stories and Recipes from an Uncommon Life in the Country *(Chronicle Books, 2011)*

Farro is always in my pantry. I love using it in this recipe for veggie burgers. In addition to protein and heart-healthy fiber, the texture it contributes is incredibly hearty. You can sandwich the burgers in a bun (top with tomato chutney or a condiment of your choice) or eat it as a cutlet with chutney and a green salad on the side.

2¼ cups water
¾ cup farro
1 pound sweet potatoes
Leaves from 1 sprig fresh rosemary
Leaves from 1 sprig fresh thyme
6 tablespoons olive oil
1 teaspoon freshly ground black pepper
1½ pounds brown mushroom caps, finely chopped
1 teaspoon kosher salt
5 to 8 tablespoons extra-virgin olive oil

3 shallots, finely chopped
1 tablespoon dry white wine, dry vermouth, or water
½ cup finely grated Parmesan cheese (about 2 ounces)
1 cup whole wheat panko bread crumbs

1. Bring the water to a boil in a medium saucepan. Add the farro, return to a boil, cover, and reduce the heat to medium-low. Cook until the farro is tender, about 30 minutes. Turn off the heat, fluff the farro with a fork, cover, and set aside.

2. While the farro cooks, bring a large saucepan of water to a boil, add the potatoes, return the water to a boil, and cook until a paring knife easily slips into the center of the largest potato, about 20 minutes. Drain and set aside. Once the potatoes are cool, peel them and place the flesh in a large bowl.

3. In a large skillet, combine the rosemary, thyme, olive oil, and pepper and heat over medium-high heat, stirring occasionally. Once the herbs start crackling, after about 1½ minutes, add the mushrooms and salt. Cook the mushrooms, stirring often, until they release their liquid and the skillet is dry again, 6 to 7 minutes. Transfer the mushrooms to the bowl with the potatoes and set aside.

4. In the same skillet, heat 1 tablespoon of the extra-virgin olive oil over medium-high heat. Add the shallots and cook until they are soft and just starting to brown, about 2 minutes. Add the wine and stir, scraping up any browned bits from the bottom of the skillet. Turn off the heat and scrape the shallots into the bowl with the mushrooms and potatoes. Add the Parmesan along with the farro. Use a potato masher or fork to mash the ingredients together.

5. Form the mixture into 10 patties. Place the panko bread crumbs in a shallow dish and press the top and bottom of each patty into the panko to evenly coat.

6. In a clean large skillet, heat 4 tablespoons of the extra-virgin olive oil over medium-high heat. Add 5 patties and cook on each side until nicely browned and crusty, 8 to 10 minutes total. Remove the patties from the skillet and place them on a plate. Repeat with the remaining patties, adding more oil between batches if necessary. Serve hot.

Yield: 10 servings

Calories: 305; Protein: 7 g; Carbohydrate: 26 g; Fiber: 4 g; Sodium: 199 mg; Fat: 20 g (Sat: 4 g, Mono: 13 g, Poly: 2 g, Trans: 0 g); Cholesterol: 4 mg

Asparagus, Tofu, Shiitake, and Cashew Stir-Fry (FAST FIX)

Roasted peanut oil has an intensely nutty flavor that adds something special to this stir-fry. It can be found in most large supermarkets or health food stores. Tamari soy sauce is a special variety that has a more concentrated soy flavor. It can be found in most supermarkets in both regular and low-sodium varieties. Consider cooking up a larger batch of the brown rice and then saving leftovers for the Pad Thai–Style Fried Rice (page 323).

> ¼ cup raw cashews
> 2 tablespoons roasted peanut oil or canola oil
> 1½ teaspoons minced fresh ginger
> 2 garlic cloves, minced
> ½ pound thin fresh asparagus, trimmed and cut on an angle into 3-inch lengths
> ½ cup sliced shiitake mushrooms (about 4 ounces)
> 1 (16-ounce) package firm or extra-firm water-packed tofu, drained and cut into 1-inch cubes
> ½ cup vegetable stock or broth
> 2 tablespoons tamari soy sauce
> 1 tablespoon rice vinegar
> 1 tablespoon cornstarch
> 2⅔ cups hot cooked brown or brown basmati rice

1. Place a large wok or nonstick skillet over medium-high heat and add the cashews and 1 teaspoon of the oil. Stir-fry for 2 to 3 minutes, or until nuts are lightly browned, stirring occasionally to prevent scorching. Remove the nuts from the wok and set aside.

2. Add 2 teaspoons of the oil to the wok. Add the ginger and garlic and stir-fry for 45 seconds. Add the asparagus and stir-fry for 3 to 4 minutes, or until crisp-tender. Transfer the asparagus mixture to a plate and keep warm. Repeat the procedure with the mushrooms and 1 teaspoon of the oil and stir-fry for 2 to 3 minutes. Transfer the mushrooms to the plate with the asparagus and keep warm. Add 2 teaspoons of the oil to the pan and stir-fry the tofu for 3 to 4 minutes, until the cubes are lightly browned. Transfer the tofu to the plate with the vegetables and keep warm. Add 6 tablespoons of the stock, the soy sauce, and the vinegar to the wok; cook over medium-low heat for 2 to 3 minutes, or until hot. Stir together the remaining 2 tablespoons stock and the cornstarch. Add to the wok and cook for 1 minute, or

until the mixture thickens. Return the tofu and vegetables to the wok and toss gently in the sauce to reheat. Serve over cooked brown rice.

Yield: 4 servings; Serving: 1⅓ cups stir-fry mixture, ⅔ cup brown rice

Calories: 420; Protein: 19.1 g; Carbohydrate: 49 g; Fiber: 7.2 g; Sodium: 604 mg; Fat: 17.04 g (Sat: 2.87 g, Mono: 6.96 g, Poly: 6.08 g, Trans: 0 g); Cholesterol: 0 mg

Portobello and Caramelized Onion Pizza

Too often pizzas are smothered with cheese, usually a bland mozzarella, and the flavors of vegetables and delicate toppings are muted. Here the vegetables dominate, a pairing of savory-sweet caramelized onions and rich, meaty-flavored portobello mushrooms. A small sprinkling of Asiago cheese holds everything together. The crust is made from part wheat and part white flour with a few whole grains thrown in for texture. Buy those grains (oat groats, flaxseed) at any health food store.

WHOLE WHEAT PIZZA CRUST

2 teaspoons active dry yeast
1 cup warm water (105° to 115°F)
2 tablespoons olive oil
1 teaspoon coarse salt
1¼ cups all-purpose flour, plus more for dusting
⅔ cup whole wheat flour
¼ cup oat groats, toasted
2 tablespoons flaxseed, ground, or 3 tablespoons flaxseed meal
Nonstick cooking spray or oil

TOPPINGS

2 tablespoons olive oil
2 cups sliced white or yellow onions (about 1 large)
Coarse salt and freshly ground black pepper
1 (6-ounce) package sliced portobello mushrooms, cut into quarters
1 (4-ounce) package sliced mushrooms
1 large garlic clove, minced
2 tablespoons chopped fresh parsley
1 tablespoon fresh thyme leaves
1 tablespoon sherry vinegar

Cornmeal, for dusting

2 tablespoons freshly grated Asiago or Parmesan cheese

1. To make the crust, dissolve the yeast in warm water in a medium bowl; let stand for 5 minutes. Add the oil, salt, 1 cup of the all-purpose flour, the whole wheat flour, oat groats, and flaxseed; stir until a soft dough forms. Turn the dough out onto a lightly floured surface. Knead until smooth and elastic, 8 to 10 minutes, adding enough of the remaining all-purpose flour, 1 tablespoon at a time, to prevent the dough from sticking to your hands. The dough will feel slightly tacky.

2. Place the dough in a large bowl coated lightly with cooking spray, turning once to coat the top. Cover with plastic wrap and let rise in a warm place (85°F), free from drafts, for 30 minutes, or until doubled in size.

3. To make the toppings, in a large nonstick skillet, heat 1 tablespoon of the oil over medium heat. Add the onions and cook, stirring occasionally to prevent scorching, for 5 minutes. Season with salt and pepper. Reduce the heat to low and cook for 20 minutes, or until the onions are soft and golden. Transfer the onions to a plate and keep warm. Add the remaining 1 tablespoon oil to the skillet and heat over medium-high heat. Add the mushrooms and cook, stirring, for 5 to 8 minutes, or until the mushrooms are nicely browned. Remove from the heat and stir in the garlic, parsley, thyme, and vinegar.

4. Preheat the oven to 450°F; put a pizza stone in the oven to preheat if you are using one.

5. Punch down the dough; cover and let rest for 5 minutes. Roll the dough into a 12-inch circle on a floured surface. Place the dough on a pizza peel or baking sheet sprinkled with cornmeal. Crimp the edges of the dough with your fingers to form a rim. Cover and let rise for 10 minutes.

6. Spread the caramelized onions over the pizza crust, leaving a ½-inch border; top with the mushroom mixture. Sprinkle with the cheese. Bake (on the pizza stone or a baking sheet) for 10 minutes, or until the crust is browned. Transfer the pizza to a cutting board and cut into 6 slices.

Notes: Toast oat groats just as you would any nut: place the oat groats on a small baking sheet and toast in the oven at 350°F for 16 to 20 minutes or until lightly browned, checking periodically to make sure they don't scorch. Remove from the oven and let cool. Flaxseed can be ground in a clean coffee grinder or purchased already ground.

Yield: 6 slices; Serving: 1 slice

Calories: 296; Protein: 8.7 g; Carbohydrate: 42 g; Fiber: 4.7 g; Sodium: 326 mg; Fat: 11.6 g (Sat: 1.72 g, Mono: 6.89 g, Poly: 1.19 g, Trans: 0.09 g); Cholesterol: 2 mg

Roasted Walnut and Brown Rice Loaf

Brown rice comes in all different colors. And Lundberg brown rice blends, since they include so many colors and varieties, give a nice appearance to this meatless loaf. To make the bread crumbs, place a slice of leftover bread into a food processor and pulse until crumbly.

- 3 tablespoons olive oil, plus more for the pan
- 1 cup brown rice blend or brown rice
- 2 cups mushroom or vegetable broth (such as Pacific)
- ½ cup dried porcini or shiitake mushroom pieces (½ ounce), diced
- 1 teaspoon salt
- 2 cups chopped walnuts
- 1 cup finely chopped white or yellow onions (about 1 medium)
- ¼ cup finely chopped celery
- 2 garlic cloves, minced
- 1 cup fresh whole grain bread crumbs
- ¼ cup chopped fresh parsley
- 2 teaspoons chopped fresh thyme, or ½ teaspoon dried
- 3 large eggs, lightly beaten

1. Preheat the oven to 375°F. Lightly coat an 8-inch square baking pan with oil.
2. Combine the rice, broth, mushrooms, 1 tablespoon of the oil, and ½ teaspoon of the salt in a large saucepan. Bring the mixture to a boil; cover, reduce the heat, and simmer for 45 minutes, or until the rice is tender. Place the rice in large bowl and let cool.
3. Place the walnuts on a baking sheet and toast in the oven for 3 to 5 minutes, or until they begin to brown lightly. Watch carefully to make sure nuts do not burn. Remove from the oven and finely chop.
4. In a large nonstick skillet, heat the remaining 2 tablespoons oil over medium heat. Add the onions and celery and cook, stirring, for 5 to 7 minutes, or until tender. Stir in the remaining ½ teaspoon salt and the garlic and cook for 1 minute. Remove from the heat and stir in the bread crumbs, parsley, and thyme. Add the bread crumb mixture to the cooled rice. Stir

in the eggs and pat the mixture into the pan. Bake for 40 to 50 minutes, or until the loaf is firm. Remove from the oven and let cool in the pan for 10 minutes before slicing.

Yield: 1 loaf, 12 slices; Serving: 1 slice

Calories: 266; Protein: 7.3 g; Carbohydrate: 20.3 g; Fiber: 3 g; Sodium: 234 mg; Fat: 18.4 g (Sat: 2.20 g, Mono: 5.03 g, Poly: 10.17 g, Trans 0 g); Cholesterol 53 mg

Lentil Nut Loaf with Red Pepper Sauce

Gail Willett, adapted from Yummly.com

LENTIL LOAF

2 tablespoons olive oil, plus more for the pan

2 cups water

1 cup lentils, rinsed and picked over

1 large white or yellow onion, chopped

1 cup chopped mushrooms (about 4 ounces)

1 cup ground nuts

1 cup bread crumbs

1 tablespoon fresh lemon juice

1 tablespoon soy sauce

1 tablespoon mixed fresh herbs

Salt and freshly ground black pepper

RED PEPPER SAUCE

1 tablespoon olive oil

1 garlic clove

1 roasted red pepper

3 tomatoes, chopped

Crushed red pepper flakes (optional)

1. To make the lentil loaf, preheat the oven to 350°F. Lightly grease a 9 × 5-inch loaf pan.
2. In a medium saucepan, bring the water to a boil. Add the lentils and cook until soft, about 30 minutes.
3. In a skillet, heat the 2 tablespoons oil over medium heat. Add the onion and mushrooms and cook, stirring, until soft. Add the nuts, bread crumbs,

lemon juice, soy sauce, herbs, and salt and black pepper to taste and cook, stirring, for a few minutes. Place the mixture in the pan and bake for 30 minutes.

4. Meanwhile, to make the red pepper sauce, in a skillet, heat the 1 tablespoon oil over medium heat. Add the garlic and cook, stirring, for 3 to 4 minutes. Add the roasted pepper and tomatoes. Cook until the mixture thickens. Serve hot or room temperature on Lentil Nut Loaf.

Yield: 4 servings

Calories: 504; Protein: 20 g; Carbohydrate: 42 g; Fiber: 10 g; Sodium: 505 mg; Fat: 31 g (Sat: 3 g, Mono: 5 g, Poly: 2 g, Trans: 0 g); Cholesterol: 0 mg

Winter Squash with Pecan Stuffing

Carnival squash is the same shape and size as the acorn variety, but the skin is an attractive speckled green or speckled orange. If you can't find it, use acorn or any variety of winter squash.

2 (14-ounce) carnival or acorn squash
1½ tablespoons olive oil
1 cup coarsely chopped yellow or white onions (about 1 medium)
1 teaspoon coarse salt
1 cup cooked brown rice
½ cup chopped pecans, toasted
2 tablespoons roasted sunflower seeds
¼ cup dried cherries
¼ cup dried currants
3 tablespoons chopped fresh parsley
2 teaspoons finely chopped fresh sage
¼ teaspoon freshly ground black pepper

1. Preheat the oven to 375°F.
2. Cut the squash in half from stem to tip and scoop out the seeds; brush the cut sides lightly with 1 teaspoon of the oil and place cut side down on a rimmed baking sheet. Bake for 30 to 35 minutes or until the squash is wrinkled and soft. Scoop out most of the squash flesh, leaving a thin border next to the skin; put the flesh in a bowl and mash with a fork. Set the squash shells aside.

3. In a large nonstick skillet, heat the remaining oil over medium heat. Add the onions and cook for 4 to 5 minutes, or until it begins to soften. Stir in ½ teaspoon of the salt. Add the rice and cook for 3 to 4 minutes, or until warmed through. Stir in the squash, the remaining ½ teaspoon salt, the pecans, sunflower seeds, cherries, currants, parsley, sage, and pepper and cook for 4 to 6 minutes.

4. To serve, spoon squash-rice mixture into the squash halves, pressing down with the back of the spoon to pack the filling tightly. Serve immediately.

Yield: 4 servings; Serving: 1 stuffed squash half

Calories: 379; Protein: 6.2 g; Carbohydrate: 52.3 g; Fiber: 7.8 g; Sodium: 482 mg; Fat: 18.5 g (Sat: 2 g, Mono: 10.4, Poly: 5.3 g, Trans: 0 g); Cholesterol: 0 mg

Butternut Squash, Apple, and Cranberry Gratin

Suvir Saran, chef, author, public speaker, hobby farmer, and author of Masala Farm: Stories and Recipes from an Uncommon Life in the Country *(Chronicle Books, 2011)*

½ cup plus 1 tablespoon olive oil

1 butternut squash, peeled, halved, seeded, and diced into 1-inch cubes

3 sweet-tart apples that will keep their shape after baking, peeled, cored, and diced into ½-inch cubes

1⅓ cups dried unsweetened cranberries

¼ cup finely chopped fresh flat-leaf parsley

½ teaspoon finely chopped fresh thyme

1 tablespoon kosher salt

1 teaspoon freshly ground black pepper

¼ teaspoon cayenne pepper

Heaping ½ cup whole wheat pastry flour

1. Preheat the oven to 350°F. Grease a 12 × 9-inch baking dish with the 1 tablespoon oil.

2. In a large bowl, toss together the squash, apples, cranberries, parsley, thyme, salt, black pepper, and cayenne. Drizzle in the ½ cup oil and stir to combine, then add the flour and mix to evenly coat the squash mixture.

3. Turn the mixture into the baking dish and bake until the top is deep golden brown and the squash is tender but not mushy (a paring knife should eas-

ily slip into the center of a piece of squash), 50 to 55 minutes. Remove from the oven and let cool for 5 minutes before serving.

Yield: 8 servings

Calories: 335; Protein: 3 g; Carbohydrate: 50 g; Fiber: 7 g; Sodium: 429 mg; Fat: 15 g (Sat: 2 g, Mono: 11 g, Poly: 2 g, Trans: 0 g); Cholesterol: 0 mg

Farro and Roasted Butternut Squash

Heidi Swanson, 101 Cookbooks (www.101cookbooks.com)

If you are pressed for time, opt for a lightly or semi-pearled farro (actually easier to find in some places), which will cut the cooking time for the grains down to about 20 minutes. Barley, both hulled and pearl, would make a nice substitution if you are having trouble finding farro. Also, I found beautiful red spring onions at the farmers' market but regular red onions will work well, and will be much easier to find.

2 cups farro, rinsed and drained
1 teaspoon fine sea salt, plus more as needed
5 cups water or stock
3 cups cubed butternut squash (½-inch dice)
1 large red onion, cut into eighths
1 tablespoon fresh thyme, minced
3 tablespoons olive oil
1 tablespoon balsamic vinegar
1 cup walnuts, deeply toasted
3 tablespoons toasted walnut oil (or more olive oil)
¼ cup crumbled goat cheese (about 1 ounce)

1. Preheat the oven to 375°F.
2. Combine the farro, salt, and water in a large, heavy saucepan. Cover and simmer over medium heat, stirring occasionally, until the farro is tender, 45 minutes to 1 hour, or about half the time if you are using semi-pearled farro. Taste often as it is cooking, you want it to be toothsome and retain structure. Remove from the heat, drain any excess water, and set aside.
3. While the farro is cooking, on a rimmed baking sheet toss the squash, onion, and thyme with the olive oil, vinegar, and a couple big pinches of

salt. Arrange in a single layer and roast for about 20 minutes. Toss the squash and onion every 5 to 7 minutes to get browning on all sides. Remove from the oven, let cool a bit, and mince just half of the red onions.

4. In a large bowl, gently toss everything except the goat cheese with the walnut oil. Taste and add a bit of salt if necessary. Serve family-style in a simple bowl or on a platter, garnished with the goat cheese.

Yield: 6 servings

Calories: 509; Protein: 14 g; Carbohydrate: 54 g; Fiber: 7 g; Sodium: 460 mg; Fat: 31 g (Sat: 4 g, Mono: 7 g, Poly: 10 g, Trans: 0 g); Cholesterol: 4 mg

SOUPS AND STEWS

Curried Winter Squash Soup (FAST FIX)

This version of winter squash soup is a snap to make. Start with frozen winter squash and add some new flavors—apple and curry—to make a delicious but quick entrée. Serve with a crusty whole grain bread and a mixed green salad for a complete cold-weather meal. If you don't have any homemade stock on hand, opt for reduced-sodium canned broth or reduced-sodium powdered stock; regular canned or powdered stocks are extremely salty. It's much better to start with a lower-sodium stock and add salt to taste.

2 tablespoons olive oil

2 cups coarsely chopped white or yellow onions (about 1 large)

1 to 2 teaspoons minced fresh ginger

1 tablespoon curry powder

2½ cups defatted chicken stock or broth, preferably low-sodium

1 cup apple cider or apple juice

2 (14-ounce) boxes frozen mashed winter squash, thawed

¼ cup unsweetened applesauce

Coarse salt

1. In a large soup pot or Dutch oven, heat the oil over medium heat. Add the onions, cook, stirring, for 12 to 18 minutes, or until the onions have softened. Stir in the ginger and curry powder and cook for 1 minute, stirring continuously. Add the stock, apple cider, squash, and applesauce. Bring

the soup to a boil, reduce the heat, and simmer for 5 to 10 minutes to blend the flavors.

2. Transfer a small amount of the soup to a blender or food processor and carefully puree on low speed, leaving the center part of the cover off so that steam can escape. Continue pureeing the soup in small batches until the mixture is smooth. Return the soup to the pot and keep warm until ready to serve. Taste for seasoning and add salt as desired.

Note: The soup will be thick. If you like a thinner soup, add more stock.

Yield: 6 cups; Serving: 1½ cups

Calories: 192; Protein: 4.8 g; Carbohydrate: 32 g; Fiber: 5.7 g; Sodium: 391 mg; Fat: 6.9 g (Sat: 0.93 g, Mono: 7.83 g, Poly: 0.61 g, Trans: 0.07 g); Cholesterol: 0 mg

Wheat Berry and Lentil Soup

Start this soup early in the day since the wheat berries take about 45 minutes to cook. Or consider cooking several cups of wheat berries to have on hand. That way you can slip them into this soup, hot cereal, or casseroles at the last minute.

1 cup wheat berries
¾ teaspoon coarse salt
9 cups water
2 tablespoons olive oil
1½ cups chopped white or yellow onions (about 1 large)
1 cup diced carrots (about 2 medium)
¾ cup diced celery
2 garlic cloves, minced
1 cup dried French green or other lentils
2 cups vegetable broth
1 tablespoon tomato paste
1 tablespoon soy sauce
3 thyme sprigs
1 bay leaf
¼ teaspoon freshly ground black pepper
4 cups baby leaf spinach

1. Place the wheat berries in a large Dutch oven or saucepan. Add ¼ teaspoon of the salt and 4 cups of the water; bring to a boil. Cover, reduce the heat, and simmer for 45 to 50 minutes, or until tender. Drain.

2. In a large Dutch oven or large saucepan, heat the oil over medium heat. Add the onions, carrots, and celery and sauté for 6 to 8 minutes, or until they begin to become tender. Stir in the garlic and ¼ teaspoon of the salt and cook for 1 minute.

3. Add the lentils, the remaining 5 cups water, the broth, tomato paste, soy sauce, thyme, and bay leaf to the pot. Raise the heat to high and bring to a boil. Reduce the heat and simmer for 15 minutes. Stir in the remaining ¼ teaspoon salt, the pepper, and the spinach and cook for 2 to 3 minutes, or until spinach is wilted. Stir in the wheat berries and cook until warmed through, 1 to 2 minutes.

Yield: 6 servings; Serving: about 1½ cups

Calories: 283; Protein: 12.4 g; Carbohydrate: 50 g; Fiber: 10.6 g; Sodium: 706 mg; Fat: 5.2 g (Sat: 0.73 g, Mono: 3.40 g, Poly: 0.73 g, Trans: 0 g); Cholesterol 0 mg

Tomato Soup

Charles Burke, MD, president of the New Hampshire Farm to Restaurant Connection

This tomato soup features fennel two ways: fresh fennel and fennel seed, augmented with Pernod or other anise-flavored liqueur. The recipe can be made without the liqueur, using double the amount of tarragon, which adds its own unique anise-like flavor. Use any rich tomato sauce, preferably without other herb flavors, or simmer a large can of whole tomatoes until thickened. This soup can be made a day or two ahead, and the flavor actually improves with time.

2½ tablespoons olive oil

1 medium fennel bulb, sliced

1 medium sweet onion, sliced

2 garlic cloves, sliced

1 tablespoon fennel seed

1 teaspoon crushed red pepper flakes

1 tablespoon fresh tarragon, chopped, or 2 teaspoons dried

¼ cup Pernod or other anise-flavored liqueur

½ cup dry white wine

2 cups tomato sauce

¼ cup grated Parmesan cheese (about 1 ounce)

3 cups water

Freshly ground black pepper

1. In a heavy-bottomed pan, heat the oil over medium heat. Add the fresh fennel, onion, garlic, and fennel seed. Cook, stirring, until the onion and fennel begin to caramelize.
2. Add the red pepper flakes, tarragon, and Pernod, reduce the heat, and simmer until the vegetables are glazed, then add the wine and cook until it has reduced to a glaze.
3. Add the tomato sauce, Parmesan, and water and boil until thickened.

Yield: 4 servings

Calories: 290; Protein: 7 g; Carbohydrate: 26 g; Fiber: 7 g; Sodium: 377 mg; Fat: 13 g (Sat: 2 g, Mono: 8 g, Poly: 1 g, Trans: 0 g); Cholesterol: 4 mg

White Bean, Chicken, and Spinach Soup

Try this quick but hearty version of chicken soup for days when you're feeling a little under the weather. Instead of refined white noodles, it's chock-full of white beans and spinach, two antioxidant-rich foods.

1 tablespoon olive oil

1 small white or yellow onion, chopped

1 celery stalk, chopped

1 large carrot, chopped

2 bay leaves

3 cups reduced-sodium chicken broth

2 cups water

12 ounces chicken breast tenders, chopped

1 (15-ounce) can small white beans, rinsed and drained

1 cup tightly packed baby spinach leaves

3 tablespoons finely chopped fresh oregano

¼ cup finely chopped fresh parsley

2 tablespoons fresh lemon juice

¼ teaspoon salt

½ teaspoon freshly ground black pepper

1. In a large saucepan, heat the oil over medium heat until hot. Stir in the onion, celery, and carrot and cook, stirring, for 6 to 8 minutes, or until they begin to soften. Add the bay leaves and cook, stirring, for 1 minute.

2. Add the broth and water and bring the mixture to a boil. Reduce the heat and stir in the chicken and beans. Simmer for 3 to 4 minutes, or until the chicken is tender. Stir in the spinach and remove from the heat. Let stand for 2 to 3 minutes, or until the spinach wilts. Stir in the oregano, parsley, lemon juice, salt, and pepper. Serve immediately.

Yield: 4 servings; Serving: about 1½ cups

Calories: 200; Protein: 26.6 g; Carbohydrate: 15.9 g; Fiber: 4.3 g; Sodium: 871 mg; Fat: 4.9 g (Sat 0.76 g, Mono: 2.77 g, Poly: 0.63 g, Trans: 0 g); Cholesterol 49 mg

Tunisian Chickpea Breakfast Stew

Author Martha Rose Shulman's latest cookbook is Spiralize This! *(Houghton Mifflin Harcourt, 2016)*

This is a traditional Tunisian breakfast dish, a simple bowl of chickpeas flavored with onion, garlic, harissa, and olive oil, served with a number of garnishes. For us, it's dinner.

STEW

1 pound dried chickpeas, washed, picked over, and soaked in 2 quarts water for 6 hours or overnight

2 quarts water

2 tablespoons extra-virgin olive oil

1 medium white or yellow onion, chopped

4 large garlic cloves, minced or pressed

1 tablespoon cumin seed, lightly toasted and ground

2 tablespoons harissa, or ½ to 1 teaspoon cayenne pepper

Salt

2 tablespoons fresh lemon juice, or more to taste

OPTIONAL GARNISHES

Lemon wedges or preserved lemon wedges

Coarse sea salt or kosher salt

Harissa

Chopped fresh tomatoes

Chopped green and red bell peppers

Chopped hard-boiled eggs

Rinsed capers

Ground lightly toasted cumin

Finely chopped fresh flat-leaf parsley

Finely chopped fresh cilantro

Croutons

Thinly sliced scallions, both white and green parts

Extra-virgin olive oil

1. To make the stew, drain the chickpeas and combine with the water in a large, heavy soup pot or Dutch oven. Bring to a boil, reduce the heat, cover, and simmer for 1 hour.

2. Meanwhile, in a heavy nonstick medium skillet, heat the oil over medium heat. Add the onion and cook, stirring, until tender, about 5 minutes. Stir in the garlic and cumin and stir together for 30 seconds to 1 minute, until the garlic is fragrant. Remove from the heat and stir into the beans.

3. After the beans have cooked for 1 hour, stir in the harissa and season with salt. Cover and cook for 30 minutes to 1 hour more, until the beans are very tender and the broth fragrant. Add the lemon juice, taste, and adjust the seasoning.

4. Serve the soup, passing your choice of condiments on a large tray, or have them laid out on a buffet to stir into the soup.

Note: The finished soup will taste great for another 3 to 4 days. Keep in the refrigerator. You will want to refresh the condiments each time you serve. You can also make a salad with the leftover beans.

Yield: 4 servings, excluding garnishes

For stew only: Calories: 501; Protein: 22 g; Carbohydrate: 74 g; Fiber: 20 g; Sodium: 140 mg; Fat: 14 g (Sat: 2 g, Mono: 7 g, Poly: 4 g, Trans: 0 g); Cholesterol: 0 mg

Oldways Sweet Potato Peanut Stew (Mafe)

Sara Baer-Sinnott, president of Oldways, a nonprofit food and nutrition organization (www.oldwayspt.org), *from* The Oldways 4-Week Mediterranean Diet Menu Plan *(Oldways, 2013)*

*M**afe*, or groundnut stew, is common throughout West and Central Africa. This traditional stew can incorporate meat, vegetables, or seafood, and it is always based on a savory sauce made from peanut butter and tomatoes. This recipe is based on one from Iba Thiam, chef and owner of Cazmance restaurant in Austin, Texas, and it is one of the recipes in Oldways's A Taste of African Heritage cooking and nutrition program. The sweet potato, a much-loved African heritage food, is a featured ingredient.

2 teaspoons extra-virgin olive oil
1 medium yellow onion, diced
2 garlic cloves, minced
1 large sweet potato (about 12 ounces), cut into medium cubes
2 large carrots, thinly sliced
2 zucchini, halved lengthwise and thinly sliced
1 (15-ounce) can diced tomatoes
2 cups low-sodium vegetable broth
1 tablespoon curry powder
¼ cup natural peanut butter
Leaves from 3 sprigs fresh thyme, minced, or 1 teaspoon dried
Sea salt

1. In a large Dutch oven or soup pot, heat the oil over medium heat. Add the onion and garlic and cook, stirring, for 3 to 4 minutes, or until translucent.
2. Add the sweet potato, carrots, and zucchini to the pot and cook, stirring, for 3 to 4 minutes.
3. Add the tomatoes, broth, and curry powder; bring to a boil. Reduce the heat, cover, and simmer for 10 minutes.
4. Add the peanut butter and thyme to the stew. Cook, uncovered, for 3 to 5 minutes, or until the vegetables are tender. Season with salt and serve.

Yield: 4 servings; Serving: approximately 2½ cups
Calories: 240 calories; Protein: 7 g; Carbohydrate: 27 g; Fiber: 7 g; Sodium: 280 mg; Fat: 11 g (Sat: 1.5 g, Mono: 6 g, Poly: 3 g, Trans: 0 g); Cholesterol: 0 mg

Chipotle Chicken Chili

Substitute 2 (15-ounce) cans of any variety of cooked legume—black bean, soybean, red kidney bean—for the dried beans if you're short on time. But do try the anasazi bean version at least once; it will be worth the extra effort. This ancient bean variety has a beautiful speckled appearance and a hint of sweetness not found in other dried beans. Chipotle peppers in adobo sauce are large, dried, and smoked jalapeño peppers rehydrated in a tomato-vinegar–based sauce. They lend a wonderful smoky flavor and a small amount of heat to this chili. You'll find them in the Mexican food section of the supermarket. Leave out the chicken if you'd like a vegetarian chili.

1½ cups dried anasazi beans
1 cup dried cannellini beans
2 tablespoons canola oil
2 garlic cloves, chopped
1 bay leaf
1 tablespoon paprika
1 tablespoon chili powder
1 tablespoon dried oregano
1 teaspoon cumin seed
1 teaspoon ground cumin
2 cups coarsely chopped white onions (about 1 large)
2 cups coarsely chopped green bell peppers (about 2 large)
4 cups water
1 canned chipotle pepper in adobo sauce, finely chopped
1 (14.5-ounce) can diced tomatoes
1 (28-ounce) can whole tomatoes, chopped, with liquid
1 cup cooked or canned hominy, drained
8 chicken breast tenders (about 12 ounces), cut into 2-inch pieces
¼ cup fresh cilantro, chopped
Coarse salt
Chopped white onions and chopped fresh cilantro, mixed together (optional)

1. Soak the beans in water to cover overnight. (Or use the quick-soak method: Place the beans in a stockpot and cover with water. Bring the water to a boil and cook for 1 minute. Remove from the heat and let stand for 1 hour. Drain the beans and proceed to step 2.)

2. In a large soup pot or Dutch oven, heat the canola oil over medium heat. Add the garlic, bay leaf, paprika, chili powder, oregano, cumin seed, and ground cumin. Cook, stirring, for 1 minute. Stir in the onions and bell peppers; cook, stirring, for 3 to 5 minutes. Add the beans, water, and chipotle pepper. Bring the mixture to a boil; reduce the heat and simmer for 60 to 75 minutes, or until the beans are soft but still somewhat firm. Add the diced and chopped tomatoes and their liquid. Stir in the hominy, chicken, and cilantro and simmer, uncovered, for 15 to 20 minutes, or until the chicken is cooked through. Season with salt. Spoon into bowls and garnish with onions and cilantro, if using.

Note: Leftovers will freeze well; freeze the chili without the onion and cilantro garnish.

Yield: 9 servings; Serving: 1½ cups

Calories: 309; Protein: 22.4 g; Carbohydrate: 46.3 g; Fiber: 13.8 g; Sodium: 315 mg; Fat: 4.9 g (Sat: 0.47 g, Mono: 3.67 g, Poly: 1.38 g, Trans: 0.01 g); Cholesterol: 22 mg

Simple Seafood Stew

Buy the peeled and deveined raw shrimp to save time. Serve leftovers over fresh spinach linguine for a different meal.

2 tablespoons olive oil
1 cup diced white or yellow onions (about 1 medium)
½ cup diced fennel or celery
2 garlic cloves, minced
½ teaspoon crushed red pepper flakes
1 bay leaf
½ cup dry white wine
1 (28-ounce) can Italian tomatoes, chopped, with liquid
1 cup water
½ cup fresh or frozen corn kernels
¼ cup fresh parsley, finely chopped
½ pound medium shrimp (about 20), peeled and deveined
⅓ pound cod or pollock, cut into 2-inch pieces
⅓ pound bay scallops

Coarse salt

Chopped fresh parsley, for garnish (optional)

1. In a large nonstick skillet, heat the olive oil over medium heat. Add the onions and fennel and sauté for 8 to 10 minutes, or until the vegetables soften. Stir in the garlic, red pepper flakes, and bay leaf and sauté for 1 minute. Add the wine and cook for 1 to 2 minutes. Stir in the tomatoes with their juice, water, and corn. Bring to a boil, reduce the heat, and simmer, covered, for 10 to 12 minutes, or until the corn is cooked.

2. Uncover and add the parsley, shrimp, and cod and cook gently for 2 minutes. Stir in the scallops and cook for 1 to 2 minutes, or until all the seafood is opaque.

3. Remove the bay leaf and discard; season the stew with salt and ladle into shallow bowls. Garnish with parsley, if desired.

Yield: 4 servings (6 cups); Serving: 1½ cups

Calories: 287; Protein: 28.5 g; Carbohydrate: 22 g; Fiber: 4.2 g; Sodium: 475 mg; Fat: 9.1 g (Sat: 1.3 g, Mono: 5.4 g, Poly: 1.5 g, Trans: 0.07 g); Cholesterol: 115 mg

Chinese Cioppino with Scallops and Shrimp

Nina Simonds, award-winning author and authority on Asian food, from Spices of Life: Simple and Delicious Recipes for Great Health *(Knopf, 2005)*

Cioppino, an Italian American fish stew invented in San Francisco in the late 1800s, is usually made with the catch of the day. I like to make a simplified Chinese adaptation, using seafood infused with the flavors of fresh ginger, sake, and chili garlic paste, as well as tomatoes, fresh basil, and oregano.

1 tablespoon canola or other oil

2 large garlic cloves, minced

1½ teaspoons minced fresh ginger

½ teaspoon chili garlic sauce, or to taste

1 medium white or yellow onion, chopped

1 large green bell pepper, seeded and chopped

1 (14.5-ounce can) diced tomatoes

1½ teaspoons tomato paste

1 (8-ounce) bottle clam juice

½ cup rice wine or sake

2 tablespoons chopped fresh basil

1 teaspoon dried oregano

Coarse salt and freshly ground black pepper

SEAFOOD AND MARINADE

4 thin slices unpeeled fresh ginger

6 tablespoons rice wine or sake

½ pound medium shrimp (about 20), peeled and deveined

½ pound sea scallops (about 5 to 10), tough muscle removed from the side, if necessary

1. In a 3½-quart casserole or Dutch oven with a lid, heat the canola oil over medium-high heat. Add the garlic, ginger, chili garlic sauce, onion, and bell pepper and cook, stirring occasionally, for 7 to 8 minutes, until the onion and bell pepper are tender. Add the diced tomatoes, tomato paste, clam juice, rice wine, basil, oregano, and salt and black pepper to taste, cover, and bring to a boil. Uncover, reduce the heat to low, and simmer for 12 to 15 minutes.

2. Meanwhile, to marinate the seafood, smash the ginger slices with the flat side of a chef's knife and place them in a bowl. Add the rice wine and pinch the ginger slices to flavor the wine. Cut the shrimp along the back to butterfly, and if the scallops are very big, halve them crosswise. Add the shrimp and scallops to the ginger-wine mixture and marinate for about 10 minutes. Remove and discard the ginger slices.

3. Add the shrimp and scallops to the tomato base, cover, and cook over medium heat for 3 to 4 minutes, or until the seafood is cooked through.

Note: You can prepare the tomato base in advance and add the seafood just before serving. Look for the chili garlic sauce in the Asian section of most supermarkets.

Yield: 4 servings; Serving: 1½ cups

Calories: 156; Protein: 26 g; Carbohydrate: 18 g; Fiber: 3 g; Sodium: 538 mg; Fat: 5 g (Sat: 0 g, Mono: 2 g, Poly: 2 g, Trans: 0 g); Cholesterol: 99 mg

SIDES

Seven-Vegetable Slaw (FAST FIX)

S tart with one of the prepackaged vegetable slaw mixes and add more vegetables to make it tastier and more unique. Here we've added red pepper, zucchini, and the less familiar fennel, a crunchy vegetable with a mild anise flavor. If you don't like the flavor of anise, substitute celery.

1 (16-ounce) package shredded broccoli slaw or cabbage slaw
1 cup shredded carrots (about 2 medium)
1 cup thinly sliced fennel or celery
1 large red bell pepper, julienned (about 1 cup)
2 small zucchini, julienned (about 2 cups)
½ cup canola or soybean oil mayonnaise
½ teaspoon grated orange zest
¼ cup fresh orange juice
1 teaspoon celery seed
Coarse salt and freshly ground black pepper

1. Place the slaw, carrots, fennel, bell pepper, and zucchini in a large bowl and toss to combine.
2. Combine the mayonnaise, orange zest, orange juice, celery seed, and salt and black pepper to taste in a small bowl and stir until blended. Pour the dressing over the slaw and toss gently to coat.

Note: For a spunkier slaw, omit the celery seed, orange zest, and orange juice from the dressing and add prepared horseradish to taste.

Yield: 8 cups (16 servings); Serving: ½ cup

Calories: 71; Protein: 1.9 g; Carbohydrate: 7.2 g; Fiber: 2.6 g; Sodium: 60 mg; Fat: 2.1 g (Sat: 0.4 g, Mono: 0.4 g, Poly: 1.3 g, Trans: 0 g); Cholesterol: 2 mg

Pear and Mixed Green Salad

A simple but elegant salad dressed with a lemon-shallot vinaigrette. Add some toasted walnuts or a little bit of blue cheese for special occasions—a little of either one of these higher-fat items can go a long way. But make sure to include at least one strong-flavored green such as arugula or endive. They make a nice match for the sweet pear.

3 tablespoons extra-virgin olive oil
1 tablespoon minced shallots or red onions
1½ tablespoons fresh lemon juice
1½ teaspoons water
Coarse salt
4 cups mixed salad greens
2 cups frisée, endive, or arugula
2 unpeeled Bosc pears, cored and sliced lengthwise into 12 sections
Freshly ground black pepper

1. In a small nonstick skillet, heat 1 tablespoon of the olive oil over medium heat. Add the shallot and sauté for 2 to 3 minutes, or until softened. Remove from the heat and let cool. Combine the shallot, lemon juice, water, and salt to taste in a small bowl; whisk to blend. While whisking, slowly add the remaining 2 tablespoons oil and whisk until well blended.
2. Combine the salad greens and frisée in a large bowl; add the vinaigrette and toss gently so that the greens are well coated with the dressing. Add the pears and toss gently to mix. Season with pepper and serve.

Note: Prepare the vinaigrette in advance, but leave the greens undressed and the pears unsliced until just before serving. That way the greens will stay crisp and the pears won't discolor. Alternatively, toss the pears with the vinaigrette and keep refrigerated; the acid in the lemon juice will help keep the pears from turning brown. Toss with the greens just prior to serving.

Yield: 8 cups; Serving: 2 cups

Calories: 176; Protein: 1.8 g; Carbohydrate: 20.1 g; Fiber: 4.9 g; Sodium: 15 mg; Fat: 11.1 g (Sat: 1.52 g, Mono: 8.18 g, Poly: 1.13 g, Trans: 0 g); Cholesterol: 0 mg

Greek Salad

This salad tastes great with or without the feta cheese. Serve it as a side salad at dinner. Or consider adding some grilled chicken to make it a substantial main dish.

VINAIGRETTE

3 tablespoons extra-virgin olive oil

2 tablespoons red wine vinegar

1 tablespoon fresh lemon juice

Coarse salt and freshly ground black pepper

SALAD

3 cups chopped romaine lettuce (about 8 leaves)

1 cup sliced radishes (about 3 ounces)

1 large yellow bell pepper, julienned (about 1 cup)

1 cup diced cucumber

½ cup thinly sliced red onions (about 1 small)

½ cup fresh mint, chopped

⅓ cup pitted Kalamata olives, cut or torn into large pieces

Feta cheese, crumbled (optional)

1. To make the vinaigrette, whisk together the olive oil, vinegar, lemon juice, and salt and pepper to taste in a small bowl.
2. To make the salad, combine all the salad ingredients in a large bowl; toss to mix. Just prior to serving, add the vinaigrette and toss gently to coat.

Yield: 6 cups; Serving: 1½ cups

Calories: 160; Protein: 2 g; Carbohydrate: 9.7 g; Fiber: 2.7 g; Sodium: 167 mg; Fat: 13.4 g (Sat: 1.83 g, Mono: 10.0 g, Poly: 1.40 g, Trans: 0 g); Cholesterol: 0 mg

Roasted Winter Vegetable Medley

Tossed with a garlicky bread crumb topping, this colorful assortment of root vegetables and winter squash makes a nice side dish for a holiday meal. Or use it as a hearty main course for a vegetarian supper. Chop vegetables in large irregular chunks, about 2 inches in length, for the best appearance.

BREAD CRUMB TOPPING

¼ cup walnuts, toasted

1 (1-ounce) slice whole wheat peasant-style bread

2 garlic cloves, minced

2 tablespoons fresh parsley leaves
½ teaspoon coarse salt

ROASTED VEGETABLES

2 cups coarsely chopped peeled parsnips (about 4 medium)
4 cups coarsely chopped peeled butternut squash (about 1 large)
3 cups coarsely chopped carrots (about 6 medium)
12 large shallots
1½ tablespoons olive or canola oil
Coarse salt and freshly ground black pepper

1. Preheat the oven to 400°F.
2. To make the bread crumb topping, combine the walnuts, bread, garlic, parsley, and coarse salt in a food processor; process until well blended and set aside.
3. To make the roasted vegetables, in a large baking dish, toss together the parsnips, squash, carrots, shallots, and olive oil. Roast for 40 to 45 minutes, or until the vegetables are tender and nicely browned. Remove from the oven and toss the vegetables with the bread crumb topping. Taste and season with salt and pepper. Serve immediately.

Yield: 7 cups (14 servings); Serving: ½ cup

Calories: 105; Protein: 2.2 g; Carbohydrate: 18.3 g; Fiber: 3.5 g; Sodium: 132 mg; Fat: 3.3 g (Sat: 0.27 g, Mono: 1.22 g, Poly: 1.43 g, Trans: 0.05 g); Cholesterol: 0 mg

Dijon-Herb Carrots

Vegetables don't have to be dripping with butter to taste great. Here we've paired olive oil with some fresh herbs and Dijon mustard for an elegant-looking and flavorful sauce.

1 cup loosely packed fresh parsley leaves
6 large fresh basil leaves
1 garlic clove, minced
1 tablespoon water
2 teaspoons Dijon mustard
Coarse salt
1 tablespoon olive oil
4 cups sliced carrots, cut thickly on an angle (about 4 large)

1. Place the parsley, basil, garlic, water, mustard, and salt to taste in a food processor and blend. Add the oil and blend until it forms a thick sauce. (Alternatively, mince the parsley and basil. Combine the herbs, garlic, water, mustard, and salt in a small bowl. Whisk in the oil until well blended.)
2. Steam the carrots in a large saucepan until tender, 8 to 10 minutes. Toss the carrots gently with the sauce and serve.

Yield: 4 cups; Serving: ½ cup

Calories: 46; Protein: 1.0 g; Carbohydrate: 6.9 g; Fiber: 2 g; Sodium: 57 mg; Fat: 2 g (Sat: 0.26 g, Mono: 0.13 g, Poly: 0.23 g, Trans: 0.02 g); Cholesterol: 0 mg

Spicy Sweet Potato Fries

Sweet potatoes have a lot more going for them nutritionally than white potatoes. Sweets are rich in beta-carotene, vitamin C, fiber, and a whole host of other nutrients. Try a small amount of these sweet-and-spicy "oven" fries with the Farro and Mushroom Burgers (page 334). Make the fries ahead if you need to, then reheat them under the broiler for 1 to 2 minutes to get them crisp.

1 tablespoon olive or canola oil, plus more if needed for the pan
Nonstick cooking spray (optional)
1 large sweet potato, cut into thin matchstick pieces (about 3½ cups)
½ teaspoon freshly ground black pepper
¼ teaspoon chili powder
¼ teaspoon ground cumin
¼ teaspoon paprika
Coarse salt

1. Preheat the oven to 450°F. Lightly coat a large baking sheet with the oil or cooking spray.
2. Place the sweet potato in a bowl and drizzle with the 1 tablespoon of oil; toss gently to coat. Combine the pepper, chili powder, cumin, paprika, and salt to taste in a small bowl and sprinkle over the sweet potatoes; toss gently to coat. Place the sweet potatoes on the baking sheet. Bake for 12 to 15 minutes, or until the ends begin to crisp. Remove from the oven and serve.

Yield: 3½ cups; Serving: ½ cup

Calories: 52; Protein: 0.6 g; Carbohydrate: 8 g; Fiber: 1.1 g; Sodium: 5 mg; Fat: 2.1 g (Sat: 0.28 g, Mono: 1.45 g, Poly: 0.21 g, Trans: 0.02 g); Cholesterol: 0 mg

Cardamom Roasted Cauliflower

Suvir Saran, American Masala *(Clarkson Potter, 2007)*

Coarse kosher salt, or even Maldon sea salt, adds a lovely crunch to this otherwise creamy and yielding roasted cauliflower.

⅓ cup extra-virgin olive oil, plus more for the baking dish
3 cardamom pods
3 dried red chilies (optional)
1 tablespoon coriander seed
1 teaspoon cumin seed
½ teaspoon whole black peppercorns
1 (2½- to 3-pound) head cauliflower, cored and broken into medium florets
1 medium red onion, halved and thinly sliced
Kosher salt, for sprinkling

1. Preheat the oven to 425°F. Grease a baking dish with olive oil and set aside.
2. Grind the cardamom, chilies (if using), coriander seed, cumin seed, and peppercorns in a coffee grinder or small food processor until a fine powder. Mix the spices with the oil in a large bowl. Add the cauliflower and onion and toss to coat. Transfer the vegetables to the baking dish and roast until tender, about 1 hour, stirring every 20 minutes. Sprinkle with salt and serve.

Yield: 8 servings

Calories: 184; Protein: 4 g; Carbohydrate: 13 g; Fiber: 5 g; Sodium: 64 mg; Fat: 15 g (Sat: 2 g, Mono: 10 g, Poly: 2 g, Trans: 0 g); Cholesterol: 0 mg

Wilted Spinach with Nuts and Golden Raisins (FAST FIX)

Buy prewashed baby spinach leaves and this colorful side dish will come together quickly. To save time and cleanup, toast the pine nuts in the same skillet used for cooking the spinach.

2 teaspoons olive oil

¼ cup thinly sliced red onions (about 1 small)

1 garlic clove, thinly sliced

¼ teaspoon coarse salt

2 (6-ounce) packages baby leaf spinach

2 tablespoons golden raisins

2 tablespoons pine nuts, toasted

Dash of freshly ground black pepper

In a large nonstick skillet, heat the olive oil over medium-low heat. Add the onions and cook, stirring, for 5 to 6 minutes, or until tender. Stir in the garlic and cook for 1 minute. Add the salt, spinach, and raisins and cook for 3 to 4 minutes, or until the spinach begins to wilt. Remove from the heat and stir in the pine nuts and pepper. Serve immediately.

Yield: 4 servings; Serving: about ¾ cup

Calories: 89; Protein: 3.3 g; Carbohydrate: 9 g; Fiber: 2.4 g; Sodium: 186 mg; Fat: 5.5 g (Sat: 0.57 g, Mono: 2.47 g, Poly: 1.83 g, Trans: 0 g); Cholesterol 0 mg

Lemony Kale with Toasted Almonds (FAST FIX)

Since kale requires a longer cooking time than many greens, it's boiled here and then combined with oil and seasonings. Any variety of kale will work, although the dark green, curly- leafed dinosaur kale looks spectacular.

2 bunches kale (about 12 ounces)

¼ cup sliced almonds

2 teaspoons olive oil

1 teaspoon grated lemon zest

½ teaspoon salt

¼ teaspoon freshly ground black pepper

1. Remove the tough inner stem from the kale and coarsely chop the leaves. Bring water to a boil in a large Dutch oven. Add the kale and boil gently for 10 minutes, or until tender. Drain well, pressing excess water out of the kale using the back of a spoon. Transfer the kale to a large bowl.
2. Place the almonds in a dry skillet over medium heat and toast, stirring continuously, for 1 to 2 minutes, or until they begin to brown lightly. Add the nuts, oil, lemon zest, salt, and pepper to the bowl with the kale and serve.

Yield: 4 servings; Serving: 1 cup

Calories: 82; Protein: 3 g; Carbohydrate: 6.5 g; Fiber: 1.7 g; Sodium: 258 mg; Fat: 5.6 g (Sat: 0.59 g, Mono: 3.57 g, Poly: 1.13 g, Trans: 0 g); Cholesterol 0 mg

Oldways Tangy Collard Greens

Sara Baer-Sinnott, author, The Oldways Table: Essays & Recipes from the Culinary Think Tank *(Ten Speed Press, 2002)*

Greens are the foundation of the African Heritage Diet Pyramid. People of African descent have been cooking with greens for centuries. In Southern cooking, greens are usually slow-cooked and flavored with pork. In Oldways's A Taste of African Heritage cooking program, we show students that cooking greens can be quick and healthy, using lemon juice and mustard as flavor-enhancing meat substitutes.

2 bunches collard greens (about 3½ pounds)
1 tablespoon extra-virgin olive oil
1 medium yellow onion, diced
4 garlic cloves, minced
1 tablespoon Dijon mustard
Juice of ¼ lemon
Salt

1. Stem the collards and cut the leaves into long, thin strips.
2. In a large skillet, heat the olive oil over medium heat. Add the onion and the garlic and cook, stirring, for 2 to 3 minutes, until the onion is golden.
3. Add the mustard and lemon juice to the skillet and stir to combine.
4. Add the greens to the skillet and toss to coat. Season with salt and add a splash of water to slightly moisten the greens. Cover and cook for 10 to 12 minutes, or until the collards are bright green and softened. Stir before serving.

Yield: 4 servings; Serving: approximately 1 cup

Calories: 120; Protein: 7 g; Carbohydrate: 16 g; Fiber: 10 g; Sodium: 280 mg; Fat: 5 g (Sat: 0.5 g, Mono: 3 g, Poly: 0 g, Trans: 0 g); Cholesterol: 0 mg

Bitter Greens with Sweet Onions and Tart Cherries

Mollie Katzen, author and illustrator of numerous cookbooks for adults and children and best known for her Moosewood Cookbook *(Ten Speed Press, 1977). Adapted from* Vegetable Heaven *(Hyperion, 1997).*

This is a great way to get some of those bitter greens into your diet, because the sweet onions and tart cherries balance out the favor. The result is surprisingly smooth. I like to use a mixture of collards, red mustard, arugula, and a little kale. The amount of greens might seem enormous, but don't forget that they will cook way down. Unsweetened sour cherries from a can work beautifully here, but if you have access to fresh sour cherries (and you have a good pitting gadget), by all means use them. Vidalia onions are terrific, but if you can't find them, just use regular ones. This dish gives off a lot of cooking liquid, but it is too pretty and delicious to let evaporate. So just include some with each serving, especially if you are pairing this dish with pasta or rice.

1 cup fresh sour cherries, pitted, or canned unsweetened sour cherries, drained
2 to 3 teaspoons sugar
1 tablespoon canola oil
3 cups sliced sweet yellow onions, such as Vidalia (about 2 large)
A few shakes of salt (optional)
3 large bunches fresh greens, stemmed, if necessary, and coarsely chopped (about 12 cups)
1 cup dried sour cherries (optional)

1. Place the fresh cherries in a small bowl and sprinkle with the sugar. Let sit for about 10 minutes.
2. In a large deep skillet or Dutch oven, heat the canola oil over high heat. Add the onions and a light sprinkling of salt, if using, and cook, stirring, for about 5 minutes. Turn the heat to medium, cover, and let the onions cook until very tender, about 10 minutes more.
3. Begin adding the greens in batches (as much as will fit), sprinkling in a little salt with each addition, as desired.
4. Stir and cover between additions, letting the greens cook down for about 5 minutes each time, to make room for the next batch.
5. When all the greens have been added and have wilted, stir in the fresh cherries and cook for just about 5 minutes more. Transfer to a platter and

sprinkle the dried cherries on top, if using. Serve hot or warm, being sure to include some of the delicious cooking juices with each serving.

Yield: 4 servings

Calories: 160; Protein: 5 g; Carbohydrate: 29 g; Fiber: 5 g; Sodium: 95 mg; Fat: 4 g (Sat: 2 g, Mono: 2 g, Poly: 1 g, Trans: 0 g); Cholesterol: 0 mg

Brazilian Greens

Jessica B. Harris, historian and cookbook author, High on the Hog: A Culinary Journey from Africa to America *(Bloomsbury, 2011)*

> 2 pounds fresh young collard greens
> 3 tablespoons olive oil
> 8 garlic cloves, minced, or to taste

1. Wash the collards thoroughly and bunch them together.
2. Take each bunch, roll it tightly, and cut it crosswise into thin strips.
3. In a large heavy skillet, heat the olive oil over medium heat. Add the garlic and cook, stirring, until it is only slightly browned.
4. Add the collard strips and cook, stirring continuously, for 5 minutes so that the greens are soft but retain their bright green color.
5. Add a tablespoon of water, cover, lower the heat, and cook for 2 minutes more.
6. Serve hot, with the hot sauce of your choice.

Yield: 4 servings

Calories: 157; Protein: 5 g; Carbohydrate: 13 g; Fiber: 3 g; Sodium: 1 mg; Fat: 11 g (Sat: 1 g, Mono: 7 g, Poly: 1 g, Trans: 0 g); Cholesterol: 0 mg

Tuscan Beans

Charles Burke, MD, president of the New Hampshire Farm to Restaurant Connection

This hearty preparation appears frequently on Tuscan tables, especially in the area around Florence. Every family and chef has a preferred preparation, but common to all are olive oil, garlic, and herbs boiled gently with the current year's crop of dried cannellini beans. They are served hot or cold with both meat and fish, even appearing in antipasti courses. With a salad, they are a filling lunch or light dinner. They can also serve as a base for broiled chicken or seafood. Place into an ovenproof pan, spread evenly, and then lightly brush the surface with olive oil. Place chicken or fish onto the beans and broil until the protein is done. The beans develop a nice crust for a one-dish main course. Finally, placed into a blender with fresh herbs and some olive oil, they make a great spread.

1 pound dried cannellini beans, soaked in cold water to cover for 6 to 8 hours or overnight
4 tablespoons extra-virgin olive oil
3 garlic cloves, thinly sliced
1 teaspoon sea or kosher salt
2 sprigs fresh sage or rosemary
Freshly ground black pepper

1. Drain the beans. In a heavy saucepan, heat the olive oil over medium heat. Add the garlic and salt and cook until the garlic softens and the oil is infused with the flavor of the garlic. Adjust the heat so that the garlic does not brown.
2. Add the sage and the beans. Add cold water just to cover the beans. Cover and bring to a slow simmer. Cook for about 1 hour, checking the beans every 20 minutes and adding water as needed to cover. The cooking time will vary, but the beans are done when they are still slightly firm but easily mashed. Mash some of the beans to thicken the liquid. Taste and season with pepper, adding more oil and herbs to taste.

Yield: 6 servings

Calories: 337; Protein: 17 g; Carbohydrate: 47 g; Fiber: 18 g; Sodium: 191 mg; Fat: 11 g (Sat: 1 g, Mono: 7 g, Poly: 2 g, Trans: 0 g); Cholesterol: 0 mg

Wild Rice–Quinoa Pilaf

Quinoa (*keen-WAH*), high in protein and other nutrients, has been dubbed a supergrain by some. But once you see it and taste it for the first time, the nutty flavor and pearly appearance are what you'll remember most. Here quinoa is paired with wild rice for a dark, rich-colored pilaf. To save time, cook the wild rice the night before, following the package directions. Resist the temptation to use instant wild rice, if possible; it doesn't look or taste quite as good as the regular variety, nor does it deliver quite as many nutrients.

> 1 tablespoon canola oil
> ⅓ cup finely chopped white or yellow onions (about 1 small)
> ⅓ cup finely chopped celery
> ¼ cup pistachios or almonds, chopped
> 1 cup quinoa, rinsed and drained
> 3 cups defatted chicken stock or vegetable broth, preferably low-sodium
> 1 cup cooked wild rice
> Coarse salt and freshly ground black pepper

In a saucepan, heat the canola oil over medium heat. Add the onions and celery and cook, stirring, for 5 to 6 minutes, or until the vegetables begin to soften. Stir in the nuts and quinoa and cook for 1 to 2 minutes. Add the stock and bring to a boil; reduce the heat to low, cover, and simmer for 18 to 20 minutes. Stir in the wild rice, cover, and cook for 2 to 3 minutes, or until the mixture is hot. Taste and season with salt and pepper as desired.

Yield: 5 cups; Serving: ½ cup

Calories: 165; Protein: 6.2 g; Carbohydrate: 26 g; Fiber: 2.6 g; Sodium: 228 mg; Fat: 4.8 g (Sat: 0.51 g, Mono: 2.62 g, Poly: 1.26 g, Trans: 0 g); Cholesterol: 0 mg

Roasted Corn Tabbouleh

A popular Lebanese salad made with cracked wheat (bulgur), tabbouleh is definitely for parsley lovers. This version cuts down a bit on the parsley and adds fresh pan-roasted corn for a new flavor twist.

> 1 cup bulgur
> 1 cup boiling water
> 6 teaspoons olive oil
> 1½ cups fresh corn kernels (about 2 ears)
> 1 cup chopped seeded tomatoes
> ½ cup thinly sliced scallions
> ½ cup fresh parsley, chopped
> 2 tablespoons white wine vinegar
> Coarse salt and freshly ground black pepper
> Extra-virgin olive oil (optional)

1. Place the bulgur in a medium bowl. Add the boiling water and let stand for 30 minutes or until the liquid has been completely absorbed.
2. In a nonstick skillet, heat 1 teaspoon of the olive oil over medium-high heat. Add the corn kernels and pan-roast, stirring occasionally to prevent scorching, for 8 to 10 minutes, or until browned.
3. Stir the tomatoes, scallions, and parsley into the bulgur. Mix the remaining 5 teaspoons olive oil, the vinegar, and salt and pepper to taste together in a small bowl and pour over the bulgur mixture. Toss gently. Drizzle with a small amount of extra-virgin olive oil just prior to serving, if using.

Yield: 5 cups; Serving: ½ cup

Calories: 100; Protein: 2.7 g; Carbohydrate: 16.7 g; Fiber: 3.7 g; Sodium: 10 mg; Fat: 3.2 g (Sat: 0.45 g, Mono: 2.11 g, Poly: 0.46 g, Trans: 0 g); Cholesterol: 0 mg

Wild Mushroom–Barley Risotto

P earl barley makes a great stand-in for Arborio rice. The whole grain has a similar chewiness and swells gradually as it cooks, just like short-grain rice. Even better, it's not as labor-intensive to cook. Periodic stirring is all that's necessary. Here the nutty flavor of the barley is complemented by the rich, almost meaty taste of dried porcini mushrooms. You'll find these mushrooms in the produce section or on the canned-vegetable aisle of most supermarkets.

¼ cup dried porcini mushrooms (about ½ ounce)
1½ cups boiling water
2 cups defatted chicken stock or broth, preferably low-sodium
2 tablespoons olive oil
¼ cup minced shallots or red onions (about 3 medium shallots or 1 small onion)
1 cup pearl barley
1½ teaspoons chopped fresh thyme, or ½ teaspoon dried
Coarse salt and freshly ground black pepper

1. Combine the dried mushrooms and boiling water in a small bowl and let stand for 30 minutes, or until the mushrooms are soft. Let cool slightly and remove the mushrooms from the liquid with a slotted spoon. Chop the mushrooms and set aside. Strain the soaking liquid through cheesecloth (to remove any grit that came with the dried mushrooms) into a

small saucepan. Add the stock and mushrooms; bring to a boil. Reduce the heat and keep the liquid at a simmer on a back burner.

2. In a large saucepan, heat the olive oil over medium heat. Add the shallots and cook, stirring, for 3 to 4 minutes, or until the shallots have softened. Stir in the barley and cook, stirring, for 1 minute. Stir in ½ cup of the mushroom-stock mixture and cook at a simmer until the liquid has been absorbed, stirring occasionally. Continue adding the hot stock ½ cup at a time until the barley is tender, 30 to 35 minutes. Stir in the thyme. Taste and season with salt and pepper as desired.

Note: Fresh or dried rosemary can be substituted for the thyme.

Yield: 3 cups, 6 servings; Serving: ½ cup

Calories: 188; Protein: 6.3 g; Carbohydrate: 30 g; Fiber: 6.2 g; Sodium: 213 mg; Fat: 5.1 g (Sat: 0.72 g, Mono: 3.48 g, Poly: 0.66 g, Trans: 0.05 g); Cholesterol: 0 mg

Pistachio-Apricot Bulgur Salad (FAST FIX)

Since bulgur cooks so quickly, this salad is a snap to put together. To add even more pistachio flavor, try using pistachio oil in place of the olive oil. Look for the rich green oil in specialty grocery stores or order it online.

1 cup fine- or medium-grain bulgur
½ cup chopped dried apricots
1 cup boiling water
1 cup chopped fresh parsley
3 tablespoons finely chopped fresh mint
½ cup chopped pistachios
⅓ cup olive or pistachio oil
3 tablespoons fresh orange juice or white wine vinegar
¼ cup minced red onions (about 1 small)
2 tablespoons thinly sliced scallions
¾ teaspoon coarse salt
¼ teaspoon freshly ground black pepper

Combine the bulgur and apricots in a medium bowl. Add the boiling water and let stand for 30 minutes, or until the liquid has been absorbed. Add the remaining ingredients and toss gently to mix.

Yield: 6 cups; Serving: ¾ cup

Calories: 267; Protein: 6.1 g; Carbohydrate: 31.6 g; Fiber: 6.8 g; Sodium: 247 mg; Fat: 14.2 g (Sat: 1.87 g, Mono: 9.21 g, Poly: 2.49 g, Trans: 0 g); Cholesterol 0 mg

DESSERTS

Easy Peach, Pineapple, and Apricot Crisp

Using frozen and precut fresh and dried fruits lets you put together this crisp in a hurry. The topping is a quick mix of oats, pecans, and wheat germ for crunch. A little pineapple juice concentrate provides sweetness.

Nonstick cooking spray or canola oil

FILLING

1 (16-ounce) package frozen unsweetened peach slices, cut into chunks
2 cups precut fresh pineapple tidbits
½ cup coarsely chopped dried unsweetened apricots
¼ cup thawed frozen unsweetened pineapple juice concentrate
¼ cup oat flour
½ teaspoon ground cinnamon
⅛ teaspoon freshly grated nutmeg
¼ teaspoon coarse salt

TOPPING

⅓ cup oat flour
⅓ cup rolled oats
¼ cup toasted wheat germ
3 tablespoons canola oil
2 tablespoons chopped pecans
2 tablespoons thawed frozen unsweetened pineapple juice concentrate
⅛ teaspoon salt

1. Preheat the oven to 375°F. Lightly coat an 11 x 7-inch baking dish with cooking spray or oil.
2. To make the filling, place all the filling ingredients in a medium bowl and toss gently to combine. Place the filling in the baking dish and spread it evenly.

3. To make the topping, combine all the topping ingredients in a small bowl. Sprinkle the topping mixture over the filling and bake for 30 to 35 minutes, or until the filling is bubbling.

Yield: 8 servings; Serving: about ¾ cup

Calories: 212; Protein: 4.3 g; Carbohydrate: 34 g; Fiber: 4.9 g; Sodium: 90 mg; Fat: 7.7 g (Sat: 0.59 g, Mono: 0.40 g, Poly: 2.23 g, Trans: 0.01 g); Cholesterol: 0 mg

Apple-Cherry Crumb Pie

Filling a whole wheat piecrust with fruit and nut toppings makes for a healthful special occasion or holiday dessert. Using a combination of tart and sweet apples can give more depth to flavor. Look for premade whole wheat crusts in whole-food supermarkets. One of the better brands, called Mother Nature's Goodies, is both sugar-free and trans-fat-free.

2 medium Granny Smith apples (about 14 ounces), peeled, cored, and thinly sliced into wedges
2 medium Rome apples (about 12 ounces), peeled, cored, and thinly sliced into wedges
1½ teaspoons fresh lemon juice
⅓ cup dried cherries
5 tablespoons whole wheat flour
½ teaspoon ground cinnamon
1 (9-inch) store-bought whole wheat pastry crust
2 tablespoons honey
⅓ cup sliced almonds
¼ cup rolled oats
2 tablespoons canola oil
1 tablespoon brown sugar
⅛ teaspoon salt

1. Preheat the oven to 350°F.
2. Combine the apples and lemon juice in a large bowl and toss to coat. Add the cherries, 1 tablespoon of the flour, and the cinnamon; toss gently to mix. Place half the apples in the crust; drizzle evenly with 1 tablespoon of the honey. Repeat the layers.
3. Combine the almonds, oats, the remaining ¼ cup flour, the oil, sugar, and salt in a small bowl. Mix with a fork until well blended. Sprinkle the nut

mixture evenly over the apples and bake for 50 to 55 minutes, or until the apples are tender.

Yield: 8 servings; Serving: 1 wedge

Calories: 271; Protein: 4.2 g; Carbohydrate: 39.6 g; Fiber: 6.8 g; Sodium: 149 mg; Fat: 11.8 g (Sat: 1.47 g, Mono: 3.38 g, Poly: 1.62 g, Trans: 0 g); Cholesterol 0 mg

Orange Juice Sorbet

This sorbet has a refreshing sweet-tart flavor rather than the overpowering sugary taste found in many commercial sorbets. Be sure to use fresh-squeezed orange juice for the best flavor. Serve it with sliced fresh strawberries for a special dessert.

1 quart fresh orange juice
2 tablespoons Cointreau or other orange liqueur
¼ teaspoon lemon extract
Sliced fresh strawberries (optional)

Place the orange juice, Cointreau, and lemon extract in an ice cream machine and churn according to the manufacturer's instructions. (Alternatively, combine the ingredients in a small bowl and pour the mixture into three large ice cube trays; freeze until firm or overnight. Remove from the freezer and let stand at room temperature for 5 to 10 minutes until the cubes begin to thaw and soften. Place the cubes into a blender or food processor and blend until smooth.) Serve immediately, garnished with strawberries, if using.

Note: Leftovers can be returned to the freezer and reblended in a food processor as needed. The sorbet texture actually becomes smoother with a second freezing and blending.

Yield: 4 cups; Serving: ½ cup

Calories: 69; Protein: 0.9 g; Carbohydrate: 14.5 g; Fiber: 0.3 g; Sodium: 1.5 mg; Fat: 0.3 g (Sat: 0.03 g, Mono: 0.05 g, Poly: 0.05 g, Trans: 0 g); Cholesterol: 0 mg

Spiced Poached Pears

Anjou or Comice pears are the best for poaching. Choose fruit that is ripe but firm. Cardamom is a sweet-spicy seasoning used frequently in desserts served in India. It adds a unique flavor to the pear syrup, but you can omit it if you like.

PEARS

4 large Anjou pears, peeled and cored
1 cup dry white wine
½ cup water
½ cup white grape juice
1 tablespoon honey
1 teaspoon pure vanilla extract
1 cardamom pod, or ⅛ teaspoon ground
2 whole cloves
Pinch of freshly grated nutmeg

TOPPING

2 tablespoons slivered almonds, toasted
2 tablespoons pistachios toasted

1. To make the pears, slice ¼ inch from the bottom of each pear so it will sit flat.
2. Combine the wine, water, grape juice, honey, vanilla, cardamom, cloves, and nutmeg in a medium saucepan; bring to a boil. Add the pears; reduce the heat, cover, and simmer for 12 to 15 minutes, or until the pears are tender. Remove the pears from the cooking liquid with a slotted spoon. Turn the heat to medium-high and bring the cooking liquid to a boil; cook for 10 to 15 minutes, or until the liquid has reduced by half and becomes syrupy. Strain the syrup through a sieve into a bowl or large measuring cup, discarding the solids. Cover and chill.
3. To make the topping, place the nuts into a mini food processor and pulse until coarse and crumbly. (Alternatively, finely chop the nuts by hand; combine and set aside.)
4. Cut each pear in half and then slice each half lengthwise from top to bottom into 5 sections, leaving the top and stem intact. Place 2 pear halves on a small dessert plate and fan the sections so that the pear lies flat (the pear

will still be connected at the stem). Spoon ¼ cup of the syrup over each pear and sprinkle with 1 tablespoon of the nut mixture.

Yield: 4 servings; Serving: 2 pear halves with nuts and syrup

Calories: 220; Protein: 2.7 g; Carbohydrate: 42 g; Fiber: 5.9 g; Sodium: 4 mg; Fat: 5 g (Sat: 0.47 g, Mono: 2.86 g, Poly: 0.95 g, Trans: 0 g); Cholesterol: 0 mg

Slow-Roasted Spiced Peaches

Rebecca Katz, author of The Healthy Mind Cookbook *(Ten Speed Press, 2015)*

These peaches are simple and absolutely intoxicating; take peaches at the height of their season and toss them with cinnamon, ginger, and just a spritz of lemon juice. You'll find yourself making excuses to be in the kitchen while these goodies roast, 'cause they just smell soooooo good.

1 tablespoon pure maple syrup
1½ teaspoons extra-virgin olive oil
1 teaspoon fresh lemon juice
¼ teaspoon sea salt
¼ teaspoon ground cinnamon
1 teaspoon grated fresh ginger, or 1½ teaspoons ground
4 peaches, peeled, pitted, and sliced
2 teaspoons very thinly sliced fresh mint

1. Preheat the oven to 300°F. Line a rimmed baking sheet with parchment paper.
2. Put the maple syrup, oil, lemon juice, salt, cinnamon, and ginger in a large bowl and whisk to combine.
3. Add the peaches and stir gently until they are well coated. Spread the peaches on the baking sheet in a single layer. Bake for about 1½ hours, until the peaches are moist and about one-third of their original size, stirring and redistributing them halfway through the baking time. Let cool for 5 minutes, then transfer the peaches and any remaining juices to a bowl.
4. Gently stir in the mint, then let sit for 5 minutes for the flavors to meld. Serve warm or at room temperature. Store in an airtight container in the refrigerator for up to 2 days or in the freezer for up to 3 months.

Yields 1 cup (2 servings); Serving: ½ cup
Calories: 189; Total Fat: 4 g (1 g saturated, 3 g monounsaturated); Carbohydrates: 20 g;
Protein: 2 g; Fiber: 3 g; Sodium: 204 mg

The Three Pleasures

Walter Willett, MD, PhD

The Three Pleasures is more of a concept than a specific recipe, developed out of frustration with dessert menus that almost always feature only various combinations of sugar, white flour, and cream. Knowing that foods can be enjoyable without destroying our health, it occurred to me that three of the healthiest foods we know are fruit, nuts, and dark chocolate. So I started asking our waiters if they had a creative chef. Of course they all said yes. To which I responded, "that's great," and asked to have the chef put together a combination of fruit, nuts, dark chocolate, and nothing more in a creative way. Almost always I've gotten something delicious. Some of these were works of art, some were elegantly laid out on a plate, and some were simply offered in a bowl. Sometimes the chocolate was a syrup, sometimes chopped pieces. I was never seriously disappointed, and I suspect that most chefs enjoy a little challenge beyond their routine. Given this experience, I thought the dessert deserved a name. At a dinner with my colleague Frank Hu and our wives, we decided to call this Three Pleasures.

I like this name because it conveys enjoyment, not decadence, from both the sensual experience of eating three wonderful foods and also from the knowledge that we have respected the bodies that we have been given. Do try ordering Three Pleasures. I hope that restaurants will start to put it on their menus. To see some stunning examples prepared by a variety of chefs, visit The Nutrition Source (www.hsph.harvard.edu/nutritionsource/2016/07/11/dessert-by-design-three-pleasures).

Because of the many types of fruits, nuts, and chocolates, the ways to create Three Simple Pleasures are almost endless. If fresh fruit is not available, dried fruit can work quite well (think dates, currants, and cranberries). A Fourth Pleasure is also an option: a sprinkle of a quality spirit such as bourbon, rum, port, or rye can add another delightful dimension. Here is a simple example that can be put together in a few minutes. It is followed by a gourmet version, mango granita with chocolate-coated macadamia nuts.

¼ cup fresh blueberries, sliced fresh peaches, or strawberries
1 ounce slivered almonds

½ ounce dark chocolate (small pieces or syrup)

Drizzle of bourbon (optional)

Put the fruit in a bowl. Add the nuts, then top with chocolate and drizzle with bourbon, if using. (Alternatively, these ingredients can be artfully displayed on a dish.)

Yield: 1 serving

Without bourbon: *Calories: 269; Protein: 7 g; Carbohydrate: 23 g; Fiber: 6 g; Sodium: 1 mg; Fat: 19 g (Sat: 4 g, Mono: 9 g, Poly: 4 g, Trans: 0 g); Cholesterol: 0 mg*

Mango Granita with Chocolate-Coated Macadamia Nuts

Joanne Burke, Weather Hill Farm, Sanbornton, New Hampshire

3 mangoes

6 ounces dark chocolate (70% to 72% cacao), such as Lindt Excellence or Godiva

4 to 5 ounces unsalted macadamia nuts

Nonstick cooking spray

Blueberries, for garnish

1. Peel, pit, and slice 2 of the mangoes. Peel and cube the third mango and set aside. Puree the sliced mangoes in a food processor until smooth. Transfer to a freezer-safe container, cover, and freeze for 3 hours.
2. Set a heatproof bowl over a saucepan of simmering water (the bottom of the bowl should not touch the water). Melt the chocolate in the bowl, stirring as it melts until smooth. Add the macadamia nuts and stir to coat with the chocolate.
3. Line a rimmed baking sheet with parchment paper. Spray a wire rack with cooking spray and set it over the baking sheet.
4. Using a spatula, lift the chocolate-covered nuts from the bowl and set them on the rack. Spread some of the melted chocolate left in the bowl on the parchment paper to make a garnish. Refrigerate the nuts until set.
5. Place the mango granita in a bowl and top with the cubed mango, blueberries, and chocolate-covered nuts. Peel the chocolate from the parchment paper, break it in small pieces, and use it as garnish. Serve.

Yield: 4 servings

Calories: 673; Protein: 8 g; Carbohydrate: 66 g; Fiber: 12 g; Sodium: 4 mg; Fat: 46 g (Sat: 16 g, Mono: 21 g, Poly: 1 g, Trans: 0 g); Cholesterol: 0 mg

Chocolate Cherry Walnut Truffles

Rebecca Katz, author of The Healthy Mind Cookbook *(Ten Speed Press, 2015)*

These truffles are filled with dates, cherries, and walnuts, smothered in dark chocolate, then rolled in coconut and curry powder. Studies suggest walnuts may boost memory, while chocolate is the ultimate mood-boosting agent. One bite of this dessert and you'd be hard-pressed to feel any stress.

2 tablespoons boiling water

2 ounces dark chocolate (64% to 72% cacao), very finely chopped

½ cup walnuts

1 tablespoon unsweetened cocoa powder

1 cup halved pitted Medjool dates

1 teaspoon pure vanilla extract

Sea salt

¼ cup finely diced dried cherries

2 tablespoons shredded coconut

¼ teaspoon curry powder

1. Place the water into a small bowl, stir in the chocolate, and let stand for 30 seconds. Using a small whisk, stir until the chocolate is completely melted and glossy.
2. Coarsely grind the walnuts in a food processor, then add the cocoa powder, dates, vanilla, and ⅛ teaspoon of the salt and process for a minute. Add the chocolate mixture and process until smooth, 1 minute.
3. Transfer to a bowl and stir in the cherries. Cover and chill in the refrigerator for about 2 hours, or in the freezer for 15 minutes, until firm.
4. On a plate, mix the coconut, curry powder, and a pinch of salt. Scoop up about 2 teaspoons of the chilled chocolate mixture and roll it into a smooth ball between your palms, then roll it in the curried coconut to coat. Repeat with the remaining chocolate mixture, then place the truffles in an airtight container and chill thoroughly before serving. The truffles will keep in an airtight container for up to 2 days.

Note: If you want to give the truffles a golden hue, toast the coconut in a pre-heated 300°F oven for 10 to 15 minutes.

Yield: 20 truffles; Serving: 1 truffle

Calories: 72; Total Fat: 4 g (Sat: 2 g, Mono: 1 g, Poly: 1 g, 1 g saturated, 1 g monounsaturated); Carbohydrates: 9 g; Protein: 1 g; Fiber: 1 g; Sodium: 16 mg

Oatmeal–Raisin and Nut Cookies

Oats and whole wheat pastry flour gives these cookies a wonderfully chewy texture. For added crunch, there's both sunflower seeds and nuts. And for sweetness, we've cut down on the sugar of traditional cookie recipes and let dried fruits add some natural sweetness.

- ½ cup canola oil
- ⅓ cup packed brown sugar
- 2 tablespoons honey
- 1 large egg
- 1 teaspoon pure vanilla extract
- 2 cups rolled oats
- ¾ cup whole wheat pastry flour
- ¾ teaspoon ground cinnamon
- 1 teaspoon baking powder
- ⅛ teaspoon salt
- ½ cup raisins
- 3 tablespoons coarsely chopped pecans
- 3 tablespoons slivered blanched almonds

1. Preheat the oven to 350°F.
2. Combine the oil, sugar, and honey in a large bowl and using a hand mixer, beat on medium speed to blend. Stir in the egg and vanilla.
3. Spoon the oats into a small bowl. Add the flour, cinnamon, baking powder, and salt and whisk until well combined. Add the oat mixture to the oil mixture; beat well. Stir in the raisins, pecans, and almonds. Cover and refrigerate for 30 minutes to chill.
4. Spoon heaping tablespoons of the dough onto a nonstick baking sheet and flatten gently with your fingers. Bake for 10 to 12 minutes, or until lightly browned. Let the cookies cool on the baking sheet for 2 minutes. Transfer to wire racks to cool completely.

Yield: 36 cookies

Calories: 79; Protein: 1.4 g; Carbohydrate: 9.2 g; Fiber: 1 g; Sodium: 33 mg; Fat: 4.3 g (Sat: 0.38 g, Mono: 2.38 g, Poly: 1.24 g, Trans: 0 g); Cholesterol 6 mg

Sweet Spiced Couscous

In Tunisia, home cooks make a breakfast meal of *farka*, a cooked couscous studded with dates and nuts and sweetened with sugar. This version is sweetened naturally with fruit juice and dried dates and makes a nice light dessert. Since it's traditionally served with milk, try it with a splash of soy milk, if you'd like.

¼ cup chopped raw cashews
¼ cup slivered blanched almonds
2 tablespoons chopped hazelnuts
1½ cups unsweetened apple juice
1 cup whole wheat couscous
1½ tablespoons hazelnut oil or canola oil
¾ cup chopped pitted dates
Soy milk (optional)

1. Place the cashews, almonds, and hazelnuts in a large nonstick skillet and toast over medium-high heat, stirring frequently, for 3 to 4 minutes, until they begin to lightly brown. Remove from the heat.
2. Bring the apple juice to a boil in a small saucepan. Stir in the couscous and cook for 1 minute. Remove from the heat, cover, and let stand for 5 minutes. Stir in the oil, dates, and toasted nuts. Spoon into bowls and serve with a splash of soy milk, if using.

Yield: 6 servings; Serving: ⅔ cup

Calories: 268; Protein: 5.6 g; Carbohydrate: 41.8 g; Fiber: 5.1 g; Sodium: 23 mg; Fat: 10.4 g (Sat: 0.99 g, Mono: 6.85 g, Poly: 1.52 g, Trans: 0 g); Cholesterol 0 mg

Further Reading

CHAPTER ONE: HEALTHY EATING MATTERS

1. Willett, W. C. "Balancing Life-style and Genomics Research for Disease Prevention." *Science* 296 (2002): 695–8.
2. Wang, D. D., et al. "Improvements in US Diet Helped Reduce Disease Burden and Lower Premature Deaths, 1999–2012; Overall Diet Remains Poor." *Health Affairs* 34 (2015): 1916–22.
3. *2015–2020 Dietary Guidelines for Americans, 8th Ed.* U.S. Department of Health and Human Services and U.S. Department of Agriculture, December 2015. www.health.gov/dietaryguidelines/2015/guidelines/
4. Pollan, M. *In Defense of Food: An Eater's Manifesto.* New York: Penguin, 2009.

CHAPTER TWO: OF PYRAMIDS, PLATES, AND DIETARY GUIDELINES

1. Foxcroft, L. *Calories and Corsets: A History of Dieting over 2,000 years.* London: Profile Books, 2012.
2. Banting, W. *Letter on Corpulence, Addressed to the Public.* London: Self-published, 1863.
3. Davis, C., and E. Saltos. "Dietary Recommendations and How They Have Changed over Time," in E. Frazão, *America's Eating Habits: Changes and Consequences.* Economic Research Service 1999: U.S. Department of Agriculture Information Bulletin AIB-750. www.ers.usda.gov/publications/aib-agricultural-information -bulletin/aib750.aspx
4. U.S. Department of Agriculture and National Institutes of Health. "History of Dietary Guidance Development in the United States and the Dietary Guidelines for Americans." 2013. www.health.gov/dietaryguidelines/2015-BINDER/meeting1 /historyCurrentUse.aspx
5. Kennedy, E. T., et al. "The Healthy Eating Index: Design and Applications." *Journal of the American Dietetic Association* 95 (1995): 1103–8.
6. McCullough, M. L., et al. "Adherence to the Dietary Guidelines for Americans and Risk of Major Chronic Disease in Men." *American Journal of Clinical Nutrition* 72 (2000): 1223–31; "Adherence to the Dietary Guidelines for Americans and Risk

of Major Chronic Disease in Women." *American Journal of Clinical Nutrition* 72 (2000): 1214–22.

7. Willett, W. C., et al. "Mediterranean Diet Pyramid: A Cultural Model for Healthy Eating." *American Journal of Clinical Nutrition* 61, Supplement 6 (1995): 1402S–1406S.

8. Trichopoulou. A., et al. "Adherence to a Mediterranean Diet and Survival in a Greek Population." *New England Journal of Medicine* 348 (2003): 2599–608.

9. Estruch, R., et al. "Primary Prevention of Cardiovascular Disease with a Mediterranean Diet." *New England Journal of Medicine* 368 (2013): 1279–90.

10. McCullough, M. L., et al. "Diet Quality and Major Chronic Disease Risk in Men and Women: Moving Toward Improved Dietary Guidance." *American Journal of Clinical Nutrition* 76 (2002): 1261–71.

11. Scientific Report of the 2015 Dietary Guidelines Advisory Committee: Advisory Report to the Secretary of Health and Human Services and the Secretary of Agriculture. health.gov/dietaryguidelines/2015-scientific-report/PDFs/Scientific-Report-of-the-2015-Dietary-Guidelines-Advisory-Committee.pdf

12. McCullough, M.L., et al. "Diet Quality and Major Chronic Disease Risk in Men and Women: Moving Toward Improved Dietary Guidance." *American Journal of Clinical Nutrition* 76 (2002): 1261–71.

13. Ibid.

14. Chiuve, S.E., et al. "Alternative Dietary Indices Both Strongly Predict Risk of Chronic Disease." *Journal of Nutrition* 142 (2012): 1009–18.

15. Purdy, C., Evich, H. B. "The Money Behind the Fight Over Healthy Eating." *Politico*, Oct. 7, 2015. www.politico.com/story/2015/10/the-money-behind-the-fight-over-healthy-eating-214517

16. Wang, D. D., et al. "Improvements in US Diet Helped Reduce Disease Burden and Lower Premature Deaths, 1999–2012; Overall Diet Remains Poor." *Health Affairs* 34 (2015): 1916–22.

CHAPTER THREE: WHAT CAN YOU BELIEVE ABOUT DIET?

1. Goodman, E. "To Swallow or Not to Swallow; That Is the New Vitamin Question." *Boston Globe* April 7, 1994: A27

2. Willett, W. *Nutritional Epidemiology, 3rd Edition*. New York: Oxford University Press, 2012.

3. Huo, Y., et al. for the CSPPT Investigators. "Efficacy of Folic Acid Therapy in Primary Prevention of Stroke Among Adults with Hypertension in China: The CSPPT Randomized Clinical Trial." *JAMA* 313 (2015): 1325–35.

4. Multiple Risk Factor Intervention Trial Research Group. "Multiple Risk Factor Intervention Trial. Risk Factor Changes and Mortality Results." *JAMA* 248 (1982): 1465–77.

5. *American Journal of Public Health.* 2016 Sep;106(9)

6. Keys, A. *Seven Countries: A Multivariate Analysis of Death and Coronary Heart Disease.* Cambridge, MA: Harvard University Press, 1980.

7. Chowdhury, R., et al. "Association of Dietary, Circulating, and Supplement Fatty Acids with Coronary Risk: A Systematic Review and Meta-analysis." *Annals of Internal Medicine* 160 (2014): 398–406.

8. Heberden, W. "Some Account of a Disorder of the Breast." *Medical Transactions of the Royal College of Physicians* 2 (1786): 59–67.

9. Ronksley, P. E., et al. "Association of Alcohol Consumption with Selected Cardiovascular Disease Outcomes: A Systematic Review and Meta-analysis." *BMJ* 342 (2011): d671.

10. Hines, L. M., et al. "Genetic Variation in Alcohol Dehydrogenase and the Beneficial Effect of Moderate Alcohol Consumption on Myocardial Infarction. *New England Journal of Medicine* 344 (2001): 549–55.

CHAPTER FOUR: HEALTHY WEIGHT

1. Kasman, M., et al. "An In-depth Look at the Lifetime Economic Cost of Obesity." Brookings Institution, 2015. www.brookings.edu/~/media/events/2015/05/12 -economic-costs-of-obesity/0512-obesity-presentation-v6-rm.pdf

2. National Center for Health Statistics. "Health, United States, 2015." Hyattsville, MD. 2015. Table 58: Normal Weight, Overweight, and Obesity Among Adults Aged 20 and Over, by Selected Characteristics: United States, Selected Years 1988–1994 Through 2011–2014.

3. Ogden, C. L., et al. "Prevalence of Overweight, Obesity, and Extreme Obesity Among Adults: United States, Trends 1960–1962 Through 2007–2008." National Center for Health Statistics (2010). www.cdc.gov/nchs/data/hestat/obe sity_adult_07_08/obesity_adult_07_08.pdf

4. Cawley, J., and C. Meyerhoefer. "The Medical Care Costs of Obesity: An Instrumental Variables Approach." *Journal of Health Economics* 31 (2012): 219–30.

5. Ng, M., et al. "Global, Regional, and National Prevalence of Overweight and Obesity in Children and Adults During 1980–2013: A Systematic Analysis for the Global Burden of Disease Study 2013." *Lancet* 384 (2014): 766–81.

6. Flegal, K. M., et al. "Association of All-Cause Mortality with Overweight and Obesity Using Standard Body Mass Index Categories: A Systematic Review and Meta-analysis." *JAMA* 309 (2013): 71–82.

7. Global BMI Mortality Collaboration. "Body-Mass Index and All-Cause Mortality: Individual-Participant-Data Meta-analysis of 239 Prospective Studies in Four Continents." *Lancet* 388 (2016): 776–86.

8. Aune, D., et al. "BMI and All-Cause Mortality: Systematic Review and Non-linear Dose-Response Meta-analysis of 230 Cohorts with 3.74 Million Deaths Among 30.3 Million Participants." *BMJ* 353 (2016): i2156.

9. Ogden, C. L., et al. "Obesity and Socioeconomic Status in Adults: United States, 2005–2008." National Center for Health Statistics Data Brief No. 50, 2010. www .cdc.gov/nchs/products/databriefs/db50.htm

10. Willett, W. C., et al. "Guidelines for Healthy Weight." *New England Journal of Medicine* 341 (1999): 427–34.

11. Cerhan, J. R., et al. "A Pooled Analysis of Waist Circumference and Mortality in 650,000 Adults." *Mayo Clinic Proceedings* 89 (2014): 335–45.

12. Willett, W. C., et al. *Thinfluence: The Powerful and Surprising Effect Friends, Family, Work, and Environment Have on Weight.* Emmaus, PA: Rodale (2014).

13. Nieuwdorp, M., et al. "Role of the Microbiome in Energy Regulation and Metabolism." *Gastroenterology* 146 (2014): 1525–33.

14. U.S. Department of Agriculture Economic Research Service. Food Availability (per Capita) Data System. www.ers.usda.gov/data-products/food-availability-(per-capita)-data-system/.aspx#26715

15. Stampfer, M. J., et al. "Primary Prevention of Coronary Heart Disease in Women Through Diet and Lifestyle." *New England Journal of Medicine* 343 (2000): 16–22.

16. Banting, W. *Letter on Corpulence, Addressed to the Public.* London: Self-published, 1863.

17. Ludwig, D.S., et al. "High Glycemic Index Foods, Overeating, and Obesity." *Pediatrics* 103 (1999): E26.

18. Mozaffarian, D., et al. "Changes in Diet and Lifestyle and Long-Term Weight Gain in Women and Men." *New England Journal of Medicine* 364 (2011): 2392–404.

19. Shai, I., et al. for the Dietary Intervention Randomized Controlled Trial (DIRECT) Group. "Weight Loss with a Low-Carbohydrate, Mediterranean, or Low-Fat Diet." *New England Journal of Medicine* 359 (2008): 229–41.

20. Schwarzfuchs, D., et al. "Four-Year Follow-up After Two-Year Dietary Interventions." *New England Journal of Medicine* 367 (2012): 1373–74.

21. *Physical Activity and Health: A Report of the Surgeon General.* Washington, D.C.: U.S. Department of Health and Human Services, Centers for Disease Control and Prevention, National Center for Chronic Disease Prevention and Health Promotion, 1996. www.cdc.gov/nccdphp/sgr/pdf/sgrfull.pdf

22. Manson, J. E., et al. "A Prospective Study of Walking as Compared with Vigorous Exercise in the Prevention of Coronary Heart Disease in Women." *New England Journal of Medicine* 341 (1999): 650–8.

23. Biswas, A., et al. "Sedentary Time and Its Association with Risk for Disease Incidence, Mortality, and Hospitalization in Adults: A Systematic Review and Meta-analysis." *Annals of Internal Medicine* 162 (2015): 123–32.

24. Ornish, D., et al. "Can Lifestyle Changes Reverse Coronary Heart Disease? The Lifestyle Heart Trial." *Lancet* 336 (1990): 129–33.

25. Tobias, D. K., et al. "Effect of Low-Fat Diet Interventions Versus Other Diet Interventions on Long-Term Weight Change in Adults: A Systematic Review and Meta-analysis." *Lancet Diabetes and Endocrinology* 3 (2015): 968–79.

26. Halton, T. L., et al. "Low-Carbohydrate-Diet Score and the Risk of Coronary Heart Disease in Women." *New England Journal of Medicine* 355 (2006): 1991–2002.

27. Larsen, T. M., et al. "Diets with High or Low Protein Content and Glycemic Index for Weight-Loss Maintenance." *New England Journal of Medicine* 363 (2010): 2102–13.

28. Eaton, S. B., and M. Konner. "Paleolithic Nutrition—A Consideration of Its Nature and Current Implications." *New England Journal of Medicine* 312 (1985): 283–89.

29. Wing, R. R., and J. O. Hill. "Successful Weight Loss Maintenance." *Annual Review of Nutrition* 21 (2001): 323–41.

30. "The Truth About Dieting." *Consumer Reports* 67 (2002): 22.

31. Tobias, D. K., et al. "Effect of Low-Fat Diet Interventions Versus Other Diet Interventions on Long-Term Weight Change in Adults: A Systematic Review and Meta-analysis." *Lancet Diabetes and Endocrinology* 3 (2015): 968–79.

CHAPTER FIVE: STRAIGHT TALK ABOUT FAT

1. National Center for Health Statistics. "Health, United States, 2015." Hyattsville, MD, 2016. Table 58: Normal Weight, Overweight, and Obesity Among Adults Aged 20 and over, by Selected Characteristics: United States, Selected Years 1988–1994 Through 2011–2014. www.cdc.gov/nchs/hus/contents2015.htm#058

2. Innis, S. M. "Dietary (n-3) Fatty Acids and Brain Development." *Journal of Nutrition* 137 (2007): 855–59.

3. Hu, F. B., et al. Dietary Intake of Alpha-linolenic Acid and Risk of Fatal Ischemic Heart Disease Among Women. *American Journal of Clinical Nutrition* 69 (1999): 890–7.

4. Wang, D. D., et al. "Association of Specific Dietary Fats with Total and Cause-Specific Mortality." *JAMA Internal Medicine* 126 (2016): 1134–45.

5. Hu, F. B., et al. "Dietary Fat Intake and the Risk of Coronary Heart Disease in Women." *New England Journal of Medicine* 337 (1997): 1491–9.

6. Hu, F. B., et al. "Diet, Lifestyle, and the Risk of Type 2 Diabetes Mellitus in Women." *New England Journal of Medicine* 345 (2001): 790–7.

7. Final Determination Regarding Partially Hydrogenated Oils: A Notice by the Food and Drug Administration. 80 Federal Register 34650 (June 17, 2015). www.federalregister.gov/articles/2015/06/17/2015-14883/final-determination-regarding-partially-hydrogenated-oils

8. Mayne, S. "Protecting Consumers from Trans Fat." June 15, 2015. blogs.fda.gov/fdavoice/index.php/2015/06/protecting-consumers-from-trans-fat/

9. Mozaffarian D. " Trans fatty acids and cardiovascular disease." *New England Journal of Medicine.* 2006 Apr 13;354(15):1601–13.

10. Mozaffarian, D., et al. "Heart Disease and Stroke Statistics—2016 Update: A Report from the American Heart Association." *Circulation* 133 (2015): e38–e360.

11. Sacks, F. M., et al. "Comparison of Weight-Loss Diets with Different Compositions of Fat, Protein, and Carbohydrates." *New England Journal of Medicine* 360 (2009): 859–73.

12. Tobias, D. K., et al. "Effect of Low-Fat Diet Interventions Versus Other Diet In-

terventions on Long-Term Weight Change in Adults: A Systematic Review and Meta-analysis." *Lancet Diabetes and Endocrinology* 3 (2015): 968–79.

13. Page, I. H., et al. "Atherosclerosis and the Fat Content of the Diet." *Circulation* 16 (1957): 164–78.

14. Appel, L. J., et al., for the OmniHeart Collaborative Research Group. "Effects of Protein, Monounsaturated Fat, and Carbohydrate Intake on Blood Pressure and Serum Lipids: Results of the OmniHeart Randomized Trial." *JAMA* 294 (2005): 2455–64.

15. USDA Economic Research Service. Food Availability (per Capita) Data System. www.ers.usda.gov/datafiles/Food_Availabily_Per_Capita_Data_System/Food _Availability/eggs.xls

16. Hu, F. B., et al. "A Prospective Study of Egg Consumption and Risk of Cardiovascular Disease in Men and Women." *JAMA* 281 (1999): 1387–94.

17. Rong, Y., et al. "Egg Consumption and Risk of Coronary Heart Disease and Stroke: Dose-Response Meta-analysis of Prospective Cohort Studies." *BMJ* 346 (2013): e8539.

18. Mensink, R. P., and M. B. Katan. "Effects of Monounsaturated Fatty Acids Versus Complex Carbohydrates on High-density Lipoproteins in Healthy Men and Women." *Lancet* 1 (1987): 122–25.

19. Knopp, R. H., et al., "Long-Term Cholesterol-Lowering Effects of Four Fat-Restricted Diets in Hyper-Cholesterolemic and Combined Hyperlipidemic Men: The Dietary Alternatives Study." *Journal of the American Medical Association* 278 (1997): 1509–15.

20. Knopp, R. H., et al. "Long-Term Cholesterol-Lowering Effects of Four Fat-Restricted Diets in Hyper-Cholesterolemic and Combined Hyperlipidemic Men: The Dietary Alternatives Study." *JAMA* 278 (1997): 1509–15.

21. Wang, D. D., et al. "Association of Specific Dietary Fats with Total and Cause-Specific Mortality." *JAMA Internal Medicine* 126 (2016): 1134–45.

22. Hu, F. B., et al. "Dietary Fat Intake and the Risk of Coronary Heart Disease in Women." *New England Journal of Medicine* 337 (1997): 1491–9.

23. de Lorgeril, M., et al. "Mediterranean Alpha-linolenic Acid-Rich Diet in Secondary Prevention of Coronary Heart Disease." *Lancet* 343 (1994): 1454–59.

24. de Lorgeril, M., et al. "Mediterranean Diet, Traditional Risk Factors, and the Rate of Cardiovascular Complications After Myocardial Infarction: Final Report of the Lyon Diet Heart Study." *Circulation* 99 (1999): 779–85.

25. Estruch, R., and the PREDIMED Study Investigators. "Primary Prevention of Cardiovascular Disease with a Mediterranean Diet." *New England Journal of Medicine* 368 (2013): 1279–90.

26. Chowdhury, R., et al. "Association of Dietary, Circulating, and Supplement Fatty Acids with Coronary Risk: A Systematic Review and Meta-analysis." *Annals of Internal Medicine* 160 (2014): 398–406.

27. Pimpin, L., et al. "Is Butter Back? A Systematic Review and Meta-analysis of Butter Consumption and Risk of Cardiovascular Disease, Diabetes, and Total Mortality." *PLoS One* 11 (2016): e0158118.

28. Chen, M., et al. "Dairy Fat and Risk of Cardiovascular Disease in 3 Cohorts of US Adults." *American Journal of Clinical Nutrition* 104 (2016): 1209–17.

29. Kim, E. H., et al. "Dietary Fat and Risk of Postmenopausal Breast Cancer in a 20-Year Follow-up." *American Journal of Epidemiology* 164 (2006): 990–7.

30. Boeke, C. E., et al. Dietary Fat Intake in Relation to Lethal Breast Cancer in Two Large Prospective Cohort Studies." *Breast Cancer Research and Treatment* 146 (2014): 383–92.

31. Toledo, E., et al. "Mediterranean Diet and Invasive Breast Cancer Risk Among Women at High Cardiovascular Risk in the PREDIMED Trial: A Randomized Clinical Trial." *JAMA Internal Medicine* 175 (2015): 1752–60.

32. Cho, E., et al. "Premenopausal Fat Intake and Risk of Breast Cancer." *Journal of the National Cancer Institute* 95 (2003): 1079–85.

33. Farvid, M. S., et al. "Premenopausal Dietary Fat in Relation to Pre- and Postmenopausal Breast Cancer." *Breast Cancer Research and Treatment* 145 (2014): 255–65.

34. Prentice, R. L., et al. "Low-Fat Dietary Pattern and Risk of Invasive Breast Cancer: The Women's Health Initiative Randomized Controlled Dietary Modification Trial." *JAMA* 295 (2006): 629–42.

35. Martin, L. J., et al. "A Randomized Trial of Dietary Intervention for Breast Cancer Prevention." *Cancer Research* 71 (2011): 123–33.

36. Bouvard, V., et al. on behalf of the International Agency for Research on Cancer Monograph Working Group. "Carcinogenicity of Consumption of Red and Processed Meat." *Lancet Oncology* 16 (2015): 1599–1600.

37. Leitzmann, M. F., et al. "Dietary Intake of n-3 and n-6 Fatty Acids and the Risk of Prostate Cancer." *American Journal of Clinical Nutrition* 80 (2004): 204–16.

CHAPTER SIX: CARBOHYDRATES FOR BETTER AND WORSE

1. National Center for Health Statistics. "Crude and Age-Adjusted Rates of Diagnosed Diabetes per 100 Civilian, Non-Institutionalized Adult Population, United States, 1980–2014." www.cdc.gov/diabetes/statistics/prev/national/figageadult.htm

2. Yang, W., et al. "Prevalence of Diabetes Among Men and Women in China." *New England Journal of Medicine* 362 (2010):1090–101.

3. Block, G. "Foods Contributing to Energy Intake in the US: Data from NHANES III and NHANES 1999–2000." *Journal of Food Composition and Analysis* 17 (2004): 439–47.

4. World Health Organization. *Guideline: Sugars Intake for Adults and Children.* Geneva, 2015.

5. Schwingshackl, L., Hoffmann, G. "Comparison of Effects of Long-Term Low-Fat vs High-Fat Diets on Blood Lipid Levels in Overweight or Obese Patients: A Systematic Review and Meta-analysis." *Journal of the Academy of Nutrition and Dietetics* 113 (2013): 1640–61.

6. Jenkins, D. J., et al. "Glycemic Index of Foods: A Physiological Basis for Carbohydrate Exchange." *American Journal of Clinical Nutrition* 34 (1981): 362–68.

7. Bhupathiraju, S. N., et al. "Glycemic Index, Glycemic Load, and Risk of Type 2 Diabetes: Results from 3 Large US Cohorts and an Updated Meta-analysis. *American Journal of Clinical Nutrition* 100 (2014): 218–32.

8. Ibid.

9. Chiasson, J. L., et al. for the STOP-NIDDM Trail Research Group. "Acarbose for Prevention of Type 2 Diabetes Mellitus: The STOP-NIDDM Randomised Trial." *Lancet* 359 (2002): 2072–7.

10. Gadgil, M. D., et al. "The Effects of Carbohydrate, Unsaturated Fat, and Protein Intake on Measures of Insulin Sensitivity: Results from the OmniHeart Trial." *Diabetes Care* 36 (2013): 1132–7.

11. Mozaffarian, D., et al. "Changes in Diet and Lifestyle and Long-Term Weight Gain in Women and Men." *New England Journal of Medicine* 364 (2011): 2392–404.

12. Bhupathiraju, S. N., et al. Glycemic Index, Glycemic Load, and Risk of Type 2 Diabetes. Op cit.

13. Liu, S., et al. "A Prospective Study of Dietary Glycemic Load, Carbohydrate Intake and Risk of Coronary Heart Disease in U.S. Women." *American Journal of Clinical Nutrition* 71 (2000): 1455–61.

14. Mirrahimi, A., et al. "Associations of Glycemic Index and Load with Coronary Heart Disease Events: A Systematic Review and Meta-analysis of Prospective Cohorts." *Journal of the American Heart Association* 1 (2012): e000752.

15. Sommers, T., et al. "Emergency Department Burden of Constipation in the United States from 2006 to 2011." *American Journal of Gastroenterology* 110 (2015): 572–79.

16. Park, Y., et al. "Dietary fiber Intake and Risk of Colorectal Cancer: A Pooled Analysis of Prospective Cohort Studies." Journal of the American Medical Association 294 (2005): 2849–57.

17. Farvid, M. S., et al. "Dietary Fiber Intake in Young Adults and Breast Cancer Risk." *Pediatrics* 137 (2016): e20151226.

18. Mozaffarian, R. S., et al. "Identifying Whole Grain Foods: A Comparison of Different Approaches for Selecting More Healthful Whole Grain Products." *Public Health Nutrition* 16 (2013): 2255–64.

CHAPTER SEVEN: CHOOSE HEALTHIER SOURCES OF PROTEIN

1. World Cancer Research Fund, American Institute for Cancer Research. *Food, Nutrition, Physical Activity, and the Prevention of Cancer: a Global Perspective.* Wash-

ington, DC: American Institute for Cancer Research, 2007. www.aicr.org/assets /docs/pdf/reports/Second_Expert_Report.pdf

2. Song, M., et al. "Association of Animal and Plant Protein Intake with All-Cause and Cause-Specific Mortality." *JAMA Internal Medicine* 176 (2016): 1453–63.

3. Bouvard, V., et al., on behalf of the International Agency for Research on Cancer Monograph Working Group. "Carcinogenicity of consumption of red and processed meat." *Lancet Oncology* 16 (2015): 1599–1600.

4. Farvid, M. S., et al. "Adolescent Meat Intake and Breast Cancer Risk." *International Journal of Cancer* 136 (2015): 1909–20.

5. Preis, S. R., et al. "Dietary Protein and Risk of Ischemic Heart Disease in Middle-aged Men." *American Journal of Clinical Nutrition* 92 (2010): 1265–72.

6. Kelemen, L. E., et al. "Associations of Dietary Protein with Disease and Mortality in a Prospective Study of Postmenopausal Women." *American Journal of Epidemiology* 161 (2005): 239–49.

7. Iocono, G., et al. "Intolerance of Cow's Milk and Chronic Constipation in Children." *New England Journal of Medicine* 339 (1998): 1100–4.

8. Smith, J. D., et al. "Changes in Intake of Protein Foods, Carbohydrate Amount and Quality, and Long-Term Weight Change: Results from 3 Prospective Cohorts." *American Journal of Clinical Nutrition* 101 (2015): 1216–24.

9. Darling, A. L., et al. "Dietary Protein and Bone Health: A Systematic Review and Meta-analysis." *American Journal of Clinical Nutrition* 90 (2009): 1674–92.

10. Estruch, R., et al. for the PREDIMED Study Investigators. "Primary Prevention of Cardiovascular Disease with a Mediterranean Diet." *New England Journal of Medicine* 368 (2013): 1279–90.

11. Song, Y., et al. "Whole Milk Intake Is Associated with Prostate Cancer-Specific Mortality Among U.S. Male Physicians." *Journal of Nutrition* 143 (2013): 189–96; Aune, D., et al. "Dairy Products, Calcium, and Prostate Cancer Risk: A Systematic Review and Meta-analysis of Cohort Studies." *American Journal of Clinical Nutrition* 101 (2015): 87–117.

12. Sorensen, A. C., et al. "Interplay Between Policy and Science Regarding Low-Dose Antimicrobial Use in Livestock." *Frontiers in Microbiology* 5 (2014): 86.

13. Food and Drug Administration. FDA's Strategy on Antimicrobial Resistance— Questions and Answers. www.fda.gov/AnimalVeterinary/GuidanceCompliance Enforcement/GuidanceforIndustry/ucm216939.htm

14. Anderson, J. W., et al. "Meta-analysis of the Effects of Soy Protein Intake on Serum Lipids." *New England Journal of Medicine* 333 (1995): 276–82.

15. Lee, S. A., et al. "Adolescent and Adult Soy Food Intake and Breast Cancer Risk: Results from the Shanghai Women's Health Study." *American Journal of Clinical Nutrition* 89 (2009): 1920–6.

16. Franco, O. H., et al. "Use of Plant-Based Therapies and Menopausal Symptoms: A Systematic Review and Meta-analysis." *JAMA* 315 (2016): 2554–63.

17. Hwang, Y. W., et al. "Soy Food Consumption and Risk of Prostate Cancer: A Meta-analysis of Observational Studies." *Nutrition and Cancer* 61 (2009): 598–606.

18. Soni, M., et al. "Phytoestrogens and Cognitive Function: A Review." *Maturitas* 77 (2014): 209–20.

19. McMichael-Phillips, D. F., et al. "Effects of Soy-Protein Supplementation on Epithelial Proliferation in the Histologically Normal Human Breast." *American Journal of Clinical Nutrition* 68 (supplement) (1998): 1431–36.

20. White, L. R., et al. "Brain Aging and Midlife Tofu Consumption." *Journal of the American College of Nutrition* 19 (2000): 242–55.

21. Morris, M. C., et al. "Association of Seafood Consumption, Brain Mercury Level, and APOE ε4 Status with Brain Neuropathology in Older Adults." *JAMA* 315 (2016): 489–97.

CHAPTER EIGHT: EAT PLENTY OF FRUITS AND VEGETABLES

1. U.S. Supreme Court. *Nix v. Hedden.* caselaw.findlaw.com/us-supreme-court/149/304.html

2. Moore, L. V., et al. "Adults Meeting Fruit and Vegetable Intake Recommendations—United States, 2013." *Morbidity and Mortality Weekly Report* 64 (2015): 709–13.

3. World Health Organization. *A Global Brief on Hypertension: Silent Killer, Global Public Health Crisis.* Geneva, 2013. www.ish-world.com/downloads/pdf/global_brief_hypertension.pdf

4. Borgi, L., et al. "Fruit and Vegetable Consumption and the Incidence of Hypertension in Three Prospective Cohort Studies." *Hypertension* 67 (2016): 288–93.

5. Joshipura, K. J., et al. "Fruit and Vegetable Intake in Relation to Risk of Ischemic Stroke." *JAMA* 282 (1999): 1233–9.

6. Huo, Y., et al. "Efficacy of Folic Acid Therapy in Primary Prevention of Stroke Among Adults with Hypertension in China: The CSPPT Randomized Clinical Trial." *JAMA* 313 (2015): 1325–35.

7. Appel, L. J., et al. "A Clinical Trial of the Effects of Dietary Patterns on Blood Pressure." *New England Journal of Medicine* 336 (1997): 1117–24.

8. Wu, J., et al. "Intakes of Lutein, Zeaxanthin, and Other Carotenoids and Age-Related Macular Degeneration During 2 Decades of Prospective Follow-up." *JAMA Ophthalmology* 133 (2015): 1415–24.

9. Aldoori, W. H., et al. "A Prospective Study of Dietary Fiber Types and Symptomatic Diverticular Disease in Men." *Journal of Nutrition* 128 (1998): 714–719.

10. Crowe, F. L., et al. "Source of Dietary Fibre and Diverticular Disease Incidence: A Prospective Study of UK women." *Gut* 63 (2014): 1450–6.

11. Bertoia, M. L., et al. "Changes in Intake of Fruits and Vegetables and Weight Change in United States Men and Women Followed for up to 24 Years: Analysis from Three Prospective Cohort Studies." *PLoS Medicine* 12 (2015): e1001878.

12. Hung, H. C., et al. "Fruit and Vegetable Intake and Risk of Major Chronic Disease." *Journal of the National Cancer Institute* 96 (2004): 1577–84.

13. Alberts, D. S., et al., for the Phoenix Colon Cancer Prevention Physicians' Network. "Lack of Effect of a High-Fiber Cereal Supplement on the Recurrence of Colorectal Adenomas. *New England Journal of Medicine* 342 (2000): 1156–62 and Lanza, E., et al., for the Polyp Prevention Trial Study Group. "The Polyp Prevention Trial Continued Follow-up Study: No Effect of a Low-Fat, High-Fiber, High-Fruit, and -Vegetable Diet on Adenoma Recurrence Eight Years After Randomization." *Cancer Epidemiology Biomarkers and Prevention* 16 (2007): 1745–52.

14. Boffetta, P., et al. "Fruit and Vegetable Intake and Overall Cancer Risk in the European Prospective Investigation into Cancer and Nutrition (EPIC)." *Journal of the National Cancer Institute* 21 (2010): 529–37.

15. Smith-Warner, S. A., et al. "Intake of Fruits and Vegetables and Risk of Breast Cancer: A Pooled Analysis of Cohort Studies." *JAMA* 285 (2001):769–76.

16. Hendrickson, S. J., et al. "Plasma Carotenoid- and Retinol-Weighted Multi-SNP Scores and Risk of Breast Cancer in the National Cancer Institute Breast and Prostate Cancer Cohort Consortium." *Cancer Epidemiology Biomarkers and Prevention* 22 (2013): 927–36.

17. Giovannucci, E. "Tomatoes, Tomato-Based Products, Lycopene, and Cancer: Review of the Epidemiologic Literature." *Journal of the National Cancer Institute* 91 (1999): 317–31.

18. Farvid, M. S., et al. "Fruit and Vegetable Consumption in Adolescence and Early Adulthood and Risk of Breast Cancer: Population Based Cohort Study." *BMJ* 353 (2016): i2343.

19. Park, Y., et al. "Dietary Fiber Intake and Risk of Colorectal Cancer: A Pooled Analysis of Prospective Cohort Studies." *JAMA* 294 (2005): 2849–57.

20. Muraki, I., et al. "Fruit Consumption and Risk of Type 2 Diabetes: Results from Three Prospective Longitudinal Cohort Studies." *BMJ* 347 (2013): f5001.

21. Ames, B. N. "Dietary Carcinogens and Anticarcinogens. Oxygen Radicals and Degenerative Diseases." *Science* 221 (1983): 1256–64.

22. Taylor, E. N., and G. C. Curhan. "Oxalate Intake and the Risk for Nephrolithiasis." *Journal of the American Society of Nephrology* 18 (2007): 2198–2204.

23. Koushik, A., et al. "Intake of Fruits and Vegetables and Risk of Pancreatic Cancer in a Pooled Analysis of 14 Cohort Studies." *American Journal of Epidemiology* 176 (2012): 373–86.

24. Borgi, L., et al. "Fruit and Vegetable Consumption and the Incidence of Hypertension in Three Prospective Cohort Studies." *Hypertension* 67 (2016): 288–93.

25. Wang, X., et al. "Fruit and Vegetable Consumption and Mortality from All Causes, Cardiovascular Disease, and Cancer: Systematic Review and Dose-Response Meta-analysis of Prospective Cohort Studies." *BMJ* 349 (2014): g4490.

26. Bhupathiraju, S. N., et al. "Quantity and Variety in Fruit and Vegetable Intake and

Risk of Coronary Heart Disease." *American Journal of Clinical Nutrition* 98 (2013): 1514–152.

27. National Potato Council/USDA, U.S. per Capita Utilization of Potatoes, by Category: 1970–2014. http://www.nationalpotatocouncil.org/files/6414/4223/8719/Pg._76_US_per_capita_Utilization_of_Potatoes_by_category_1970-2014.pdf

28. Muraki, I., et al. "Potato Consumption and Risk of Type 2 Diabetes: Results from Three Prospective Cohort Studies." *Diabetes Care* 39 (2016): 376–84.

29. Borgi, L., et al. "Potato Intake and Incidence of Hypertension: Results from Three Prospective US Cohort Studies." *BMJ* 353 (2016): i2351.

CHAPTER NINE: YOU ARE WHAT YOU DRINK

1. Valtin, H. " 'Drink at Least Eight Glasses of Water a Day.' Really? Is There Scientific Evidence for '8 x 8'?" *American Journal of Physiology—Regulatory, Integrative and Comparative Physiology* 283 (2002): R993–1004.

2. Food and Nutrition Board, National Academy of Sciences. *Recommended Dietary Allowances, Revised 1945.* National Research Council, Reprint and Circular Series, no. 122, 1945 (August), p. 3–18.

3. Food and Nutrition Board, Institute of Medicine. *Dietary Reference Intakes for Water, Potassium, Sodium, Chloride, and Sulfate.* Washington, D.C: National Academies Press, 2004.

4. Imamura, F., et al. "Consumption of Sugar Sweetened Beverages, Artificially Sweetened Beverages, and Fruit Juice and Incidence of Type 2 Diabetes: Systematic Review, Meta-analysis, and Estimation of Population Attributable Fraction." *BMJ* 351 (2015): h3576.

5. Fung, T. T., et al. "Sweetened Beverage Consumption and Risk of Coronary Heart Disease in Women." *American Journal of Clinical Nutrition* 89 (2009): 1037–42.

6. Ferraro, P. M., et al. "Soda and Other Beverages and the Risk of Kidney Stones." *Clinical Journal of the American Society of Nephrology* 9 (2013): 1389–95.

7. Food and Drug Administration. "Additional Information About High-Intensity Sweeteners Permitted for Use in Food in the United States." www.fda.gov/Food/IngredientsPackagingLabeling/FoodAdditivesIngredients/ucm397725.htm

8. Burke, M. V., and D.M. Small. "Physiological Mechanisms by Which Non-Nutritive Sweeteners May Impact Body Weight and Metabolism." *Physiology and Behavior* 152 (2015): 381–8.

9. Mozaffarian, D., et al. "Changes in Diet and Lifestyle and Long-Term Weight Gain in Women and Men." *New England Journal of Medicine* 364 (2011): 2392–404.

10. de Ruyter, J. C., et al. "A Trial of Sugar-Free or Sugar-Sweetened Beverages and Body Weight in Children." *New England Journal of Medicine* 367 (2012): 1397–406.

11. Chen, M., et al. "Effects of Dairy Intake on Body Weight and Fat: A Meta-analysis of Randomized Controlled Trials." *American Journal of Clinical Nutrition* 96 (2012): 735–47.

12. Adebamowo, C. A., et al. "High School Dietary Dairy Intake and Teenage Acne." *Journal of the American Academy of Dermatology* 52 (2005): 207–14.

13. Aune, D., et al. "Dairy Products, Calcium, and Prostate Cancer Risk: A Systematic Review and Meta-analysis of Cohort Studies." *American Journal of Clinical Nutrition* 101 (2015): 87–117.

14. Ganmaa, D., et al. "Milk, Dairy Intake and Risk of Endometrial Cancer: A 26-Year Follow-up." *International Journal of Cancer* 130 (2012): 2664–71.

15. Missmer, S. A., et al. "Meat and Dairy Food Consumption and Breast Cancer: A Pooled Analysis of Cohort Studies." *International Journal of Epidemiology* 31 (2002): 78–85.

16. World Cancer Research Fund/American Institute for Cancer Research. *Food, Nutrition, Physical Activity, and the Prevention of Cancer: A Global Perspective.* Washington, D.C.: American Institute for Cancer Research., 2007.

17. Berkey, C. S., et al. "Milk, Dairy Fat, Dietary Calcium, and Weight Gain: A Longitudinal Study of Adolescents." *Archives of Pediatric and Adolescent Medicine* 159 (2005): 543–50.

18. Hemenway, D., et al. "Risk Factors for Hip Fracture in US Men Aged 40 Through 75 Years." *American Journal of Public Health* 84 (1994): 1843–5.

19. Feskanich, D., et al. "Milk Consumption During Teenage Years and Risk of Hip Fractures in Older Adults." *JAMA Pediatrics* 168 (2014): 54–60.

20. Thoma, G., et al. "Greenhouse Gas Emissions from Milk Production and Consumption in the United States: A Cradle-to-Grave Life Cycle Assessment." *International Dairy Journal* 31 (2013): S3–S14.

21. Ferraro, P. M., et al. "Caffeine Intake and the Risk of Kidney Stones." *American Journal of Clinical Nutrition* 100 (2014): 1596–603.

22. Ding, M., et al. "Caffeinated and Decaffeinated Coffee Consumption and Risk of Type 2 Diabetes: A Systematic Review and a Dose-Response Meta-analysis." *Diabetes Care* 37 (2014): 569–86.

23. Lucas, M., et al. "Coffee, Caffeine, and Risk of Completed Suicide: Results from Three Prospective Cohorts of American Adults." *World Journal of Biological Psychiatry* 15 (2014): 377–86.

24. Qi, H., and S. Li. "Dose-Response Meta-analysis on Coffee, Tea and Caffeine Consumption with Risk of Parkinson's Disease." *Geriatrics and Gerontology International* 14 (2014): 430–9.

25. Petrick, J. L., et al. "Coffee Consumption and Risk of Hepatocellular Carcinoma and Intrahepatic Cholangiocarcinoma by Sex: The Liver Cancer Pooling Project." *Cancer Epidemiology Biomarkers and Prevention* 24 (2015): 1398–1406.

26. Ding, M., et al. "Association of Coffee Consumption with Total and Cause-Specific Mortality in 3 Large Prospective Cohorts." *Circulation* 132 (2015): 2305–15; Freedman, N. D., et al. "Association of Coffee Drinking with Total and Cause-Specific Mortality." *New England Journal of Medicine* 366 (2012): 1891–904.

27. Zhang, Y. F., et al. "Tea Consumption and the Incidence of Cancer: A Systematic Review and Meta-analysis of Prospective Observational Studies. *European Journal of Cancer Prevention* 24 (2015): 353–62.

28. Chen, W. Y., et al. "Moderate Alcohol Consumption During Adult Life, Drinking Patterns, and Breast Cancer Risk." *JAMA* 306 (2011): 1884–90.

29. Mukamal, K. J., et al. "Roles of Drinking Pattern and Type of Alcohol Consumed in Coronary Heart Disease in Men." *New England Journal of Medicine* 348 (2003): 109–18.

CHAPTER TEN: CALCIUM: NO EMERGENCY

1. Tai, V., et al. "Calcium Intake and Bone Mineral Density: Systematic Review and Beta-analysis." *BMJ* 351 (2015): h4183.

2. Bischoff-Ferrari, H. A., et al. "Dietary Calcium and Serum 25-hydroxyvitamin D Status in Relation to BMD Among U.S. Adults." *Journal of Bone and Mineral Research* 24 (2009): 935–42.

3. Hegsted, D. M. "Calcium and Osteoporosis." *Journal of Nutrition* 116 (1986): 2316–9.

4. Bischoff-Ferrari, H. A., et al. "Calcium Intake and Hip Fracture Risk in Men and Women: A Meta-analysis of Prospective Cohort Studies and Randomized Controlled Trials." *American Journal of Clinical Nutrition* 86 (2007): 1780–90.

5. Jackson, R. D., et al., for the Women's Health Initiative Investigators. "Calcium Plus Vitamin D Supplementation and the Risk of Fractures." *New England Journal of Medicine* 354 (2006): 669–83.

6. Moyer, V.A., et al. for the U.S. Preventive Services Task Force. "Vitamin D and Calcium Supplementation to Prevent Fractures in Adults: U.S. Preventive Services Task Force Recommendation Statement." *Annals Internal Medicine* 158 (2013): 691–96.

7. Booth, A. O., et al. "Effect of Increasing Dietary Calcium Through Supplements and Dairy Food on Body Weight and Body Composition: A Meta-analysis of Randomised Controlled Trials." *British Journal of Nutrition* 114 (2015): 1013–25.

8. Larsson, S. C., et al. "Dietary Calcium Intake and Risk of Stroke: A Dose-Response Meta-analysis." *American Journal of Clinical Nutrition* 97 (2013): 951–7.

9. Michaëlsson, K., et al. "Long Term Calcium Intake and Rates of All Cause and Cardiovascular Mortality: Community Based Prospective Longitudinal Cohort Study." *BMJ* 346 (2013): f228.

10. Feskanich, D., et al. "Calcium, Vitamin D, Milk Consumption, and Hip Fractures: A Prospective Study Among Postmenopausal Women." *American Journal of Clinical Nutrition* 77 (2003): 504–11.

11. Bischoff-Ferrari, H. A., et al. "Fracture Prevention with Vitamin D Supplementation: A Meta-analysis of Randomized Controlled Trials." *JAMA* 293 (2005): 2257–64.

12. Utiger, R. D. "The Need for More Vitamin D." *New England Journal of Medicine* 338 (1998): 828–29.

13. Shea, M. K., Booth, S. L. "Update on the Role of Vitamin K in Skeletal Health." *Nutrition Reviews* 66 (2008): 549–57.

14. Feskanich, D., et al. "Vitamin K Intake and Hip Fractures in Women: A Prospective Study." *American Journal of Clinical Nutrition* 69 (1999): 74–9.

CHAPTER ELEVEN: TAKE A MULTIVITAMIN FOR INSURANCE

1. Hennekens, C. H. "Micronutrients and Cancer Prevention." *New England Journal of Medicine* 315 (1986): 1288–9.

2. Smithells, R. W., et al. "Vitamin Deficiencies and Neural Tube Defects." *Archives of Diseases in Childhood* 51 (1976): 944–50.

3. MRC Vitamin Study Research Group. "Prevention of Neural Tube Defects: Results of the Medical Research Council Vitamin Study." *Lancet* 338 (1991): 131–7; Czeizel, A. E., et al. "Prevention of the First Occurrence of Neural-Tube Defects by Periconceptional Vitamin Supplementation." *New England Journal of Medicine* 327 (1992): 1832–5.

4. Williams, J., et al. "Updated Estimates of Neural Tube Defects Prevented by Mandatory Folic Acid Fortification—United States, 1995–2011." *Morbidity and Mortality Weekly Report* 64 (2015): 1–5.

5. Feskanich, D., et al. "Vitamin A Intake and Hip Fractures Among Postmenopausal Women." *JAMA* 287 (2002): 47–54.

6. Whelan, A. M., et al. "Herbs, Vitamins and Minerals in the Treatment of Premenstrual Syndrome: A Systematic Review." *Canadian Journal of Clinical Pharmacology* 16 (2009): e407–29.

7. Gaskins, A. J., et al. "Dietary Folate and Reproductive Success Among Women Undergoing Assisted Reproduction." *Obstetrics and Gynecology* 124 (2014): 801–9.

8. Jacques, P. F., et al. "The Effect of Folic Acid Fortification on Plasma Folate and Total Homocysteine Concentrations." *New England Journal of Medicine* 340 (1999): 1449–54.

9. Li, Y., et al. "Folic Acid Supplementation and the Risk of Cardiovascular Diseases: A Meta-analysis of Randomized Controlled Trials." *Journal of the American Heart Association* 5 (2016): e003768.

10. Zhang, S. M., et al. "Plasma Folate, Vitamin B_6, Vitamin B_{12}, Homocysteine, and Risk of Breast Cancer." *Journal of the National Cancer Institute* 95 (2003): 373–80.

11. Nan, H., et al. "Prospective Study of Alcohol Consumption and the Risk of Colorectal Cancer Before and After Folic Acid Fortification in the United States." *Annals of Epidemiology* 23 (2013): 558–63.

12. Huo, Y., et al. "Efficacy of Folic Acid Therapy in Primary Prevention of Stroke Among Adults with Hypertension in China: The CSPPT Randomized Clinical Trial." *JAMA* 313 (2015): 1325–35.

13. Hemilä, H., and E. Chalker. "Vitamin C for Preventing and Treating the Common Cold." *Cochrane Database of Systematic Reviews* (2013): CD000980.

14. Kalyani, R. R., et al. "Vitamin D Treatment for the Prevention of Falls in Older Adults: Systematic Review and Meta-analysis." *Journal of the American Geriatrics Society* 58 (2010): 1299–310.

15. Bischoff-Ferrari, H. A., et al. "Monthly High-Dose Vitamin D Treatment for the Prevention of Functional Decline: A Randomized Clinical Trial." *JAMA Internal Medicine* 176 (2016): 175–83.

16. Feldman, D., et al. "The Role of Vitamin D in Reducing Cancer Risk and Progression." *Nature Reviews Cancer* 14 (2014): 342–57.

17. Ford, J. A., et al. for the RECORD Trial Group. "Cardiovascular Disease and Vitamin D Supplementation: Trial Analysis, Systematic Review, and Meta-analysis." *American Journal of Clinical Nutrition* 100 (2014): 746–55.

18. Munger, K. L., et al. "Serum 25-Hydroxyvitamin D Levels and Risk of Multiple Sclerosis." *JAMA* 296 (2006): 2832–8.

19. Munger, K. L., et al. "Vitamin D Intake and Incidence of Multiple Sclerosis." *Neurology* 13 (2004): 60–5.

20. Mokry, L. E., et al. "Vitamin D and Risk of Multiple Sclerosis: A Mendelian Randomization Study." *PLoS Medicine* 12 (2015): e1001866.

21. Chandler, P. D., et al. "Impact of Vitamin D Supplementation on Inflammatory Markers in African Americans: Results of a Four-Arm, Randomized, Placebo-Controlled Trial." *Cancer Prevention Research* 7 (2014): 218–25.

22. Jackson, R. D., et al. "Calcium Plus Vitamin D Supplementation and the Risk of Fractures." *New England Journal of Medicine* 354 (2006): 669–83.

23. Lee, I. M., et al. "Vitamin E in the Primary Prevention of Cardiovascular Disease and Cancer: The Women's Health Study: A Randomized Controlled Trial." *JAMA* 294 (2005): 56–65.

24. Ames, B. N., et al. "The Causes and Prevention of Cancer." *Proceedings of the National Academy of Sciences of the United States of America* 92 (1995): 5258–65.

25. Watson, J. "Oxidants, Antioxidants and the Current Incurability of Metastatic Cancers." *Open Biology* 3 (2013): 120144.

26. Age-Related Eye Disease Study Research Group. "A Randomized, Placebo-Controlled, Clinical Trial of High-Dose Supplementation with Vitamins C and E, Beta-carotene, and Zinc for Age-Related Macular Degeneration and Vision Loss: AREDS Report No. 8." Archives of Ophthalmology 119 (2001): 1417–36; Age-Related Eye Disease Study Research Group. "A Randomized, Placebo-Controlled, Clinical Trial of High-Dose Supplementation with Vitamins C and E and Beta-carotene for Age-Related Cataract and Vision Loss: AREDS Report No. 9." Archives of Ophthalmology 119 (2001): 1439–52.

27. Age-Related Eye Disease Study 2 Research Group. "Lutein + Zeaxanthin and Omega-3 Fatty Acids for Age-Related Macular Degeneration: The Age-Related

Eye Disease Study 2 (AREDS2) Randomized Clinical Trial." *JAMA* 309 (2013): 2005–15.

28. Wu, J., et al. "Intakes of Lutein, Zeaxanthin, and Other Carotenoids and Age-Related Macular Degeneration During 2 Decades of Prospective Follow-up." *JAMA Ophthalmology* 133 (2015): 1415–24.

29. Grodstein, F. A., et al. "A Randomized Trial of Beta Carotene Supplementation and Cognitive Function in Men: The Physicians' Health Study II." *Archives of Internal Medicine* 167 (2007): 2184–90.

30. Glynn, R. J., et al. "Effects of Random Allocation to Vitamin E Supplementation on the Occurrence of Venous Thromboembolism: Report from the Women's Health Study." *Circulation* 116 (2007): 1497–503.

31. Forbes, S. C., et al. "Effect of Nutrients, Dietary Supplements and Vitamins on Cognition: A Systematic Review and Meta-analysis of Randomized Controlled Trials." *Canadian Geriatrics Journal* 18 (2015): 231–45.

32. Wang, H., et al. "Vitamin E Intake and Risk of Amyotrophic Lateral Sclerosis: A Pooled Analysis of Data from 5 Prospective Cohort Studies." *American Journal of Epidemiology* 173 (2011): 595–602.

33. Miller, E. R., et al. "Meta-analysis: High-Dosage Vitamin E Supplementation May Increase All-Cause Mortality." *Annals of Internal Medicine* 142 (2005): 37–46.

34. *Dietary Reference Intakes for Vitamin C, Vitamin E, Selenium, and Carotenoids: A Report of the Panel on Dietary Antioxidants and Related Compounds, Subcommittees on Upper Reference Levels of Nutrients and of Interpretation and Use of Dietary Reference Intakes, and the Standing Committee on the Scientific Evaluation of Dietary Reference Intakes, Food and Nutrition Board, Institute of Medicine.* Washington, D.C.: National Academy Press, c2000.

35. Booth, S. L., et al. "Food Sources and Dietary Intakes of Vitamin K-1 (Phylloquinone) in the American Diet: Data from the FDA Total Diet Study." *Journal of the American Dietetic Association* 96 (1996): 149–54.

36. Sacks, F. M., et al. for the DASH-Sodium Collaborative Research Group. "Effects on Blood Pressure of Reduced Dietary Sodium and the Dietary Approaches to Stop Hypertension (DASH) Diet." *New England Journal of Medicine* 344 (2001): 3–10.

37. Clark, L. C., et al. "Effects of Selenium Supplementation for Cancer Prevention in Patients with Carcinoma of the Skin. A Randomized Controlled Trial. Nutritional Prevention of Cancer Study Group." *JAMA* 276 (1996): 1957–63.

38. Lippman, S. M., et al. "Effect of Selenium and Vitamin E on Risk of Prostate Cancer and Other Cancers: The Selenium and Vitamin E Cancer Prevention Trial (SELECT)." *JAMA* 301 (2009): 39–51.

39. Singh, M., and R. R. Das. "Zinc for the Common Cold." *Cochrane Database of Systematic Reviews* (2013): CD001364; Science, M., et al. "Zinc for the Treatment of the Common Cold: A Systematic Review and Meta-analysis of randomized controlled trials." *Canadian Medical Association Journal* 184 (2012): E551–61.

40. Gaziano, J. M., et al. "Multivitamins in the Prevention of Cancer in Men: the Physicians' Health Study II Randomized Controlled Trial." *JAMA* 308 (2012): 1871–80.

41. Sesso, H. D., et al. "Multivitamins in the Prevention of Cardiovascular Disease in Men: The Physicians' Health Study II Randomized Controlled Trial." *JAMA* 308 (2012): 1751–60.

CHAPTER TWELVE: THE PLANET'S HEALTH MATTERS TOO

1. U.S. Environmental Protection Agency. *Inventory of U.S. Greenhouse Gas Emissions and Sinks, 1990–2015.* April 2017. www.epa.gov/sites/production/files/2017-02/documents/2017_complete_report.pdf

2. Nelson, M. E., et al. "Alignment of Healthy Dietary Patterns and Environmental Sustainability: A Systematic review." *Advances in Nutrition* 7 (2016) 1005–25.

3. City of Boston, Greenovate Boston, Massachusetts Office of Coastal Zone Management, Boston Green Ribbon Commission. *Climate Ready Boston.* December 2016. www.boston.gov/sites/default/files/20161207_climate_ready_boston_digital2.pdf

4. United Nations Department of Economic and Social Affairs. *The World Population Prospects: 2015 Revision.* www.un.org/en/development/desa/news/population/2015-report.html

5. United Nations Treaty Collection. Environment, Chapter XXVII. 7. d Paris agreement. 12 December 2015. treaties.un.org/pages/ViewDetails.aspx?src=TREATY&mtdsg_no=XXVII-7-d&chapter=27&lang=en

6. EAT Foundation. *EAT-Lancet Commission on Healthy Diets from Sustainable Food Systems.* December 9, 2016. eatforum.org/article/eat-lancet-commission-on-healthy-diets-from-sustainable-food-systems/

7. Heller, M. C., Keoleian, G. A. Greenhouse Gas Emission Estimates of U.S. Dietary Choices and Food Loss. *Journal of Industrial Ecology* 19 (2014): 391–401.

8. Culinary Institute of America and Harvard T.H. Chan School of Public Health. *Menus of Change: 2016 Annual Report.* www.menusofchange.org/images/uploads/pdf/CIA-Harvard_MenusOfChangeAnnualReport2016_(7-1)1.pdf

9. Brower, M., and W. Leon. *The Consumer's Guide to Effective Environmental Choices.* New York: Three Rivers Press, 1999.

10. Dietary Guidelines Advisory Committee. *Scientific Report of the 2015 Dietary Guidelines Advisory Committee.* February 2015. health.gov/dietaryguidelines/2015-scientific-report/

11. Burwell, S. M., Vilsack, T. "2015 Dietary Guidelines: Giving You the Tools You Need to Make Healthy Choices." HHS.gov blog, Oct. 6, 2015. www.hhs.gov/blog/2015/10/06/2015-dietary-guidelines.html

12. U.S. Department of Health and Human Services and U.S. Department of Agri-

culture. *2015–2020 Dietary Guidelines for Americans*. 8th edition, December 2015. health.gov/dietaryguidelines/2015/guidelines/

13 U.S. Department of Agriculture, Economic Research Service. *Cattle and Beef, Statistics and Information*. April 2017. www.ers.usda.gov/topics/animal-products/cattle-beef/statistics-information/

14. Vogliano, C., Brown, K. "The State of America's Wasted Food and Opportunities to Make a Difference." *Journal of the Academy of Nutrition and Dietetics* 116 (2016): (2016): 1199–1207.

CHAPTER THIRTEEN: PUTTING IT ALL TOGETHER

1. Willett, W. C. "Balancing Life-style and Genomics Research for Disease Prevention." *Science* 296 (2002): 695–8.

2. Keys, A. *Seven Countries: A Multivariate Analysis of Death and Coronary Heart Disease*. Cambridge, MA: Harvard University Press, 1980.

3. Keys, A. B., and M. Keys. *How to Eat Well and Stay Well the Mediterranean Way*. Garden City, NY: Doubleday, 1975.

4. Stampfer, M. J., et al. "Primary Prevention of Coronary Heart Disease in Women Through Diet and Lifestyle." *New England Journal of Medicine* 343 (2000): 16–22; Chomistek, A. K., et al. "Healthy Lifestyle in the Primordial Prevention of Cardiovascular Disease Among Young Women." *Journal of the American College of Cardiology* 65 (2015): 43–51.

5. de Longeril, M., et al. "Mediterranean Diet, Traditional Risk Factors, and the Risk of Cardiovascular Complications After Myocardial Infarction: Final Report of the Lyon Diet Heart Study." *Circulation* 99 (1999): 779–85.

6. Estruch, R., and the PREDIMED Study Investigators. "Primary Prevention of Cardiovascular Disease with a Mediterranean Diet." *New England Journal of Medicine* 368 (2013): 1279–90.

7. U.S. Department of Health and Human Services and U.S. Department of Agriculture. *2015–2020 Dietary Guidelines for Americans*. 8th Edition, December 2015. www.health.gov/dietaryguidelines/2015/guidelines/

8. Anand, S. S., et al. "Food Consumption and Its Impact on Cardiovascular Disease: Importance of Solutions Focused on the Globalized Food System: A Report from the Workshop Convened by the World Heart Federation." *Journal of the American College of Cardiology* 66 (2015): 1590–614.

9. Drewnowski, A. "Obesity and the Food Environment: Dietary Energy Density and Diet Costs." *American Journal of Preventive Medicine* 27 (2004): 154–62.

10. Stewart, H., et al. "The Cost of Satisfying Fruit and Vegetable Recommendations in the Dietary Guidelines." U.S. Department of Agriculture, Economic Research Service, February 2016. www.ers.usda.gov/media/2023016/eb27.pdf

11. Frazão, E. "High Costs of Poor Eating Patterns in the United States." In Frazão E.,

ed. America's Eating Habits: Changes & Consequences. Washington, D.C.: Economic Research Service, U.S. Department of Agriculture, 1999. http://www.ers.usda.gov/publications/aib750

CHAPTER FOURTEEN: HEALTHY EATING IN SPECIAL SITUATIONS

1. National Research Council. *Maternal Nutrition and the Course of Pregnancy*. Report of the Committee on Maternal Nutrition, Food and Nutrition Board. Washington, D.C.: National Academy of Sciences, 1970.

2. American College of Obstetricians and Gynecologists. "Weight Gain During Pregnancy." www.acog.org/Resources-And-Publications/Committee-Opinions/Committee-on-Obstetric-Practice/Weight-Gain-During-Pregnancy

3. Centers for Disease Control and Prevention. "Folic Acid: Recommendations." http://www.cdc.gov/ncbddd/folicacid/recommendations.html

4. Brigham and Women's Hospital. "The Pregnancy Food Guide." www.brighamand womens.org/publicaffairs/images/bwh_pregnancy_food_guide.pdf

5. Lucas, M., et al. "Coffee, Caffeine, and Risk of Completed Suicide: Results from Three Prospective Cohorts of American Adults." *World Journal of Biological Psychiatry* 15 (2014): 377–86.

6. Chang, S. C., et al. "Dietary Flavonoid Intake and Risk of Incident Depression in Midlife and Older Women." *American Journal of Clinical Nutrition* (2016): ajcn124545. Published online, July 13, 2016.

7. Johnson, G. H., and K. Fritsche. "Effect of Dietary Linoleic Acid on Markers of Inflammation in Healthy Persons: A Systematic Review of Randomized Controlled Trials." *Journal of the Academy of Nutrition and Dietetics* 112 (2012): 1029–41.

8. Tsai, A. C., et al. "Suicide Mortality in Relation to Dietary Intake of n-3 and n-6 Polyunsaturated Fatty Acids and Fish: Equivocal Findings from 3 Large US Cohort Studies." *American Journal of Epidemiology* 179 (2014): 1458–66.

9. Satizabal, C. L., et al. "Incidence of Dementia over Three Decades in the Framingham Heart Study." *New England Journal of Medicine* 374 (2016): 523–32.

10. Morris, M. C., et al. "MIND Diet Slows Cognitive Decline with Aging." *Alzheimer's & Dementia* 11 (2015): 1015–22.

11. Valls-Pedret, C., et al. "Mediterranean Diet and Age-Related Cognitive Decline: A Randomized Clinical Trial." *JAMA Internal Medicine* 175 (2015): 1094–103.

CHAPTER FIFTEEN: SHOPPING TIPS, RECIPES, AND MENUS

1. Smith-Spangler, C., et al. "Are Organic Foods Safer or Healthier Than Conventional Alternatives? A Systematic Review." *Annals of Internal Medicine* 157 (2012): 348–66.

Credits

The Healthy Eating Plate on pages 4, 19, and 252 is from Harvard Health Publications and the Harvard T.H. Chan School of Public Health.

MyPyramid on page 17 is from the U.S. Department of Agriculture and the U.S. Department of Health and Human Services.

The Harvard Healthy Eating Pyramid on pages 16 and 251 is illustrated by Christopher Bing and Heather Foley.

The Food Guide Pyramid on page 11 is from the U.S. Department of Agriculture and the U.S. Department of Health and Human Services.

MyPlate on page 18 is from the U.S. Department of Agriculture and the U.S. Department of Health and Human Services.

The graph on page 39 is adapted from Willett, W.C., et al., *New England Journal of Medicine*, vol. 341, no. 6 (August 5, 1999): p. 430.

The table on page 41, courtesy of Harvard Health Publications, is adapted from the National Heart, Lung, and Blood Institute's "Body Mass Index Table." https://www.nhlbi.nih.gov/health/educational/lose_wt/BMI/bmi_tbl.htm

The chart on page 43, courtesy of Harvard Health Publications, is adapted from the National Heart, Lung, and Blood Institute's "Body Mass Index Table." https://www.nhlbi.nih.gov/health/educational/lose_wt/BMI/bmi_tbl.htm

The illustration on page 47 is from "Metabolic Syndrome: Putting the Heart in Harm's Way." *Harvard Heart Letter*, vol. 12, no. 9 (May 2002): 2.

The illustration on page 62 is from "Low Carb vs. Low Fat," *Harvard Health Letter*, vol. 29, no. 10 (August 2004): 4.

The graph on page 92 is adapted from *Nutritional Epidemiology* by Walter Willett, page 419.

The graph on page 95 is adapted from deLorgeril et al., *Circulation*, vol. 99, no. 6 (February 16, 1999): 781.

The illustration on page 113 is from Harvard Health Publications.

The illustration on page 119 was adapted from Salmeron, J., et al., *JAMA*, vol. 277, no. 6 (February 12, 1997): 476.

The illustration on page 123 is from "Heart Gains from Whole Grains," *Harvard Heart Letter*, vol. 13, no. 3 (November 2002): 3.

The graph on page 197 is adapted from Hegsted, D. M., *Journal of Nutrition*, vol. 116, no. 11 (November 1986): 2317.

The tables on pages 237–239 are adapted from the Dietary Reference Intakes of the Institute of Medicine's (now National Academy of Medicine) Food and Nutrition Board.

The illustration on page 213 is adapted from *Nutritional Epidemiology* by Walter Willett, page 451.

Index

INDEX

Recipe Index

About the Authors

Walter C. Willett, MD, DʀPH, is Professor of Epidemiology and Nutrition at the Harvard T.H. Chan School of Public Health and Professor of Medicine at Harvard Medical School. A world-renowned researcher, he is a lead investigator of the landmark Nurses' Health Study and Health Professionals Follow-Up Study. Dr. Willett has received many awards, including the Medal of Honor of the American Cancer Society.

Coauthor Patrick J. Skerrett, the former Executive Editor of Harvard Health Publications, is the editor of First Opinion at STATnews.com.